THE FERTILITY DOCTOR

The Fertility Doctor

JOHN ROCK

AND THE REPRODUCTIVE REVOLUTION

Margaret Marsh and Wanda Ronner

THE

JOHNS HOPKINS

UNIVERSITY PRESS

BALTIMORE

© 2008 The Johns Hopkins University Press
All rights reserved. Published 2008
Printed in the United States of America
on acid-free paper

2 4 6 8 9 7 5 3 1

The Johns Hopkins University Press
2715 North Charles Street
Baltimore, Maryland 21218-4363
www.press.jhu.edu

Library of Congress Cataloging-in-Publication Data

Marsh, Margaret S., 1945–
     The fertility doctor : John Rock and the reproductive revolution / Margaret Marsh,
Wanda Ronner.
       p. ; cm.
     Includes bibliographical references and index.
     ISBN-13: 978-0-8018-9001-7 (hardcover : alk. paper)
     ISBN-10: 0-8018-9001-2 (hardcover : alk. paper)
     1. Rock, John Charles, 1890–1984. 2. Gynecologists—United States—Biography.
3. Oral contraceptives—United States—History. 4. Oral contraceptives—Religious
aspects—Catholic Church. 5. Human reproductive technology—United States—
History. 6. Infertility—Treatment—United States—History. 7. Reproductive health—
United States—History. I. Ronner, Wanda. II. Title.
     [DNLM: 1. Rock, John Charles, 1890–1984. 2. Physicians—United States—Biography.
3. Contraceptive Agents—history—United States. 4. History, 20th Century—United
States. 5. Reproductive Medicine—history—United States. 6. Reproductive Techniques,
Assisted—history—United States. WZ 100 R682M 2008]
     RG76.R63M37 2008
     618.10092—dc22   2008006552

A catalog record for this book is available from the British Library.

Special discounts are available for bulk purchases of this book. For more information,
please contact Special Sales at 410-516-6936 or specialsales@press.jhu.edu.

The Johns Hopkins University Press uses environmentally friendly book materials, including
recycled text paper that is composed of at least 30 percent post-consumer waste, whenever
possible. All of our book papers are acid-free, and our jackets and covers are printed on paper
with recycled content.

For Howard, Peter, and Lukas

Contents

THE FERTILITY DOCTOR

INTRODUCTION

The ethics, medical consequences, costs, and social implications of various forms of reproductive technology are hotly debated subjects today. In state and national legislatures, in the courts, and even around the dinner table, we argue about the safety of the hormones and procedures used to induce ovulation, preimplantation genetic screening of embryos, sex selection, selective pregnancy termination after in vitro fertilization, gay and lesbian couples' use of assisted reproduction, the fate of unused embryos, and human cloning. We talk about these issues as if they are new problems, forgetting that they have a long and fascinating history.

As the field of reproductive medicine was developing, a physician named John Rock played a pivotal role in uncovering knowledge about how human reproduction occurs as well as in calling attention to the problems facing both women who were infertile and women who were all too fertile. This book is about John Rock—his life and his work, and the consequences of that work.

Rock, with the help of his research assistant Miriam Menkin, was the first researcher to achieve human in vitro fertilization in the 1940s. Later, as a Catholic who challenged his church on the subject of birth control—and nearly won—he contravened church teachings while claiming to adhere to its bedrock principles. Knowingly or not, Rock subverted conventional sexual attitudes in the name of perpetuating conventional family values. Although the technologies have multiplied over the years, the scientific and medical issues with which he and his colleagues wrestled were as ethically, culturally, and politically contested in their time as scientific and medical intervention in reproduction is today. And they are controversial for much the same reason: They separate sex from reproduction, and such a separation challenges deeply held societal beliefs about the nature of family life, the relationship of sexuality to morality, and even the basis for ascribing gender roles.

John Rock was born in 1890 in Marlborough, Massachusetts. His grandparents were Irish immigrants. His father owned a liquor business, dabbled in horse racing, and speculated in real estate. His mother raised five children. John was the next-to-youngest child and youngest son. When he was nineteen, his father, facing financial difficulties, shipped him off to Guatemala to work for the United Fruit Company as a timekeeper on a banana plantation. Frank Rock hoped his youngest son would aspire to a business career, but John rebelled and eventually attended Harvard College and Medical School. When his medical residencies were completed, he married a Boston socialite in 1925 and seemed bound for a lucrative career in private practice.

His ambitions, however, led him in a different direction. One of the most intriguing aspects of John Rock's personal life is how this often directionless and sometimes feckless boy and young man—a socially ambitious undergraduate and an average medical student who took several years even to decide what kind of doctor he wanted to be—transformed himself into a leading medical researcher and practitioner who ultimately became one of the most recognized figures of the twentieth century. His experiences can help us all answer the questions, How do we become who we are? And how do we make peace with the relationship between what we once were and what we have become?

Rock finished medical school just before the end of World War I and retired during the waning days of the war in Vietnam; he became a medical resident just before the culmination of the first women's rights movement and ceased actively practicing medicine at the height of the sexual revolution. He spent most of his career at the Harvard-affiliated Free Hospital for Women and retired from medical practice at the age of eighty-two. The impact of his life's work, which engendered profound changes in American sexual and reproductive behavior, can be compared to that of only a few others, perhaps Alfred Kinsey or Margaret Sanger.

Today, women expect to control their reproductive behavior. They assume that they can avoid pregnancy if that's what they want. Hormonal contraception, either the once revolutionary but now tried-and-true birth-control pill or the newer patches and vaginal rings, can virtually guarantee that a woman will not conceive. And conversely, if a woman hopes that she *has* conceived, she can buy an over-the-counter pregnancy test and have the answer immediately. If she is pregnant, her physician will monitor her pregnancy with ultrasound and prenatal diagnostic testing. She has access to books and videos that illustrate the development of the embryo into a fetus and ultimately a baby. She can even choose to have what is called a keepsake ultrasound, the provision of which has become a lucrative boutique business catering to the couple who wants to keep a record of every moment of their potential child's existence.

Nowadays, if a woman wants to conceive but is having difficulty, she can count on specialists in reproductive endocrinology to employ multiple technologies to visualize her reproductive organs. A surgeon skilled in laparoscopy can operate through a tiny incision without opening her abdomen. Several tests can tell if she is ovulating regularly; if not, she can take medication to promote ovulation. If her fallopian tubes are blocked, her doctor will most likely recommend IVF as the first line of treatment.

John Rock was a leader among that small group of influential researchers and practitioners whose work made all these things possible. And while Rock was not the only clinical researcher or practitioner in this field, his specific professional circumstances and intellectual predilections gave him matchless opportunities to observe and treat a range of reproductive conditions. It is impossible to comprehend fully the medical and cultural meanings of the twentieth-century transformation of ideas about reproduction and sexuality without knowing about the work of John Rock.

When Rock became director of the sterility clinic at Harvard's Free Hospital for Women in Brookline in 1926, surgeons could view a woman's pelvic organs only if they cut open her abdomen, by performing a major surgical procedure called a laparotomy. Doctors had no way to predict accurately when a woman would ovulate. Medical researchers and practitioners understood only dimly the process in which a human sperm fertilized an egg. They knew even less about such things as the length of time it took the newly fertilized egg to find its way into the uterus and successfully implant. And although scientists knew about the existence of the so-called female sex hormones, estrogen and progesterone, they had not yet figured out how to isolate the latter or synthesize either of them.

The first two decades of Rock's career coincided with the emergence of a new era of clinical investigation. In the mid-1930s, shortly after the discovery and isolation of estrogen and progesterone, Rock and his young colleague Marshall Bartlett devised a procedure to "date" the lining of the uterus through microscopic evaluation of the tissue lining the uterus. This was the first time clinicians had any way of figuring out, albeit after the fact, if a woman had ovulated—bedrock knowledge without which a workable reproductive technology could not exist. Then, from 1938 until 1950, working with pathologist Arthur Hertig, Rock engaged in a remarkable (and much later controversial) set of experiments that provided scientists and clinicians with the first visual record of early human fetal development. This research brought the two men professional accolades, helped lay the groundwork for human IVF, and earned both men a secure place in the history of obstetrics and gynecology.

Rock had his first brush with fame in 1944 when he announced that he and his research assistant Miriam Menkin had achieved the first successful fertilization in vitro of human ova. He became a media darling for the first—but by no means the last—time. Journalists mobbed him, convinced that the era of the "test tube baby" was imminent, in spite of his repeated insistence that it would be at least a decade, maybe longer, until the technology could produce successful pregnancies. (It would be three more decades before the first IVF baby, Louise Brown, was born in England in 1978.)[1]

As director of one of the first infertility clinics in the nation, in the 1930s and 1940s Rock became known as a leader in both the treatment of infertility and research on problems of fertility. He cared as much about women who had more children than they wanted as about those who wanted them in vain. When he created the first free birth-control clinic in his state in the late 1930s, his staff could provide women only with instruction in the "rhythm method" of contraception. Anything else was banned in Massachusetts, one of two states that would outlaw the prescription and use of birth control by married couples as late as the 1960s. Rock endorsed proposals for changes in that law and clandestinely subverted it. As early as the 1930s, under the guise of lecturing about the reproductive behavior of primates, he taught a course to Harvard medical students on human sexuality and reproduction. This course included, in contravention of the law, information on how to prescribe appropriate contraceptive devices.

In his medical practice, he treated infertile women from Boston and its suburbs and those from around the world, from Hollywood movie stars to at least one African princess, from proper Boston society matrons to working-class Irish Catholics, from the upper crust to the indigent. By the end of the 1940s, he had achieved national prominence. His relationships with his patients and others who sought his advice helped to shape his evolving ideas about sexuality and reproduction. By the early 1950s, from all over the world, young doctors vied for the opportunity to train and work with him, and established physicians asked to observe his methods.

In the 1960s Rock became an international celebrity because of his prominent role in the development and promotion of the oral contraceptive. In those years he was the face and voice of the pill. He was articulate. He was reassuring. He was handsome. Almost everyone, it seemed, knew the name of America's distinguished Catholic physician who urged the Church to change its mind about the legitimacy of birth control. Later, during the backlash against the pill in the late 1960s, he drew the ire of female health activists mistrustful of medical authority. And by the 1970s and 1980s, he had become a target of both fundamentalist Christians and some feminists, the former of whom considered some of his research, especially his early embryo studies, immoral, while the latter charged him—falsely, the record shows—with taking advantage of the many low-income women who came to him for medical treatment when he persuaded them to participate in his research studies.

We see this book as serving three purposes. It is the first full-scale historical biography of Rock, one of the leading figures in twentieth-century medicine; it tells the story of the development of the new field of reproductive medicine; and it examines the role that John Rock and this new field played in the dramatic changes in sexual and reproductive behavior that occurred during the twentieth century.[2] As we probe the workings of clinical research (the scientific, intellectual, and cultural milieu in which Rock worked), we also recapture the voices of his patients and research volunteers.[3] Our exploration of the life and work of John Rock illuminates the emergence of a medical specialty in the context of the dramatic changes that transformed American sexual behavior and reproductive practices in the twentieth century.

Chapter 1

FAMILY MATTERS

Marlborough, Massachusetts, December 1908. Frank Rock, fifty-one-year old saloon keeper, liquor store owner, speculator, and local Irish American politico, is facing the most serious crisis of his occupational life. His town is about to go "dry" and his income about to go up in smoke. Calling together his five children—two sons out in the world, one daughter in college, a second at home, and a third son in his last year of commercial school—Frank unveils his plan to save the family fortune. The three sons will support everyone else while Frank figures out what to do next. The two older boys are already doing what they can. The third son, eighteen-year-old John, will have to take up any slack. "My intentions are good," John writes in his diary.

Quirigua, Guatemala, July 1909. Acting on his good intentions, John arrives in the Guatemalan jungle to oversee two hundred Jamaican and indigenous workers on one of United Fruit Company's banana plantations. It is unbearably hot. Mosquitos swarm. It never seems to stop raining. Living conditions are primitive for the white timekeepers and overseers, even worse for the Caribbean and indigenous workers. During the next nine months, John will learn a great deal about himself. The experience will change his life, although hardly in ways either he or his family anticipate.

John Rock was born into a second-generation Irish American family in Marlborough, Massachusetts, a thriving small manufacturing city about thirty miles from Boston. In the mid-nineteenth century, his grandfather, John Roche, had immigrated to Boston, where he married and had a family. Sometime in the 1860s, the Roches moved to Marlborough. In the city directory in 1869, he was listed as John Roche, tailor. Prospering in his new hometown, by 1883 Roche had become John Rock and had advanced to the status of merchant tailor, with enough downtown real estate that the directory listed his business address simply as Rock's Block.

Marlborough suited the Rocks. Its principal industry was shoe manufacturing, and in the late nineteenth century the city had about ten thousand residents, more than one Catholic church, and a population of Irish and Irish American Catholics, French Canadians, and New England Protestants. At least two of John and Mary's children, Frank and John, remained in Marlborough. Like many of their fellow Irish Catholics in Massachusetts, whose occupational choices tended to be limited, the brothers became involved in the liquor business and politics. John, a "saloon-keeper," was also the chief of police by the end of the nineteenth century. The two brothers were entrepreneurs, together and separately. Frank's business interests ranged from liquor to race horses to real estate. He was a speculator, convivial and fast-talking, who delighted in risky ventures.[1]

Frank Rock had a wide-ranging circle of friends and associates who hailed from Marlborough, Boston, and nearby Hudson, where he owned and leased vacation cottages on Lake Boone. Handsome and hearty, he was given to what he liked to call "bluff."[2] Maintaining a fierce sense of family pride, he expected strict obedience from his children even after they became adults. The older ones, at least while their mother was alive, appear to have gone along. So did John, at first, but after trying for years to be what his father expected him to be, he would eventually rebel.

When John Rock was born on March 24, 1890, the third John in as many generations, Frank had been married since October 1883 to the former Ann Jane Murphy, like him a child of Irish Catholic immigrants. A year younger than her husband, she bore him five children in seven years, the first about ten months after their wedding, when she was twenty-five. That was Charlie, who was born in August 1884. Harry followed in 1886, Mary (called Maisie) in 1887, and the twins, John and Ellen (Nell), in 1890. John was not quite the youngest; he came into the world a few minutes before his twin sister.[3]

Ann Jane Rock—Annie to her friends—was a conventional late nineteenth-century middle-class matron. With the help of one or more servants, depending on how well her husband was doing financially at any one time, she looked after the family, cooked and sewed, visited with her friends, and belonged to at least two women's clubs. She loved her husband, faults and all, and her few letters to him that survive illuminate both her devotion and her recognition of his underlying insecurities. She expressed her faith in his business abilities. When the local prohibitionists threatened to undermine the family's economic security, she offered reassurance and expression of love.[4] She tactfully offered him business advice without making it apparent that she was doing so. Just as he believed he was keeping her from knowledge of his occasional financial reverses, she protected him from knowing she was helping him out of them. Theirs was a typical marriage of the era, built on affection and mutual dissimulation.

Annie gave birth for the last time when she was thirty-two. It is impossible to know why there were no more children. She may have had a difficult labor with the twins, requiring a cesarean section, which at this time often involved a simultaneous hysterectomy. Or perhaps the couple successfully engaged in contraception or abstinence. They left no record, so we will never know.[5] This was an era for which we have evidence that American Protestant couples were limiting their births through contraceptive practices and even abortion.[6] But we know less about the habits of Catholics. According to a recent biography of President John F. Kennedy, his mother Rose, once she had borne what she considered her fair share of children, moved out of her husband's bedroom and ended their intimate life.[7]

Annie and Frank may have used contraceptives, she may have had surgery, or perhaps she was of the same mind as Rose Kennedy. All that remains after all this time is a strong whiff of suspicion that at least by the time his youngest children were adolescents, Frank may have become romantically involved with another woman—Delia Flynn, the wife of one of his Boston business associates. Annie disliked her. So did the children, especially Nell and John. In years to come, Delia would play an even more significant, and unwelcome, role in the lives of the Rock children.

· · ·

His occasional reverses notwithstanding, Frank Rock was a successful businessman while his children were growing up. The family lived in relative affluence. Frank loved to take risks in business, and in these years, the risks generally paid off. He dealt with financial difficulties, whenever they arose, simply by taking out another mortgage or borrowing on his life insurance. Somewhat later, dogged by business reverses and plagued by the local antiliquor forces, he told John that he thought he'd be a great subject for a book. It should be called *How to Live on Bluff*, he told his son only half jokingly. "No man lives who could furnish you with more or better material to fit that title than your own dear dad."[8]

Almost always recovering from the occasional reverse, Frank thrived as a speculator and entrepreneur. He gloried in his large and lively family and took enormous pleasure in a host of friends and acquaintances. Every summer, the family went to Lakeside, a summer colony on Lake Boone. Although only about five or six miles from Marlborough, Lake Boone seemed a world away. At their cottage, Alabama, he and Annie hosted frequent parties for relatives and friends, some of whom occupied nearby cottages that Frank rented out. Rock and Murphy cousins, friends from Boston and its suburbs, and other Marlborough families paddled canoes and swam, fished and relaxed, and danced on Saturday nights. Most of them, at least the ones who figure in young John's correspondence, were fellow Irish Catholics. In his early years, John was cocooned within a social circle of his own faith and ethnicity. He may have known about anti-Catholicism and anti-Irish prejudice, but in Marlborough and Lakeside at least, he did not experience them.[9]

Frank Rock had much in common with his two older boys, Charlie and Harry. Both were avid and capable athletes, whose triumphs earned them plaudits in the local newspaper. The senior Rock also seemed to have a particularly close bond with his elder daughter, Maisie, a striking and clever girl. Both Charlie and Maisie were close to their father, John and Nell to their mother. As for Harry—he was a genial soul who cared for his parents about equally. Perhaps as befits the stereotypical middle child, he took things as they came and accepted more or less cheerfully whatever life had to offer.

Charlie and Harry went to work after high school, young men seeking their fortunes in various businesses, at first with only moderate success. Maisie, the pampered older daughter, wanted to go to college, and so she did, choosing Simmons College in Boston, a women's college founded in 1900. Simmons graduated its first class in the spring of 1906, just before Maisie began her freshman year. Offering degrees in household economics, teaching, library science, secretarial studies, general science, nursing, and science teaching, the college also had a joint social work program with Harvard. Maisie majored in household economics, was active in the student government, and enjoyed these years enormously, graduating in 1910.[10] Frank was extraordinarily proud of Maisie's cleverness, and she in turn had a high opinion of herself. She expected her father to cater to her, and he did.

Frank was never quite sure what to make of John, who much later implied that he had not been the kind of boy likely to earn the admiration of men like his father or older brothers. He remembered being much fonder as a child of doing "girls' things" than "boys' things." He was a relatively quiet, introspective boy who preferred the company of his twin sister, Nell, to that of almost anyone else. His older brothers thought of him as a "sissy." Nell's tastes ran to the frilly and the feminine, and John often chose to be with her rather than do other things. He played the piano, apparently quite well. His daughters say he could sew and cook, skills definitely not considered manly among his brothers' friends and acquaintances at the turn of the twentieth century.[11]

At thirteen, John began to keep a diary, which reveals a serious boy with a mischievous streak.[12] Adolescents have a reputation, deservedly or not, for self-absorption, and John's diary was indeed mostly about himself and his small world. His opinions were conventional, and he subscribed to the full range of prejudices common to white males of his generation. He did, however, possess a strong capacity for friendship and a genuinely kind manner toward his family and friends. His writings also evince—as many adolescent diaries have done for the past century—an urge toward self-improvement. Unlike some of his friends, however, John did not seem to possess any particular intellectual curiosity or passionate interest—whether in science, sports, or girls—except perhaps for music. Besides what seems to be an unusual gift for empathy, there is little indication in these youthful reflections of what he would choose to do with his life.[13]

At thirteen and fourteen, John's life revolved around school, social life, and the Church. His interest in music—which would remain a lifelong avocation—led him to found a musical club he and his friends called Orpheus, which continued to meet regularly for as long as he remained in Marlborough.[14] He tended to be a worrier. He was a good Catholic, attending Mass, confessing regularly, observing Lent by giving up something that he enjoyed, commemorating the saints' days—having his throat blessed on St. Blaise's day, for example—and occasionally commenting on a particularly affecting sermon. He was devout rather than simply observant, noting on one Holy Thursday that he had attended church three times, in two different parishes.[15] He also had a devilish side, although he sometimes tried to chastise his prankish self, for example, by apologizing to his regular teacher for plaguing the substitute or by fretting over having teased a friend into losing his temper.[16]

The family's prosperity notwithstanding, all the Rock children had their domestic responsibilities. By the time he was fifteen or so, with Harry and Charlie already in the work force, John's chores included cleaning the grate and lighting the fire at around 5:30 in the morning, dusting his and Harry's rooms, sometimes cooking the family breakfast, and at least occasionally pressing his own pants and drying the dishes. For some of the chores he was paid—the dusting was worth twenty-five cents. A few months before he turned sixteen, he acquired a part-time job clerking in a retail store in town.[17]

In early adolescence John's greatest pleasures came from rambling walks, music, reading, and the theater, the last a taste the whole family enjoyed. The family continued to spend its summers at Lakeside in the family cottage, John's father and older brothers commuting, his sisters, he, and his mother staying for most of the summer. Like his friends in Marlborough, his Lakeside companions were largely Catholic, from Boston and its suburbs as well as from home. At Lakeside, he swam and read and walked with his friends and had crushes on one girl or another. Although John never seemed to think it unusual that the Catholics and the Protestants had their own social circles along the lake, Harry, out in the world and therefore more sensitive to anti-Catholic biases, was known to comment sarcastically on the "Lakeside 400," a reference to the affluent Protestant families who chose not to mix with the equally affluent Catholics on the lake.[18]

Many of John's closest friends—boys and girls alike—came from the families who summered on the lake. Even as a teenager, he seems to have had a surprising number of nonromantic friendships with young women and girls his own age, some of whom wrote to him as a girl might write to a female friend. His sisters too expected him to be interested in the details of their lives, even sending him swatches of fabric for dresses they were having made. And like many a youth, he idolized one of his young teachers—Clara Johnson, who taught English at Marlborough High School. In an impassioned diary entry, John exclaimed that Miss Johnson "did more for me towards shaping my character than either she, or I, perhaps, can tell." His feelings about her were a bit more complicated than that. After he moved to Boston at sixteen, he learned she had been ill and sent her flowers. Then he agonized over whether he should have done so. Finally, in the throes of this internal debate in his diary, he added, "I hold the deepest, tenderest, most sincere feelings toward Miss Johnson."[19]

His friendships with girls and women did not mean that he avoided making friends with boys his age. Both in Marlborough and at Lakeside, he had several close friends. But although he attended high school football games and talked with his male friends about sports, in Marlborough he was at best lukewarm about a pastime that can sometimes amount to an adolescent male obsession. He would show more interest in athletics when he left home to complete high school in Boston; but even then, he gave the impression that his interest in sports was less an interest in the sport itself than pleasure in the companionship of his friends, several of whom were excellent athletes.

· · ·

Adolescence struck with a vengeance when John turned fifteen. He was restless, dissatisfied at home. He didn't know any more what he thought or felt. He stopped writing in his diary; he was unhappy at school. And to make everything worse, his summer romance with a girl named Ella went awry in the fall. She and her family, who lived in the Boston suburb of Charlestown, summered at Lakeside. She was pretty and lively—by Rock family standards, even a bit wild—a willful girl who stayed out late and carefully calibrated just how much she could defy her father without incurring serious paternal wrath. And in twenty-first-century parlance, she was a classic "mean girl," who persuaded her classmates to ostracize and ridicule a young Indian woman who spoke English with an accent. In spite of her teacher's scoldings and even harsher punishment, Ella persisted in tormenting the unfortunate girl. Whether John ended the romance because of her cruel streak, or whether he found himself a victim of it, their romance had died, and he felt depressed.[20]

Eager to escape Marlborough, John persuaded his parents to let him finish school in Boston. Conflicts with his father contributed to his desire to leave, and he wanted to get away from the shadow of his older brothers, who often teased him for his lack of interest in the muscular pursuits they enjoyed.[21] One of his close Lakeside friends, Eddie Gately, was attending Boston Latin and urged John to join him there. Throughout 1905 and 1906, Eddie and John had kept up a steady correspondence, visited each other, and exchanged Christmas gifts. Although much more intense about sports than John was, Eddie was like him in other ways—sweet and serious, kindhearted, and religiously observant. Very focused on his studies and determined to go to Harvard (although in the end he had to settle for Tufts), Eddie persuaded John to visit Boston Latin.[22]

John did so, but when he went to school in Boston in the fall of 1906, he went neither to Boston Latin nor to Boston English. Whether he was not admitted into either of them, or whether, despite his need to get away from his father and brothers, he still wanted to please them by training for a business career, he matriculated at the newly opened Boston High School of Commerce. It's more than possible that his father, a business-minded man if there ever was one, made attending the High School of Commerce a condition of allowing him to move to Boston.

It is easy to understand that John would have wanted to appease his father even as he sought to get away. Frank Rock seems to have been determined that John would become a successful businessman, and the High School of Commerce was designed to enable its students to become just that. Its found-

ers—prominent Boston businessmen—intended it to be an elite public institution much like Boston Latin but with a strong business curriculum modeled
on the recently created Harvard Graduate School of Business Administration. The High School of Commerce hoped to prepare young men (only boys
were admitted) to become the city's next generation of business leaders and
executives.[23]

When John went to Boston, hoping to be liberated at least in part from his
adolescent anxieties, his father insisted that he board with Tom and Delia
Flynn. But John's active dislike for Delia had not abated, and he did not want
to live in her house.[24] After enduring the situation for less than a month, he
packed up and left, moving to a boardinghouse in Boston where a fellow student lived. His father was displeased but chose not to make an issue of it.

Once out from under the Flynns, John settled in happily. He was popular
with his schoolmates, who elected him president of his graduating class. He
developed close bonds with several students, none of which was as important
to him that first year as his friendship with Ray Williams, the captain of the
basketball team. In the spring semester of 1907, John's diary is full of references to Ray, who seems to have visited John almost every evening. They studied, sometimes a lot, sometimes "a bit," and after one visit, John noted shyly,
"I like to have him come."[25]

John was much taken with Ray. The diary shows a sense of wonder and
excitement, barely suppressed, about the budding friendship. Then, suddenly,
the relationship took a different turn. In mid-March, after nearly a month of
frequent entries about Ray, John tore out a section of his diary. We suspect
that something sexual happened between John and Ray. (Although the rip-
ping of the diary entry alone might not cause suspicion, as an old man Rock,
musing on the dawning of his sexual consciousness, mentions sleeping in the
same bed with his friend "Ben" Williams and waking up to an erection and
an orgasm.)[26] Did John merely experience an adolescent nighttime erection in
Ray's presence? Or did Ray make a sexual advance? Or did they have a mutual
encounter? Whatever happened, the religious and sexually innocent Rock was
clearly shaken. One can imagine how he felt on hearing, almost immediately
thereafter, that Ray had become dangerously ill. Of the illness, John says only
that "I little expected when I wrote the last entry (which I tore out) that I would
have such bad news about Ray W. as I write now."[27]

For two months afterward, John wrote almost daily about Ray's illness, but
soon worry over Ray gave way to musings over Madeleine O'Connell, a girl on
whom John had developed a crush. Anyway, by then Ray appeared to be recov-

ering. Diagnosed at the time as cerebral meningitis, Ray's exact illness isn't clear. Rock later said it was polio. As Ray began to recover, he and John settled into a much calmer friendship, and Ray's later fate is something of a mystery. In the course of the following year, John often mentioned his friend "Ben" Williams, and over the next couple of years, he seems to have become friends with Ben's sister Mary and their mother as well. But the name Ray—and perhaps Ray in reality—simply disappeared from diaries and correspondence after the fall of 1907.[28]

We do not want to make too much of whatever happened between John and Ray. John continued to moon over Madeleine and his former teacher Clara Johnson. Before the night of the ripped-out diary entry, he had written matter-of-factly and without envy that Ray had another "best friend . . . along with me." But John's experience with Ray and its aftermath seem to have had an impact. In his later life, Rock was remarkably tolerant of the varieties of sexual behavior in others and always interested in understanding them. His friendship with Ray as an adolescent may have helped him to think this way.

In his senior year at Commerce, John continued to work at his studies, hang out with his friends, and spend time both being with and thinking about girls. In the spring of 1908, along with classmate Paul Tardival, he was awarded a traveling scholarship—the Latin American Fellowship—for a three-month tour of Latin America. The purpose of the scholarships, funded by a group of Boston business leaders, was for a few talented graduates (two from the High School of Commerce, two from Boston English) to observe Latin American business practices and potential opportunities and to make the kinds of contacts that would serve the young men well in their future lives as men of commerce.

Central and Latin America represented the new frontier for American business interests in the early twentieth century. Their ambitions were supported by the views of political leaders such as Theodore Roosevelt, whose expansionist dreams took shape in the 1890s when he was assistant secretary of the navy and could be implemented all the more readily once President William McKinley's assassination put him in the White House in 1901. The 1904 Roosevelt Corollary to the Monroe Doctrine justified American political and military intervention in Latin America to protect U.S. business investments, making doing business in Central America in particular an attractive opportunity. Except for a small minority of dissenters, most Americans believed that propping up repressive and often brutal regimes in those nations was simply one of the necessary costs of doing business.[29]

Frank Rock was not a supporter of the Republican Roosevelt but was an ardent Democrat who served as a delegate to the party's 1908 convention in Denver. Still, he was in favor of American expansionism. Delighted that John was following the family plan for him to become a businessman, Frank was more than happy that his son's future success might lie in the southern hemisphere. As his father was cheering the Democratic candidate in Denver, John was spending the summer of 1908 traveling with Paul in South America.

Never having been outside the United States, perhaps never having left New England, John was determined to make the most of this trip and to remember it well. He wrote frequent letters to his family, promising his father that he would develop more initiative and ambition, describing to his brothers the countryside and the various business establishments he visited, and detailing for his sister Maisie the richly furnished households on the estates of the American and European expatriates he encountered in his travels.[30]

John often referred to his "work" in these letters, but little actual work seems to have occurred. He and Paul spent their time touring factories and other businesses, eating numerous meals at exclusive clubs, and enjoying visits at the lavish estates of the North Americans and a few Britons who had made Latin America their home. He learned a great deal about the lives of well-to-do expatriate families and observed the work world of others. Although kind and considerate to people he knew personally, John expressed little sympathy for native workers or the poor as a group. (In fact, throughout his life he would continue to exhibit prejudice toward classes or groups of people while demonstrating kindness toward individuals within such groups.) He was scornful of the crew members and dockworkers, in his opinion "the lowest class of civilization." Stuck in port on an early leg of his trip, he groused, "I don't know when we'll get out of this old hole," the ship's departure having been delayed because the crewmen were sleeping off their hangovers in the local jail.[31]

Although some of his letters include observations on the business climate of his host countries, for the most part his remarks simply echoed the commonplaces he must have been hearing at home and in school. Parroting what his teachers had taught him, he informed his family that South America was a great place for American businessmen. While he was in Argentina, he repeated what he had already learned at Commerce: Argentina needed immigrants from among those then called the "northern races" to become workers and entrepreneurs. Detailed accounts of the extravagant lifestyles of the expatriates, including elaborate descriptions of their lavish estates and clubs, seemed calculated to impress his father and older sister in particular. Whether he wrote so much about richly furnished houses and luxuriously appointed clubs only because he thought it would interest his family, or because he was impressed so much himself, is hard to tell—probably a bit of both.

John came back from South America for a postgraduate year at the High School of Commerce. To help support himself, he held down a job as a clerk. His family—especially his father and brothers—expected him to commence his business career in earnest once he left school. His father hoped that with more training than either of his brothers, John would achieve considerable success. "Hoped" is the operative word here, since John seemed reluctant to embrace his projected future with the zeal his father and brothers expected. John wanted to please them, but his relationship with his father was never smooth and had worsened during John's adolescence. His frequent attempts to mollify Frank with promises of greater initiative and ambition only seemed to end up in some sort of self-sabotage. Although no one in the family would admit it, John did not want to follow in his father's footsteps, did not *ever* want to go into business with Charlie and Harry (his father's often-expressed dream), did not, in fact, want at all to take the path so explicitly laid out for him, but he was not ready to rebel openly.

At eighteen John was unsure of what he wanted to do with his life. Today, we're more surprised when eighteen-year-olds do have a clear set of career goals than when they don't. But in the early twentieth century, most young men were already working at eighteen. John's family apparently considered his high school education sufficient for him, although many of his Lakeside friends had either begun college or soon would. Three of the young men were at Tufts, and a fourth was about to matriculate at Harvard. Several of the young women were also college bound. One was headed to the University of Vermont, known in New England for its progressive attitudes toward women.[32] John's cousin Lizzie had been accepted at Simmons, where his sister Maisie had just finished her sophomore year. Others were heading off to local normal schools to prepare to teach.

Like their Protestant counterparts, these young Catholic women did not think of themselves as out of the ordinary for attending college. Their Catholicism, not their gender, often was the greater stumbling block, as John's friend Mae Conway discovered when anti-Catholic prejudice severely hampered her social life at Boston University. Most hurtfully, she was rushed by several sororities only to be dropped when her religion became evident. "Now you wouldn't think there would be much of a chance of passing by the name

'Conway,' would you?" She complained to John, figuring people ought to have known that her name would identify her as Irish Catholic. The sorority girls, learning her religion when she refused to eat meat at a Friday supper, immediately dropped her as a friend. "Oh, John," she finished her letter angrily, "I really never met such narrow-minded people."[33]

...

John may not have been sure of his future, but family troubles would soon mark one out for him. In the fall of 1908, Frank Rock suffered a serious, and he feared maybe permanent, financial setback. The town of Marlborough voted to go dry. Frank owned a liquor store, his brother a saloon. On May 1, 1909, Frank would be out of the business that provided most of the family's income. Something would have to be done, and in December, Frank gathered the family and gravely informed everyone of the family's difficulties. "We'll all have to work pretty hard. My intentions are good," John resolved.[34] A good thing too, since Frank's solution for these problems, unless or until he could devise another business venture, was simply to have his three sons support the rest of the family.

There was no question of sending the daughters out to work. Maisie was a junior at Simmons and had no intention of dropping out. Nor would her father have asked it of her. Nell, who seemed to live for dancing and partying, was living at home. Frank and Annie did not encourage her to take a job either, although they did try—unsuccessfully—to persuade her to consider college or secretarial school. After all, they reasoned, if at some point she did have to work, she'd fare better with some skills.

That left the boys. Charlie and Harry were working already and doing what they could. Now it was up to John to get a decent position and help support the family.[35] He was ready to oblige. In July 1909, shortly after leaving the High School of Commerce and just a few months past his nineteenth birthday, John sailed for Guatemala to work for United Fruit Company as a timekeeper on a banana plantation.

Nothing survives today to tell us why John—or more likely his father—chose United Fruit as the vehicle to bring back the Rock family fortunes. Maybe it seemed an obvious choice for a young man whose education had been made possible by businessmen with an eye to economic expansion in Central and South America, a young man who had been to Latin America, had written about its economic prospects, and who spoke a bit of Spanish. He might have even been recommended by his headmaster or one of the teachers.

If we know little of why he or his father chose United Fruit and Guatemala, we know even less about what John expected to find once he arrived there. The countries in which he had traveled the previous year offered a study in contrasts. He had seen poor workers and wealthy landowners, and he surely observed that while ordinary people had little, the expatriate businessmen were exceptionally well off. John had been struck by the wealth and culture of the well-to-do North Americans in Argentina and Brazil. He may have imagined Guatemala to be similar. And perhaps if he had been going to work for United Fruit fifteen or twenty years later, when the company built communities for their white expatriate managers and executives complete with country clubs and other amenities, such an image might have had some basis in reality. But in the summer of 1909, the conditions were much more primitive.

The United Fruit Company, founded in 1899, owed its early good fortune to the entrepreneurial spirit of Minor C. Keith, a somewhat eccentric engineer and entrepreneur whose major accomplishment until that time had been the construction of a railroad from central Costa Rica to Limón. Keith grew and marketed bananas to have a cargo that would supply a steady income for the railroad. At the end of the nineteenth century, Keith owned 200,000 acres of land and 112 miles of railroad. Although this doesn't seem like much of a rail line in the abstract, it had been hacked through the jungle and was considered a remarkable engineering experiment for its day.[36]

Keith's passion was for railroads, not bananas. So when his banana business foundered, he turned to Andrew Preston, a Boston fruit importer who, with his ship-captain partner Lorenzo Dow Baker, had operated the Boston Fruit Company since 1885. Together, the three of them founded United Fruit and began building on Keith's holdings in Central America. From its inception, United Fruit intended to expand in Central America and dominate the banana exportation business. Although an early history of the region's banana industry indicated that in 1904 United Fruit acquired, as its first holdings in Guatemala, only 4,000 acres of jungle near Quirigua, that figure is misleading. Historian Paul Dosal describes a different arrangement between Guatemala's dictator Manuel Estrada Cabrera and Minor Keith in the same year, which actually gave Keith at least 168,000 acres of land, 50,000 acres of which were deeded to United Fruit. The banana company, in turn, made a commitment to plant at least 5,000 acres in bananas by the beginning of 1908.[37]

Estrada Cabrera had taken over the presidency of Guatemala at gunpoint in 1898 and held office for the next twenty-two years. A brutal dictator, he purged the army, had his rivals assassinated, and terrorized the people using a network of spies. He exploited his office for as much personal gain as possible, and in return for bribes and other compensations, provided United Fruit with tax exemptions, land, and freedom from regulation. His arrangements were with Keith and his railway company, the Guatemala Railway Company, not directly with United Fruit. But Keith was also vice president of United Fruit. Although his railroad holdings in Guatemala were ostensibly independent of his connection to United Fruit, the railroad and United Fruit were functionally integrated.[38]

United Fruit was willing to do business with Estrada Cabrera, but Andrew Preston envisioned a company run rather differently from Minor Keith's banana and railroad empire. Keith's undertakings had attracted adventurers and others from the United States who might be called questionable characters, often drifters and misfits who found living at home too confining or conventional. Under Andrew Preston's leadership, United Fruit sought a different type of employee to oversee and supervise its Central American empire, educated men like Victor Cutter, who would later succeed Andrew Preston as president of United Fruit. Much later, Cutter recalled, "when I went into the tropics a quarter of a century ago I was one of the first of a group of young Americans sent in to replace the white riff-raff which had previously filled minor executive posts."[39] By 1909 Cutter, at the age of twenty-eight, had already been elevated to the post of superintendent of the Guatemala division and hence would be John's new boss.

A Massachusetts native, Victor Cutter was the son of a market gardener and grew up, if not in poverty, certainly without middle-class refinements. An exceptionally bright young man, he graduated Phi Beta Kappa from Dartmouth in 1903, then spent an additional year acquiring a master's degree in business from the same institution. He immediately went to work for United Fruit, beginning as a timekeeper in Costa Rica. Advancing rapidly, he became the head of the company's new division in Guatemala, where he would remain until 1914. Charles Morrow Wilson, author of a 1947 study of the American banana business, says of this operation that by around 1920, "the Guatemala division proved to be one of the first truly cosmopolitan farming centers of the Americas. It began with United States management, Yankee railroading, and the English pattern of tropical plantations," its "workers and craftsmen . . . taken from many nations."[40]

From the start, Cutter shone as a rising star within the company. He had just the combination of education and talent that Andrew Preston had envisioned managing his company. The High School of Commerce had been created to develop just such talent. It seems only natural that United Fruit would have considered the school an obvious place to find the next generation of managers for its holdings in Central and South America. John Rock, president of the first graduating class and winner of the inaugural Latin American Fellowship, with a family determined to have him succeed in business, would have seemed a natural.

...

Whatever John expected when he arrived in Guatemala, nothing in his experience had prepared him for the reality. Conditions, described as "extremely primitive" in 1906, when workers had first begun the backbreaking work of clearing the jungle, were still primitive three years later. By then, however, workers had dug the drainage ditches; felled countless trees, some of them 150 feet tall; and of course, planted the bananas. The first fruit was cut in 1908, the year before John arrived. The area was wet, fertile, and disease ridden. We do not have a record of John's initial reaction, but it could only have been shock and dismay. Still, he reported for work and was assigned first as a timekeeper on the Dartmouth plantation (no doubt named by Cutter himself), then was promoted to overseer (the next step up from timekeeper) within a few months.[41]

The timekeeper and overseer were the entire on-site management of each plantation (or "farm," as good New England terminology would have it) in Guatemala. Only whites—either North Americans or Europeans—held these positions. They ordinarily supervised two hundred or more West Indian and indigenous workers.[42] The young white men who managed the plantations lived in better quarters than the workers, but no one escaped the weather, the insects, the diseases. Timekeepers and overseers worked hard, typically rising at five in the morning and finishing their duties around eight in the evening. And it was surely lonely in those early years. Even in the 1920s, when United Fruit provided considerably more amenities to its expatriate managerial work force, fewer than half the timekeepers lasted a year. Surely the retention rate was no better, and may have been worse, in the decade before the Great War.[43]

The Guatemalan tropics have two seasons, wet and dry, although judging from John's descriptions of the weather during his stay, "dry" was a relative term that year. One woman who had grown up in Guatemala in the 1920s, the child of a United Fruit executive, remembered the "sauna-like temperatures that prevailed year round."[44] The dry season was dusty and hot, she recalled, the wet season, humid and hot. Arriving in the middle of the wet season, truly far away from home for the first time and apparently knowing no one when he arrived, John at nineteen found himself the boss of two hundred or so Jamaican and Guatemalan workers. A host of letters to John from his family and friends, a few drafts of his own letters, and even fewer diary entries survive to document John's experience in Guatemala, which lasted only about nine months—but those nine months were pivotal in shaping his future.

John must have quickly realized that he was not cast in the same mold as Victor Cutter. Cutter loved the tropics and prided himself on his rugged masculinity. He was an excellent marksman, pushed himself to his physical limits, and occasionally demonstrated a "ferocious temper." He apparently had to be dragged back to Boston for occasional visits. It soon became obvious that John hated the tropics. He did not take to several of his fellow clerks and managers and was distressed by the way many of them treated the black workers. He wouldn't have been bothered by the knee-jerk racial prejudice that existed at home, since he no doubt shared it, but such blatant racial domination as was practiced here—what one historian calls United Fruit's "Jim Crow framework of 'negro management'"—he found appalling.[45]

Still, John's salary was substantial for someone of his age and lack of experience, and he knew that his father was counting on nearly all of it to be sent home to Marlborough. Besides, John realized he had to do *something* with his life; right now he didn't think he had alternatives. So, he tried to stick it out, and at least for the first few months tried not to complain too often to his family.

John's duties required that he spend a great deal of time on "his" farm, but there were several other farms, plus a central office in "Virginia"—all linked by a trolley system—where still more of the American and European clerical workers and managers lived. He told his diary that he "found the Negroes very interesting, [and got] along well with them." Writing to his mother and father into the fall of 1909, he convinced them that he was settling in nicely. His parents expected John to spend a year or so in Guatemala, then apply for a position in the Boston headquarters of the company.[46]

Annie resigned herself to her son's proposed year-long absence, while Frank reminded John in nearly every letter how desperately the family needed him to earn money. From Frank's reiteration of his trials with the "drys"—"Business is rotten and has been since May 1st"—to reminders about "the aid I expect to receive from my Charlie and my John," in every letter Frank let John know how dependent the family was on his and Charlie's contributions from afar. (Harry still lived at home, so the family had access to him and his money at all times.) "I expect my boys will send me every dollar they can spare over and above their needed expenses," Frank repeatedly reminded him, though he did occasionally fall back on a polite fiction that John's contributions should be viewed merely as loans. "The best way for you to save," he told John, "is to send your savings to me, and then when you want it I will give it back to you. It would be much safer and will be handy for me to use until such time as you need it." And every once in a great while, "Papa" seemed to think, momentarily, that he might have gone too far: "I do so hope you are not taking out of your body and bones by your pluck and grit in staying there to make good." But the thought never lasted long: "However nothing worth getting is to be had without some sort of hardship." In other words, John, if you have malaria or another dreaded and potentially fatal tropical disease, come home. If not, tough it out![47]

John couldn't figure out how to tell his parents how miserable he was. His mother had not wanted him to go in the first place, and his father needed the money. So at first he confided his unhappiness only to Maisie. She said that if he really could not stand it, he should tell her, and she would explain it all to their parents.[48] John must have been tempted, because he wrote to ask Charlie, who not only firmly discouraged him, but also upbraided him for lacking perseverance. So, John stayed and tried to live up to his family's expectations.

Although he did not seem to have much in common with most of his fellow timekeepers and overseers, he did make one important friendship—with Neil MacPhail, the young Scots physician who ran the hospital on the Dartmouth plantation. MacPhail had founded the hospital in 1908, when he was just twenty-six years old and its only doctor. We know little about Neil MacPhail's early life. Born in either Argyllshire or Aberdeenshire, he earned his medical degree in Scotland, most likely at Edinburgh. His first job in the tropics was as a medical quarantine officer in what is now Belize, though he soon made his way to Guatemala and United Fruit. He would go on in 1913 to build a modern hospital in Quirigua, where young doctors would come from leading American medical schools as well as from Edinburgh to work with him and learn to diagnose and treat tropical diseases, and nurses would receive training in specialized care. He would enjoy a long and distinguished career as an innovator and expert in the treatment of tropical diseases. Aldous Huxley, who visited MacPhail in 1933 on a trip to the Mayan ruins of Quirigua, called him "charming" and described him as "the universal godfather of Guatemala" for his work on those diseases, especially malaria.[49]

Like Victor Cutter, Neil MacPhail loved the tropics and spent his entire career with United Fruit in Guatemala. MacPhail was an independent spirit who knew full well that he would have felt trapped in a more "civilized" environment. Refusing to be confined by conventional standards of behavior, MacPhail never married but apparently had more than one local mistress. He drank and frequented prostitutes; John accompanied him at least once, maybe more often. Perhaps more important for John, MacPhail deeply loved the practice of medicine and made sure that his hospital provided care for employees of United Fruit and the local population alike. Early on, John began taking his evening meal with the doctor at the hospital, and soon he came to spend most of his free time there. MacPhail, who was running the little hospital virtually single-handedly, in turn got in the habit of asking John to assist him during surgery. John came to know his way around the operating room, administering anesthesia and learning how to suture.[50] They came to depend on each other and developed a close bond.

Their friendship became even more important to John once he found himself at odds with the company at the end of 1909. In December, timekeeper W. W. Smith was appointed acting superintendent to replace Victor Cutter temporarily, while Cutter was on vacation in the United States. Smith informed the overseers on all the Guatemala farms that the company was paying too much to the fruit cutters and ordered the overseers to reduce the prices. In short, this was a wage cut.

Every overseer but John complied. Although he did not seem to understand at the time how seriously his defiance would be viewed, he was clearly determined to make an independent judgment about how to manage his "own" farm. Rock openly defied Smith's orders, complaining that the amounts to be offered were no more than "arbitrary prices for this or that kind of work." He thought the cut was unfair, and he was not about to let Smith tell him what to do. John expressed conviction when describing his response: "I knew what I was about" and decided simply to take Smith's "orders merely as suggestions and went on with my work." In outrage, the cutters on every farm but John's Dartmouth refused to cut fruit; and before long, the Dartmouth workers joined their fellow workers in the wildcat strike.[51]

Violence broke out a few days before Christmas.[52] The Guatemalan government deployed troops, further angering the mostly Jamaican workers. Records of dispatches between John at Dartmouth farm to Acting Superintendent Smith at headquarters make clear that John did not approve of such actions. John thought Smith had the soldiers brought in, not realizing that Cutter, still out of the country, had asked Estrada Cabrera directly to send troops.[53] It may not have mattered to John who had asked for the troops. He was furious. In one dispatch, he directed Smith (at the time his boss, let us not forget) to release one of the Dartmouth workers being held by soldiers on another farm. In another, he said, "Soldiers are not wanted. Their presence here will make a mess."

Besides these twenty-odd dispatches, there survives a never-sent letter in which John provides additional details. Although the work stoppage was the direct result of the wage cut, the ensuing violence, John wrote, was provoked by a white timekeeper, who without provocation shot "Turner, the crackerjack Jamaican foreman," and two other workers at one of the farms. A riot broke out, and one of the other Americans sent word to the hospital asking both the doctor and John to come to the scene.

Allowing for a tiny bit of dramatization (this must have been the most terrifying experience of the young man's life, and after it was over, he surely wanted to think of himself as strong and brave), John's account and the dispatches are in accord. He and MacPhail arrived on the farm to find the story of the shooting true: The timekeeper Daniels, a recent arrival in Guatemala, something of a hothead who had drifted into the company town flat broke and needing work, had lost his temper over something relatively inconsequential and started shooting. Daniels then fled for the coast, leaving behind about seventy-five very angry Jamaican workers. Their foreman had been shot, though not mortally, and another worker had been "grazed," but a third worker had been critically wounded by three bullets in his abdomen. While MacPhail, with the help of some of the workers, transported the wounded men to the hospital, John was asked to stay behind to help restore order.[54]

John had now earned the enmity of the acting superintendent and at least some of his fellow overseers and timekeepers. He had defied a direct order and had taken the part of the workers over the managers. Although he was still not above using such epithets as "black devils" for the rioters, he defended the workers, and himself, in another letter he intended to mail to Victor Cutter but never did. If the workers had been treated better, if the price cuts hadn't been so arbitrary, if one of his own workers had not been so hastily arrested and removed from the farm, and if Daniels had kept his temper, John insisted unrepentantly, the situation would not have gotten so out of hand.[55]

With the help of the soldiers, the strike was broken. John, although not immediately fired, was removed from Dartmouth and demoted to an office job. He was depressed and unhappy, and his letters home must have conveyed enough of his feelings that his father decided to come see for himself what was going on. He came, he visited, and he left convinced that John's difficulties would not be fatal to his long-term prospects at United Fruit. He was wrong. By now the company was just looking for a pretext to get rid of him. So, when John decided to see his father off, and his father's departure was somewhat delayed, John overstayed his leave by a day. The company fired him for that act, and he remained with MacPhail for a week, waiting for the next ship home. Working with MacPhail had provided John with the only happy experiences he'd had in Guatemala. MacPhail tried to cheer him up, reminding John that he "left a whole lot of warm friends behind" in Guatemala. But MacPhail also suggested that under the current circumstances, his friend would probably be better off back in the States.[56]

MacPhail's encouraging words were not enough. John came home from Guatemala a failure in his father's eyes and likely in his own. Frank could not conceal his apprehension over his youngest son's prospects. An extended adolescence was only for the privileged, and for the son of a striver still to be drifting at twenty was a cause for worry.

And as John looked around at what his friends were doing, he could see his father's point. Most of John's Lakeside and Marlborough friends had already embarked on their adult lives. Many of the boys among his childhood friends were about halfway through college. One was already a schoolmaster. John's fellow High School of Commerce alumni were settling into their careers, beginning their climbs toward business success as clerks or accountants for local and regional manufacturing or engineering firms.[57] Some of the young women were engaged or already married. Others were in college, or had taken jobs as stenographers, clerical workers, or teachers. Victor Cutter had achieved the title of superintendent of the Guatemala division in his mid-twenties, and Neil MacPhail at roughly the same age was well on his way to becoming a leading expert in tropical diseases.

But John was still floundering, and until he had met Neil MacPhail, he hadn't seen among the adults he knew any models for the kind of career he wanted to have. His father was a businessman, his father's friends were businessmen, and the people he came to know on his trip to Latin America in 1908 were businessmen, albeit in dramatically different contexts. It wasn't until MacPhail befriended him that John came not simply to long for a different kind of life but actually to envision one.

John had never known anyone like MacPhail, who was passionate about medicine but at least in those days indifferent to the kinds of material markers of success that so dazzled Frank Rock and his two other sons. MacPhail at twenty-seven found his pleasures in the profession of medicine (especially surgery), pursuing women (lots of them), and ending the day with a good stiff drink (and preferably more than one), in that order. John, miserably unhappy in United Fruit's tropical jungle, had little else in his life beyond his occasionally interesting but more often tedious and lonely work on the plantation, or his hated office job once he was demoted. So, John had his thoughts to keep him unhappy company, his letter writing to link him to friends and family, and MacPhail. It was MacPhail who brought John together with the young prostitute to whom John lost his virginity. And it was MacPhail who introduced him to surgery and to medical practice.

The hospital had become a refuge for John, and he and the doctor's friendship would last until the older man died four decades later.[58] MacPhail showed John that a career in medicine would suit him. Medicine, as MacPhail practiced it, required a steady hand, quick judgment, and confidence in one's decisions. It offered ever-constant but also ever-changing challenges. And John appreciated his kinship to MacPhail in another way as well. In so many ways different from the rugged Scot, John resembled him in his inability—or unwillingness—to conform to the life that others had planned for him, or to accept what others told him. His friendship with the young doctor was the happiest outcome of his nine months with United Fruit. Many years hence, in late middle age, the distinguished Dr. Rock would take his wife, Nan, on a sentimental journey to Guatemala, revisiting the place that had changed his life—not immediately, but irrevocably.

John decided, while spending his last days in Guatemala with MacPhail, that he wanted to pursue a medical career. After that last week of brooding and fretting and talking to Neil MacPhail about his future, John sailed for home in April 1910. Once he was home, Frank, with Charlie's help, talked John into taking yet another job as a clerk. Halfheartedly, he did his father's bidding and made his last attempt to become a businessman, working for the engineering firm of Stone and Webster. As yet unwilling to resist openly his father's ambitions for him, he nevertheless managed to get himself fired—again—in less than a year.[59]

· · ·

Much, much later in John Rock's life, when he was in the midst of his world-wide campaign to persuade the Catholic Church to change its ban against contraception, journalists and others invariably asked him how he could consider himself a good Catholic while repudiating the pope's teaching on birth control. In answer to this question, he always told a story about a conversation with a favorite priest during his adolescence. The story went like this: One day, when John was fourteen, he was leaving the church after Mass and met up with Father Finnick, one of the parish priests, who was getting ready for his weekly visit to the "poor farm." Father Finnick invited John to join him in his horse and buggy and go along for the visit. During the course of the ride, as the eminent Dr. Rock would tell the story, Father Finnick began speaking of the importance of conscience, telling young John, "Always stick to your conscience. Never let anyone else keep it for you . . . And I mean *anyone* else." Rock claimed that this buggy ride left him with an indelible impression of the way a Catholic conscience ought to function.

Journalists loved the story. When David Brinkley hosted an hour-long television program in 1963 featuring Rock and his work on the oral contraceptive, the opening scene showed Rock and Brinkley riding along a dirt road in a horse-drawn buggy, Rock recounting his visit to the poor farm with Father Finnick. The thing is, there isn't any evidence it actually happened, or if it did, that it made any impression at the time. In the diary that John kept regularly as an adolescent, beginning at age thirteen, he wrote about those people and occasions that were important to him at the time. There is no mention of a Father Finnick, or a poor farm, or any dramatic lesson imparted by a priest.

But the story did serve as a way for Rock to illustrate in a dramatic fashion his unwillingness to let others make his moral decisions. And it was surely easier to make up a story like this than to try to explain the process of growth that created the kind of person he would become—a fiercely independent man who, right or wrong, held to his own ethical standards and rejected the idea that others could dictate morality to him. His early life suggests that like most of us, John Rock took considerable time to figure out what he believed, and in part he learned what he believed from the way he acted when unhappy or threatened.

Although John seems to have tried sincerely to follow the family's plan for him, he rebelled in subtle ways from an early age. As a child, he rejected the athletic pursuits that were such a large part of the lives of his father and brothers. (Considering his growing interest in sports at the High School of Commerce and, eventually, his letter in track at Harvard, his lack of involvement in sports as a child suggests an act of quiet nonconformity, rather than a deficiency in athletic ability.) And while he did attend the High School of Commerce to prepare for a business career, probably in deference to his father's wishes, he defied his father's demand that he board with Delia Flynn. He went to Guatemala to aid the family's ailing fortunes, but when he got there, he took up with a maverick physician instead of befriending his fellow timekeepers and overseers.

His refusal to carry out his supervisor's orders to cut the wages of the Jamaican field workers provides the most dramatic evidence that he would never make a company man. He was told to cut wages, knew it was an order, and created the not-so-subtle fiction that if the *real* superintendent had been there, these orders would not have been given, and hence were not binding. (To the contrary, Cutter possibly wanted the cut to come when he was out of the country so that his fingerprints would not be on the decision.) By refusing to reduce wages, John showed the workers that management was divided, but the workers were already angered by the cut and had walked off the job at the other farms. His sympathies for the workers may not have had much influence, for good or ill, except that they likely made it easier for him and MacPhail to bring the wounded Jamaicans to the hospital.

John seemed in no doubt then or later that he had done the right thing. Ambivalent as he was about the labor force (they were interesting "Negroes" when they were working, "black devils" when they were rioting), he expressed admiration for several of the individual workers and particularly the Jamaican foremen. Whatever his opinion of the workers as a group, he was not willing to participate in or sanction what he considered an unfair and arbitrary cut in their pay.

By revealing to him what his values were and what he was prepared to do to live up to them, John's Guatemala experience was crucial in helping him to chart a course in life, even if it took him a while to do so. It is mostly in novels, and not always even there, that a life-changing experience results in a swiftly altered life. But at last, in the spring of 1911, John found himself where he had decided he wanted to be a year earlier, sitting for Harvard College's entrance examination. He had just turned twenty-one. His father, whatever his inner feelings, had conceded defeat in his quest to turn John into a businessman.

Perhaps Frank was worn down by trying to cast John into the mold of his older brothers, or perhaps he more readily agreed to John's decision because he was once again making money. Having gone dry for a year beginning in May 1909, Marlborough soon repented its collective decision. After it repealed its prohibition ordinance, in May 1910 Frank's wholesale and retail liquor business cranked up again. By 1911, with a year of profits behind him, he was not feeling the pinch of financial need quite so much. Then, too, brother Charlie, with the promise of some assistance from their father, agreed to finance John's Harvard education. They had no idea what they were letting themselves in for.

Chapter 2

CHOOSING MEDICINE, COMING OF AGE

Cambridge, Massachusetts, late spring 1917. The United States is at war with Germany. Several third-year Harvard medical students, including John, decide to drop out of medical school and enlist in the military. Their plans fall apart when the older brother of one of them, now serving in France, insists that they wait until they can be commissioned as medical officers.

Marlborough, Massachusetts, January 1919. John's world is upended when his beloved mother dies suddenly, dissolving the glue that held the Rock family together.

Boston, January 1921. John completes his final residency and takes a position as assistant in surgery at Massachusetts General Hospital. He is beginning his career at last.

In September 1911, freed from the depressing prospect of a career in business, John Rock entered Harvard College as a member of the class of 1915. Part of an elite triumvirate of colleges—Yale and Princeton were the others—Harvard was nevertheless unique. Its stature, which came from a combination of its history, the reputation of its undergraduate college, and even more important, its standing as a graduate institution, had enabled it to attract unprecedented financial contributions from industrialists and financiers, among them some of the notorious robber barons of the Gilded Age whose gifts made possible the growth of existing graduate and professional schools and the creation of new ones.[1] The largest university in the United States by the time John matriculated, Harvard enrolled four thousand students throughout its schools, enjoyed a $12 million endowment, boasted a faculty that was "the envy of other institutions," and provided the "best-funded financial aid program of any private [college or university]" in the United States.[2]

Charlie had promised to pay for John's undergraduate education, with Frank agreeing to pitch in if he could. Now all John had to concern himself with was being accepted. His good fortune held here, too. John just happened to apply to Harvard at exactly the time when the university embarked on a concerted effort to admit a broader range of students. The typical Harvard undergraduate came from one of a few private New England preparatory schools: Andover, Exeter, Milton, Groton, St. Mark's, and Middlesex. But Harvard's new president, Abbot Lawrence Lowell, who took office in 1909, had declared his intention to diversify the undergraduate population. In a deliberate attempt to attract talented students who had not attended these favored preparatory schools, Lowell developed what he called the "New Plan" for admissions.

The New Plan, inaugurated in 1911, called for prospective students, in addition to providing documentation of an "approved" high school course, to take a specific set of entrance examinations. Applicants took four examinations: in English; Latin (for a BA), German or French (for a BS); mathematics, physics, or chemistry; and one choice from this list. For example, if an applicant were examined in English, German, and physics, he could choose for his fourth subject French, mathematics, or chemistry. Of course, the New Plan was created not to recruit young men like Rock (local or near-local young men from Catholic families), but to attract promising Protestant students from beyond New England and the Mid-Atlantic. As Lowell explained his plan to a skeptical New England headmaster, he wanted to increase the absolute numbers of undergraduates and admit "boys from schools in other parts of the country which did not hitherto fit our requirements."[3]

Although the university's graduate and professional schools had already succeeded in drawing a more cosmopolitan student body, Lowell believed that the undergraduate college was still too parochial.[4] Attracting a greater number of students from a broader array of backgrounds was just one part of Lowell's vision. He also initiated the construction of freshman dormitories and mandated that first-year students live in them instead of segregating themselves by social class. And finally, he had intellectual ambitions for the undergraduate college, promoting a series of curricular revisions designed to make it more difficult for undergraduates to avoid serious study.

To attract prospective students from around the nation, Harvard orchestrated a national recruitment campaign conducted by the Harvard Federation of Territorial Clubs. (Geographically based, territorial clubs included students and alumni who came from a particular city, state, or region.) The federation took its responsibilty seriously and among other initiatives sponsored an illustrated book-length publication that advertised Harvard's intellectual, athletic, and social advantages—not to mention its scholarship program—for promising young men from all over the country.[5]

As a result of these efforts, in the early Lowell years Harvard would emerge as a more intellectually rigorous and cosmopolitan college than either Yale or Princeton. That is not to say that the university renounced or even discouraged racism, nativism, and anti-Semitism. Diversity under Lowell was of a particular kind, which would allow for the inclusion of some middle-class Protestant boys who had not attended elite New England prep schools. What Lowell was seeking was to broaden the ranks of the next generation of the Protestant elite by incorporating other young men into it, imbuing them with a common set of values and beliefs.[6] Lowell's changes had other, unintended consequences. The meritocratic elements of the New Plan provided a greater chance of admission for a small number of Irish Catholics, Jews, and African Americans. Just because students from disparate races and social circumstances were now in college together, however, did not guarantee that they would actually interact outside the classroom. The planned freshman dormitories had not yet been constructed in 1911, when John entered Harvard, so freshmen lived as they could, the wealthy and socially connected in expensive "gold coast" rooms and apartments, less well-off students in shabby college dormitories, at home, or in cheap lodgings around town. Jews and Catholics created their own separate religious organizations: the St. Paul's Catholic Society and the Menorah Society. There was even a fledgling Zionist group.

It isn't clear exactly how John viewed his Irishness. Until he left Marlborough, John had lived in a mostly Irish Catholic world; but unlike several of his friends and his brother Harry, John seems to have paid little conscious heed to the ongoing anti-Irish and anti-Catholic prejudice in which Massachusetts had been steeped for half a century. The High School of Commerce brought him into greater contact with Protestants; a number of his new friends were non-Catholics. In Guatemala, religion had been the least of John's problems. The country itself was Catholic, but John had little contact outside United Fruit, and few clerks and managers, if any, shared his religion. Still, once he arrived at Harvard, John found a social situation unlike any he had previously encountered.

John's class entered the university during the first flush of the Lowell administration. Theirs was the first class to enjoy being admitted under the New Plan and only the second to follow the new curriculum. But even though the class of 1915 was part of a new order of things, in many ways the new order looked a great deal like the old. Harvard College in this era—and long afterward—continued to encourage both exclusivity and exclusion. The sons of privilege, many from New England, still arrived at Harvard from their eastern prep schools (or, less often, midwestern country day schools) to be with others of their social circle. Most of them showed little interest in anyone else. Such students may not have dominated the college in numbers, but they certainly perceived themselves as the elect. The rest of the class was made up of several different kinds of young men, some of them the kinds of students that President Lowell deliberately courted—public school boys from the South, Midwest, and West, supported both morally and financially by the alumni members of the territorial clubs, and the sons of ministers and small-town lawyers. There were also a few self-styled intellectuals and bohemians; some bright Irish Catholics from Massachusetts; a cohort of talented young Jewish men from New York, Washington, and parts of the Midwest; and a *very* tiny sprinkling of gifted young African Americans, mostly from the eastern states.[7] Of the class's six hundred eighty-eight members, about thirty were obviously Irish Catholic students, most of them from Boston and its suburbs. Another twenty-nine students appeared to be Jewish, and between two and four were African American.[8] Taken altogether, such students accounted for less than 10 percent of the class.

The upper-class students lived in convivial luxury in private dormitories complete with servants, squash courts, and swimming pools. They summered in Newport or Bar Harbor, escorted Boston's debutantes to social events, and took tea with society matrons. The luckiest among them could look forward to election into the college's exclusive "final" clubs, of which Porcellian and A.D. were the most select. Samuel Eliot Morison, a Harvard historian whose fond chronicle of the college's first three hundred years appeared in 1936, did his best to minimize the college's social class divisions but conceded that "since 1890, it has been almost necessary for a Harvard student with social ambition to enter from the 'right' sort of school and be popular there, to room on the 'Gold Coast' and be accepted by Boston society his freshman year, in order to be on the right side of the social chasm."[9]

These were the favored few; the rest of the college's students sorted themselves out in various ways. How much it mattered to them that they lived more modestly, had middle- or working-class friends, and would have no chance to be considered for the exclusive "waiting" and final clubs no doubt depended on their pre-Harvard expectations as well as on their satisfactions in whatever other compensations their Harvard education brought them. Perhaps many didn't even notice and were perfectly happy with their lives. However they experienced their undergraduate years, their Harvard was clearly different from the Harvard of Boston society.

The first of the modern new dormitories did not open until 1914. Before then, in addition to living in run-down dorms, rooms in town, or with their families, the non-elect were "feeding in a mob at Memorial Hall," as Morison phrased it, or taking their board in cheap restaurants. There were attempts at the college to provide some amenities for such students that would approximate those of the selective clubs. The Harvard Union, for example, was an institution made possible through the generosity of Major Henry Lee Higginson, a Boston philanthropist who had attended Harvard briefly in the 1850s. Designed as "a house of fellowship" that would "bring democracy to Harvard," it was a club for the "unclubbed." Opened in 1901, for a fee of five dollars a term it provided a clublike atmosphere so that those without one could have a place to relax, listen to visiting speakers, and have parties. Although not successful in achieving its lofty purpose of democratizing the undergraduates, the union did provide accommodations for student organizations, dining rooms, reading rooms, and entertainment facilities. The territorial clubs took full advantage of the union, holding their meetings, dances, and dinners there.[10]

The several different Harvards coexisted separately, but the lines that divided them could be permeable, as they were for John, whose undergraduate life did not unfold entirely predictably. Here he was, a product of an on-again-off-again-affluent Irish Catholic family, who had attended public school, had virtually no social connections when he arrived at Harvard, and was older than most of his fellow freshmen. He would certainly seem destined to attend the Harvard of the non-elite. We should expect to see him as a denizen of a shabby dormitory in Harvard yard, eating his meals with the masses in Memorial Hall, and joining the rest of the unclubbed at social events in the Harvard Union. And to some extent, his experiences conform to that picture. In his first year, John lived in college-owned rooms, for which he paid about two hundred dollars, and took his meals at Memorial Hall, although his college bill shows no membership in the Harvard Union.[11] But while John never became a member of a waiting or a final club—the sine qua non for anyone with society connections or aspirations—he had considerably more social success in the Harvard of high society than one might expect.

He might have owed some of his social success to athletics. After having disdained sports in Marlborough, he developed some interest—at least as a spectator—at the High School of Commerce. But not until Harvard did he become an athlete. Joining the freshman track team his first year, he persevered in the sport for all three of his years as an undergraduate, enjoying enough success to earn a letter. Sports can often be something of a leveler in college. But doubtless more important for John's acceptance in the upper crust was his close friendship with Sherman "Shermie" Thorndike, grandson of General William Tecumseh Sherman and son of a prominent and socially connected Boston physician. Shermie's sister Nan would one day become John's wife.[12]

In his sophomore year, John scaled an important rung of the social ladder when he was elected to the Institute of 1770. The Institute's original purpose had been literary study and cultivation, but by the last quarter of the nineteenth century, its members no longer even pretended to be interested in intellectual pursuits. Rather, as historian Morison expressed it, the society had become "the first social sifting of the sophomores," electing to membership, in groups of ten, a hundred second-year students. In John's day, the first eight of those "tens" would be invited to join the Dickey (officially, D.K.E.), and out of the Dickey were chosen the members of the selective final clubs. "Of those socially eligible," said Morison, "it was a major catastrophe not to make the Dickey, or at least the Institute."[13]

John did not make the D.K.E. Instead he was invited to join Pi Eta and Sigma Alpha Epsilon, two of the four second-tier exclusive societies. (The others were Acacia and Delta Upsilon.) These four clubs, which according to Morison "elect[ed] about seventy-five members from outside the Institute Circle," were virtually the only Harvard clubs to which "graduates from high schools and the sons of country lawyers and ministers . . . could hope to be chosen." John joined Sigma Alpha Epsilon.[14]

In later years, Rock told at least one journalist that at Harvard he had been active in the Newman Club (a national Catholic student organization) and a member of Hasty Pudding. Neither is mentioned in his yearbook entry, but John may have been involved in the St. Paul's Catholic Society, in which several of his fellow Irish Catholic students were active, but failed to note the fact for the yearbook. As for Hasty Pudding, there is no record that he was a member as an undergraduate; however, during John's undergraduate years, Institute of 1770 members took part in Pudding productions, linking the two groups informally. In 1926 the two groups would merge, keeping the Pudding name.[15]

Underscoring the complexities of the institution and his personality, John navigated Harvard with one foot in the social set (as a member of the Institute of 1770 and a friend of Sherman Thorndike), and the other in a less socially exalted environment (as a member of Sigma Alpha Epsilon). He was admitted to some elite circles because of his friendships, but he was not fully a part of the socially elect. His Harvard experience foreshadowed his life in general. In the 1920s, he would marry a socialite (albeit a Catholic one with some unconventional interests). His marriage would elevate his social status, but his Irish Catholic heritage remained a part of him that he would never attempt to repudiate.

. . .

John knew he was lucky to be at Harvard, and he also knew to whom he was indebted for having this privilege. Unlike his friends from wealthy families, who could take the experience for granted, or his classmates among the "scholarship boys" beholden to one or another philanthropist or alumni group for their opportunities, he was being supported mostly by his hardworking older brother. And since Charlie was sending him to college at least as much for their parents' sake as for John's, he expected that John's moral indebtedness to the family would incline him to go along with the family's wishes.

John's mother was happy simply because John was doing what he wanted, but John's relationships with the men in the family continued to be strained. His father believed that his youngest son did not understand him and worse, that John never made the effort to do so. John in turn considered his father to be aggressive, controlling, and driven by the quest for wealth. Frank was perfectly aware of that fact but believed he was justified in telling his grown children what to do. Even though "because of my attitude you frequently misunderstood me," he insisted once, "I did what I thought best even if it hurt both you and myself knowing that it was only for the time being."[16]

Frank wanted his son to know that he loved and valued his children for what they were, and not for the money they could earn for the family. Unfortunately for his relationship with John, Frank was constitutionally unable to downplay his reverence for the dollar. When each of his children succeeded at something, he told John, "[I] felt fully paid for all the expenses [my children] had been to me." He "cleared off [their] slate," and "called [their] account squared." Money was the metaphor even for his expressions of happiness. Figures of speech? Perhaps. But Frank truly did place an extraordinarily high value on money and what money could do. He chased it when he didn't have it and exploited its power when he did. He constantly talked about it to his children. And even when he was trying hard to deny that he "measured, and valued, men and things by a money standard, instead of by a love and affection rule," all of his explanations came with analogies to expenses, accounts, and "slates."[17]

Their occasional attempts to connect notwithstanding, the fact was that Frank and his youngest son, no matter how hard either of them tried, could not understand each other. John may not have openly expressed his disdain for Frank's values, but his total disregard for the world of financial wheeling and dealing that so consumed the elder Rock sent the same message. Frank was not an uncaring father. He felt the chasm between himself and John, and he wanted desperately to bridge it. But he did not seem to realize the effect of his attempts to control John's life. "Keep in close touch with me, John," he wrote to his now twenty-one-year-old son, "by word and letter—I want to know your every thought, your every ambition, and your every want and desire."[18]

Frank had a much better understanding of, and relationship with, his older sons. Charlie had inherited his father's business ambitions. Harry was a willing and steady worker. John preferred his mother, whom he loved deeply and who had always had an especially strong attachment to him and his twin sister, Nell. And during John's undergraduate years, he began to feel closer to Charlie. The two brothers began to respect, if not entirely to comprehend, each other's talents and strengths.

Beyond an occasional family drama, we know a lot less than we would like about John's personal life during his undergraduate years. He left only a few letters. He was living in Boston, surrounded by friends and classmates, with his family only a forty-minute train ride away. If he fell in love, which, given his history, he probably did, the romance left no trace. If he felt disappointment in his grades or in his social life, or if conversely he was exceptionally happy, those feelings are lost in time.

We do know that he was a much greater social success at Harvard than his background would have led us to expect. And as he became comfortable in his new world, he no longer had much in common with his business-oriented pals from high school and let most of those friendships lapse. Most of his old High School of Commerce friends had entered the work force right after school. Now, whether in sales or accounting, in small businesses or substantial firms, they were looking for a steady climb up the economic ladder. They had already begun their adult lives—Ben Williams would be a father by the time John finished his formal education—while John was just beginning to find his way. In spite of the physical distance between them, he remained close to Neil MacPhail, who wrote him regularly about both personal and medical matters and came to see him whenever he could when he was in the United States.[19] The inspiration for John's ambitions, MacPhail continued to encourage John in his pursuit of a medical career. He was delighted with John's decision to attend Harvard Medical School.

. . .

Although John did not officially receive his BS until 1915, graduating along with his class, his postgraduate year at the High School of Commerce had allowed him to enter Harvard with advanced standing, and he completed his undergraduate requirements in three years. He began his studies at Harvard Medical School in the fall of 1914, while still technically a senior in college. The generous Charlie agreed to foot the bill for John's medical education.

By the time he entered the class of 1918, Harvard Medical School had become one of the finest in the nation, its success more than forty years in the making. When Charles Eliot had become president of Harvard in 1869, the medical school was, like many others in the United States, an undistinguished proprietary school, privately run and owned by physicians in Boston, and financially independent of the university. Eliot set out to change that situation, viewing the transformation of medical education as key to the creation of a modern university. Some changes he instituted quickly, if not painlessly, making the medical school part of the university within two years of assuming office, emphasizing the laboratory sciences, and expanding the time to degree from two terms of four months each to three years. Other changes were more difficult and took longer to accomplish, but by 1892 the medical curriculum took four years to complete, students were comprehensively trained in basic science, and almost half the students came in with bachelor's degrees. By 1901 the bachelor's degree was required.[20]

Harvard Medical School was not the most innovative of the modern medical schools—the medical school founded at Johns Hopkins University in 1893 would boast that distinction—but along with Hopkins and the medical schools at the Universities of Michigan and Pennsylvania, it was now a leader in the transformation of medical education.[21] Just before the turn of the century, with enrollment rising and the need for faculty in new areas of specialization reaching a critical stage, an ambitious plan for a new medical campus took shape. Dedicated in 1906, the campus gave Harvard the largest medical complex in the country.[22]

John was twenty-four when he began medical school. In choosing Harvard, he had chosen well. Having already achieved distinction in the laboratory sciences, the medical school had now managed to cement the necessary alliances with local hospitals that would enable the school to provide clinical clerkships at a range of institutions, from the venerable Massachusetts General Hospital to the new Peter Bent Brigham.[23]

John was a decent but not outstanding medical student (just as he had been a decent but not outstanding undergraduate). In his first year, he earned two Bs (very good) in physiology and biochemistry (biochemistry had recently come under the direction of Otto Folin, generally considered to be the nation's "foremost analytical biochemist"); one C (good) in histology; and a D (fair) in anatomy. In his second year, he earned a B in bacteriology, a C grade in pharmacology, and once again a D, this time in topographical anatomy. His general examination in clinical subjects posed complex diagnostic questions in the fields of medicine and surgery, obstetrics and pediatrics, psychiatry, and opthamology.[24] It was a very good education.

When he began medical school, John didn't know exactly what he wanted to do, but he had no intention of becoming a generalist in private practice. It was a good thing he didn't tell his father or oldest brother, however, since that was exactly what they intended for him. Charlie and Frank were eager for him to stop learning and start earning. Occasionally, Charlie was delegated to deliver the official family exhortation to that effect. In so doing, he always fervently expressed his expectation that when John graduated, he would begin to bring in a respectable income rather than seek additional training. After all, internships and residencies were unsalaried in these years (and long afterward), and if John wanted to study a specialty, this would just be a further drain on his generous older brother.[25]

Charlie was even more concerned for the well-being of his parents. In 1914 Frank had embarked on a new venture, a theater in downtown Marlborough. To lay his hands on the necessary capital, however, he had to cash in an insurance policy he had purchased to provide for his wife, Annie, should she be widowed. Shrewd in the ways of business herself, Annie saw the theater as a good investment and encouraged him to do so. With her blessing, Frank plunged ahead in partnership with fellow Marlborough businessman John Hayes, intending the income from this enterprise to supplement his other operations for now. And should the prohibitionists win, he reckoned, it could replace the income he would lose if forced to close his profitable wholesale and retail liquor businesses. Although his livelihood had been saved once before by Marlborough's 1910 revocation of its 1909 antiliquor ordinance,

Frank rightly feared that the drys could not be contained forever. Wisely, he planned to be prepared for the next prohibition campaign. But as usual with Frank, even with the proceeds of Annie's insurance policy, building the theater would leave him short of funds. Once again, as he had in 1909, he expected his sons to take up any slack in his and Annie's income.[26]

As a result, Charlie became even more directive in charting his youngest brother's future. During John's second year of medical school, Charlie told John that he would be expected to provide for himself, and help to provide for his parents, once he earned the MD. Charlie laid it all out: Immediately after graduation, John should take a paid position and save money for their parents. Later, much later, he could consider additional training. In the back of Charlie's mind was the idea that once John started earning money, he wouldn't want to give up an established practice to go back into training.

The next year, with a year and a half to go until John's graduation, Charlie again forcefully reminded his youngest brother of his family obligations. "I have given your future after finishing at Harvard considerable thought," he declared, "and have about arrived at a conclusion that it would be much better if you started active work as soon as possible." As the eldest son who felt responsible for everyone in the family, Charlie told John that "our first consideration, of course, is Pa and I feel that when you are actively engaged it will make him and Ma wonderfully happy." And since Pa's happiness always depended on money, John's ability to help support their parents financially would become increasingly important once liquor was outlawed, which Charlie believed likely "within the next three years." At that point their parents would be dependent on the income from Frank's movie theater, "which will never, to my way of thinking, be the money maker the store was."[27]

John was unwilling to disagree flat out, so he equivocated, apparently replying that Charlie's advice had started him on a "new line of thinking."[28] What he didn't say was that his "new line" had nothing to do with following Charlie's directions, although that was how Charlie interpreted it. Instead, John was playing for time. He could always fall back on Neil MacPhail's standing offer to work for him in Guatemala. Or he could go to war.

Within a few months of his exchange with Charlie, John was seriously considering leaving medical school and joining the military. In early 1917 war talk was everywhere; although Charlie wrote optimistically of "affairs [being] adjusted and settled in Europe" soon, the United States was on the brink of entering World War I.[29] As soon as President Woodrow Wilson declared war, in April 1917, John and his friends were ready to go. Eager to serve, and loath to wait until they finished medical school in order to be commissioned as medical officers, they considered simply enlisting in the army. Prudently, however, before rushing off to do so, the group sought advice from one of their number's brother, already serving overseas, who quashed their plans. Describing the reality of the war and its horrors, especially for enlisted troops, this older brother—an officer—urged them to wait until they could receive commissions. Agreeing with John that "of course" he and the others "must take your parts in it, but having been there and knowing what hell it is, I don't want to see you go into it as you seem to want to—as privates or as helpers in the medical corps." Fully respecting the desire "to get into it just as quickly as you can regardless of how you do it," he nevertheless insisted that "for the love of all you hold as good sense don't first of all go in the infantry, and second don't go in anything else unless you have the rank of an <u>officer</u>."[30] John took this advice and decided not to enlist immediately.

He waited, but his heart remained set on serving in the war. After graduation, he applied for a commission, even though he had just been offered an internship at Massachusetts General Hospital. Years afterward, Rock told journalist Loretta McLaughlin that his fate was decided otherwise as he completed his interview with the Harvard Medical School professor whose signature was the last required to approve the commission. "Almost as an afterthought," Rock remembered, the professor asked "what I would have done had I not got my commission. I told him I had an appointment for residency training in surgery at Massachusetts General Hospital. He called me back and took back the approval papers. 'You're not going into the service,' he said, 'Go back to MGH and learn something first.'"[31]

John ended up not going at all, although several of his close friends did sign up and serve as medical officers. When he read their letters, despite his earlier longings, John probably felt he had missed out on little. Rusty McIntosh wrote, "[my] unit got over here about the middle of Sept. [1918], was immediately dismembered—or disemboweled—and out of the wreckage a Capt. and I found that we had been assigned [to the Central Medical Laboratory] here, he in Serology and I in Path[ology]." So much for seeing combat or treating the wounded. By early 1919 John's friends were all waiting to come home, writing to John about dealing with bureaucracy, chafing under the orders of medical superiors in their "dotage," and one of them commenting jokingly of "not having a chance of getting wounded unless I laid my neck on a railroad track." Of the service itself in these immediate postwar days, Rusty referred to another friend who was waiting to be sent home as "the victim of that prevalent army disease which is so active post-bellum, namely buck-passing on the part of the superiors over him. He doesn't know how long" it would be before he could leave.[32]

From the accounts of his friends, John no doubt became reconciled to having been denied the military experience he had wanted so earnestly. He remained determined, however, to ignore his brother Charlie's instructions that he go into practice. He knew that Charlie was being shortsighted. Rock intended to specialize, and for that he would need to complete an internship and at least one residency.

By 1919 most of his friends who had gone to war had come home. Even those who had complained to John of feeling "stranded"—Frank Berry, forgotten by the military bureaucracy in Dijon, and Rusty McIntosh, detailed to the Paris Peace Conference—were now starting their medical careers. Rusty had gotten his wish and was off to a residency at Columbia Presbyterian Hospital, one of the teaching hospitals of Columbia's medical school. Showing how important the new laboratory-based medicine was to the younger generation (and how resistant the older generation could sometimes be), Rusty wrote John about the value of taking "a few months of pathology before doing clinical medicine" and being amazed that while the "attendings" claimed to be interested in pathology, "I don't think the majority know much. [We] even have one old duffer who still believes in 'a touch of pneumonia'; but fortunately there aren't as many quite as bad as that."[33] Rusty would go on to specialize in pediatrics. John's other friends and classmates from medical school scattered; some stayed in or around Boston, others went home, and still others sought good residencies wherever they were.

John, like Rusty, did not know right away which field to choose as a specialty. He would later tell reporters that he had originally hoped to become a neurologist, although he was also attracted to obstetrics and gynecology. In mid-life he often joked that he had lingered so long in obstetrics and gynecology that by the time he was ready to go into practice, he was too old to do anything else. But whatever he would do, he had rejected a career as a general practitioner.

When John graduated from medical school, although the dividing lines between the specialist and generalist, and between academic medicine and private practice, were much less distinct than they would later become, an aspiring specialist of Rock's generation still required advanced training through internships and residencies. At the end of World War I, internships came in three varieties and were becoming almost a routine extension of medical

school. The most popular, the rotating internship, allowed the new physician to spend some time in all clinical areas. A second type was referred to
as "mixed," and the interns divided their time between medicine and surgery.
And finally, there was the "straight" internship, offered primarily in hospitals
affiliated with medical schools, which enabled the intern to choose medicine
or surgery. The most desirable internships, from the point of view of a young
physician with ambitions, were in teaching hospitals like Massachusetts General. John signaled his ambition with his choice of a straight internship in
surgery, which he began on July 1, 1918.[34]

Then as now, hospitals offering internships and residencies regarded them
as educational as well as work experiences.[35] The incumbents lived in the
hospital and were given room and board but not a salary. Sometimes they received small stipends, up to ten dollars a month for interns, and from ten to
twenty-five dollars a month for residents.[36] Seminars, conferences, lectures,
and rounds (where specific cases were observed and discussed) were a regular
part of their experience. But the interns and residents were expected to learn
much by doing, and they performed a substantial number of service functions.
Although the purpose of their training was to provide them with increasing
levels of responsibility for patient care, in most major teaching hospitals (and
Massachusetts General was no different) interns and residents drew blood,
transported patients, and performed basic urinalyses and blood counts. However, in such hospitals they also received the clinical experience they sought.
John would be trained to perform general surgery and manage postoperative
care. He would routinely arise in the middle of the night to admit patients or
deal with an emergency. He would learn to think and act quickly.

John was in the middle of his internship when his mother suddenly died at
the age of sixty in January 1919. It is possible she had a heart attack or a stroke;
both Charlie and Nell would later suffer from severe hypertension, and both
would die from strokes or stroke-related complications. Annie Rock's death
devastated her children, permanently altering the dynamics of the Rock family. She had been its heart and soul, keeping everyone together and softening
her husband's sharp edges. After her death, everything changed.

Charlie, Nell, and John were most deeply affected by their mother's death.
Charlie reacted by getting as far away as he could. When Annie died, he had
been working in New England for the Gillette Safety Razor Company. He now
accepted an assignment that would take him to Egypt, India, and the Far East.
He wrote affectionate letters home but was out of touch for months at a time.
Frank and Nell took an apartment with John in Cambridge. Still at home at

twenty-nine when her mother died, Nell faced a particularly uncertain future. She had shown little interest in marriage and considered herself to be without marketable skills.[37]

Harry grieved but had worries of his own. Not only had he married a young woman who, according to his brothers and sisters, had a difficult personality, but he also had to contend with a demanding mother-in-law. Even though he took his troubles in his usual accommodating stride, his wife and her mother absorbed significant emotional energy. And although Maisie often declared in the months after her mother's death that she was an emotional wreck, she had always been her father's favorite child. She still had him, and she had a family of her own, which blunted the pain somewhat.

Devastated by his mother's death, John nevertheless had little time to devote to grieving. As a surgical house officer (i.e., intern), his daily life was one of long hours, little rest, even less money, and virtually no free time. With his mother gone, however, John turned his thoughts more seriously to joining Neil MacPhail in Guatemala. He had earlier passed up an opportunity to spend a summer during medical school with him to see if he would like it. One of his classmates did go, but John stayed in Massachusetts. Perhaps his memories were still too raw. As MacPhail continued to press him to come after Annie's death, John started to think it was not a bad idea.

By this time MacPhail was presiding over a well-equipped hospital in Quirigua, with a medical staff that had been educated in such preeminent medical schools as Edinburgh and Johns Hopkins. Skilled nurses from the United States and other countries came for training, and some stayed. The professionals and managers who worked for United Fruit, in contrast to their situations in 1908, lived in comfortable compounds with touches of luxury. MacPhail and his staff provided medical care for them all—United Fruit Company managers and white-collar employees and their families, the Guatemalan and Caribbean workers, and the local population.[38]

MacPhail often wrote to John during these years about his interesting cases. He may have been building his international reputation as an expert in tropical diseases, but he remained a surgeon at heart. He relished the tricky operation; the more complicated the problem, the happier he was. And he often described his cases in detail to John, including the harrowing but ultimately safe delivery of the first child of Rock's former boss (and soon to be president of the company) Victor Cutter. As early as 1917 MacPhail had urged John, "Go in for surgery son," he wrote, "and stick hard to it, and when you have had one year in a good hospital then come down here to be my right hand."[39] It was a genuine offer, and John had at least heeded MacPhail's advice to "go in for surgery."[40]

Still, only after his mother's death did going to work for MacPhail become a real option for John. He told his father of his intentions, and Frank in turn wrote to consult Charlie, who had mixed feelings about encouraging his youngest brother to return to Guatemala. Now traveling in such exotic locations as Egypt, India, and the Far East, Charlie was enthralled by distractions and temptations much more alluring than the picturesque sights and spectacular scenery he had been describing to his family. Projecting his own feelings onto his younger brother, he became worried that John too would be drawn to what many Americans might have considered a dissolute expatriate life. As he wrote John from Kuala Lumpur, "Since arriving East I know what an attraction and hold [such locales] can get on a person and how hard to cut the bonds and go back to civilization again and be happy." Wondering whether John had "carefully weighed all sides of the problem," he told him not to worry about money, that financial questions could all be worked out. "Don't rush away just to be doing something," he cautioned, but if it really is what you want, then "'go to it.'"[41]

John, rather more conventional than the gregarious, flirtatious, and commitment-phobic Charlie, may have been less tempted by the "exotic" possibilities of which his older brother hinted than he was by a desire to flee his family now that his mother had died. For John, Guatemala was an escape from his current life. It also had the advantage of at least being a decision about his future. But he still didn't know what he wanted, and ultimately he didn't go. This time he really did anger the patient MacPhail, who truly believed that John had accepted his offer.[42]

. . .

Instead of going to Central America at the conclusion of his internship, John moved on to a gynecological residency at the Free Hospital for Women. The Free, as it was often called, was just that, a charity hospital that specialized in the diseases of women, or as its bylaws read, a hospital for "poor women afflicted with diseases peculiar to their sex." The Free Hospital had been founded in 1875 on the model of J. Marion Sims's Woman's Hospital in New York, begun two decades earlier.[43] The Woman's Hospital, which opened its doors in 1855, had been the first of its kind, a marked departure from the "lying in" hospitals to which poor women usually turned for their health needs. There was no maternity ward. The hospital took only surgical cases involving the reproductive organs, and it exerted an enormous influence on the early development of the field of gynecology.[44]

Like the Woman's Hospital, the Free Hospital did not take obstetrical cases. Its founder, William Baker, was consciously perpetuating the legacy of Sims's Woman's Hospital. When the Free Hospital opened what Baker believed to be the nation's first cancer ward for women, treating breast as well as gyneco-logical malignancies, Sims himself spoke at the dedication. By 1895 the Free Hospital had outgrown its original quarters in Boston and moved to Brook-line. Sims was then dead; Oliver Wendell Holmes was the keynote speaker.[45]

By the early 1920s, most of the Free Hospital's surgeons were trained in both general surgery and gynecology. The women who availed themselves of their services were simultaneously patient and "teaching material."[46] John would come back to the Free Hospital for good in a few more years, but at this time he felt he needed more surgical training. Therefore, after completing his training here, he returned to Massachusetts General in 1920 for a four-month residency on the genitourinary service (urology and urological surgery).[47]

Finally, John made his last residency stop, from July 1920 to January 1921, as a house physician at the Boston Lying-In Hospital, where he received ad-ditional training in obstetrics. And in spite of his longstanding joke about having to go into obstetrics and gynecology because he was getting too old to do anything else, his real reason, his daughters remembered, was more seri-ous. Although he seemed headed in this direction already, as his residency at the Free Hospital suggested, his experiences in this residency would seem to confirm his future. One of the tasks of a resident of the Lying-In was to deliver babies at the homes of patients. Many of these deliveries were in the slums of Boston. Appalled at the conditions he saw, his service at the Boston Lying-In made him keenly aware not only of these women's medical problems, but also of their social and economic situations. John Rock was not Margaret Sanger. He did not immediately set out on a crusade. But he was affected, and he would think back to his months at the Lying-In as he shaped his own medi-cal practice.[48]

Charlie, back home in Boston for several months when John entered his final residency, had taken something of a financial beating while away. He had, unfortunately, put his financial affairs in his father's hands. Frank, still fancying himself a shrewd judge of the market, had ignored a directive from Charlie to sell Charlie's Gillette stock, only to see the stock plummet and Char-lie lose a bundle. True to form, however, Charlie did not hold a grudge; he was delighted that his father and Nell traveled all the way to San Francisco to meet his ship when he arrived home in February 1920. John was sharing an apartment with Nell and their father in Cambridge, and Charlie had no plans to leave the country again. Everyone was happy when John completed his formal training on January 3, 1921. Two weeks later he took his first postresidency professional position, as an assistant in surgery at Massachusetts General Hospital. At last, they rejoiced, John had finished training. He was just shy of his thirty-first birthday.

· · ·

It seemed that John's father was waiting only for him to finish his training before dropping a bombshell on the family. About two weeks later, Frank revealed to Charlie that he had been keeping a major secret and that he was going to marry Delia Flynn. This was the Delia so disliked by Annie, the Delia John hated and from whose house John had fled as a sixteen-year-old in Boston. Frank knew how much his children loathed her, but he intended to marry her anyway.

He had been sixty when Annie had died. Active, vigorous, and not ready to be turned out to pasture, he wanted Delia. A decade and a half his junior and now widowed, she was working as a buyer for a department store in Boston. How long their courtship had been going on is not clear. Perhaps their romance began only after Annie's death, but it may have been going on for many years. Whenever it started, Frank knew better than to mention her to his children—at least not until he decided to marry her.

As far as Frank was concerned, he was simply claiming a right to his own happiness. Charlie, he reasoned, was earning a good living and able to support himself and help his siblings; John was (at long last) ready to stop costing money and beginning to earn it. And Nell, he figured, could always be supported by her brothers if she decided not to marry. His children would probably have been reconciled to their father's remarrying—but to the dashing Delia? Their relationship was probably not a total surprise (which is likely why they so disliked her), but to learn that she would be their stepmother was a blow.[49]

Frank told only Charlie, whom he expected to take care of all his financial matters. The elder Rock's last act before getting married was to turn over the Rock and Hayes Trust (the profits from the theater) to Charlie. He told Charlie to manage the money to provide financially for Frank and Delia during Frank's lifetime.[50] Frank remained so worried about how his other children would take the news of his marriage that he couldn't bring himself to confide in anyone but the worldly Charlie, whom Frank delegated to tell the others. "I am depending on you," he wrote his eldest son, "to make it as easy for me with Harry, Mary, John, and Nell as you can," and to "put the best possible face on my offense to the senseabilities [sic] of my dear family."[51]

The family, Charlie included, took the news badly indeed. Frank beseeched Charlie "for my sake" to "receive Delia in as kindly a spirit as you can, and induce the others to do the same." Although not to be swayed in his decision by family antipathy to his intended bride, he asked Charlie, "<u>Please</u> write to Nell and John, I can't bear to tell them."[52] Nell later remembered that she "was so upset" when Charlie told her that she for one made sure her father knew how distraught she was. Because of the children's attitude toward Delia, the couple married in a private ceremony. "We have asked no one to stand up with us as witnesses and won't have anybody present but the priest and whomever he calls in as witnesses," Frank told Charlie. If his daughters thought that he expected them to acknowledge the event by their attendance or in any other way, he went on, Charlie should assure them that their father did not expect either of them "to pretend any thing—they may suit themselves and they will suit me."[53] Married on February 4, 1921, the newlyweds left immediately for a month's honeymoon in Cuba.

For John, who had expressed his loathing of Delia with a ferocity he rarely displayed, his father's marriage only exacerbated the wedge that had long existed between them in spite of the efforts of both. John's mother had been his constant defender, always convinced that her feckless youngest son, in spite of his early missteps, would make his mark in the world.

But however Frank's children reacted, he did not think he was being unreasonable. He was old enough to please himself and too old for his children to object, regardless of whether Delia had been his mistress when Annie was still alive. Frank no doubt believed that he had stayed around for his children as long as he was needed. So Frank headed off to his honeymoon with a clear conscience.

Charlie beat his father to the altar by just four days. After years of evading the many women he had courted and left behind, Charlie proposed in December to Kathryn Green, a young woman whom he had known before going abroad, and whose sister had at one time worked for him. Charlie loved women but had assiduously resisted marriage. Now, with his mother's death, his travels, his age—he turned thirty-six in 1920—adding incentives to Kathryn's own charms, he changed his mind. Nell too would marry within a few months; her groom was Charlie Molloy, whom she had known for years. John

was now the only unmarried one, and he had a while to go before he could afford to support a family. It is possible, however, that even now he had begun
to turn his romantic thoughts to Sherman Thorndike's twenty-six-year-old
sister Anna, whom everyone called Nan.

. . .

In the years to come, John and Charlie would become quite close. While John
was at Harvard studying medicine but not knowing where it would take him,
Charlie was working through some uncertainties of his own about the future.
Since he had been a young man, Charlie had worked for others, making a solid
income and enjoying financial success. But he wanted to work for himself,
not others. Once, when John was a beginning medical student, Charlie, in a
rare departure from their usual relationship, had asked John's opinion about
whether he (Charlie) should train to become a chiropractor. John had discouraged him, and Charlie, like John, would not truly come into his own until
comparatively late.

After Annie's death and especially following Frank's remarriage, even
though Charlie would continue to provide financial support to his father, the
intense family bonds loosened. As John's ties to his father became much more
distant, those to Charlie would grow ever closer. As happens more often than
children (or parents) might like to admit, when parents die, or take on a new
life, it can liberate their sons and daughters to rethink their own lives. Now
that he had no obligations to his parents and finally had a profession, John's
hopes would turn to a family—and a life—of his own. But first, he needed to
ensure that he had a future in medicine.

Chapter 3

NEW DISCOVERIES IN HUMAN REPRODUCTION

New York City, 1921. Dr. I. C. Rubin develops a nonsurgical technique to diagnose blocked fallopian tubes, which requires only a simple apparatus that can be set up easily in a physician's office.

St. Louis, Missouri, 1923. Scientists Edgar Allen and Edward Doisy isolate estrogen. A revolution in our understanding of human reproduction begins.

Brookline, Massachusetts, 1926. John Rock becomes director of the sterility clinic at the Free Hospital for Women. He has no way of knowing what either Rubin's technology or Allen and Doisy's discovery will mean for the lives of the women who stream into the clinic each week seeking a cure for their infertility. He is simply hoping he has made the right professional decision.

Any reasonable observer would think a doctor with four residencies completed—surgery, gynecology, urology, and obstetrics—surely would have figured out which field to pursue. Not John Rock. Either he simply could not decide what to do or he was keeping his options open. First, he took a position as assistant in surgery at Massachusetts General Hospital. For the next couple of years he performed gynecological, urological, and general surgery, at the same time attempting to develop a private practice in obstetrics and gynecology. The practice of medicine was less specialized in the 1920s than it later became, but not because practitioners necessarily wanted it that way. Like many of his colleagues, Rock was forced to be more of a generalist than he would have preferred because he couldn't afford to pass up paying patients.

In 1924, when he was offered the opportunity to reopen the defunct sterility clinic at Massachusetts General Hospital (MGH) and to participate in the creation of another clinic at the Free Hospital for Women, he was pleased to accept both opportunities. The MGH clinic had once been directed by Edward Reynolds, who along with his colleague Donald Macomber had a longstanding interest in the treatment of infertility.[1]

[50]

Gynecologists had been tackling the problem of sterility since the creation of the field in the mid-nineteenth century. Unfortunately, they had not enjoyed much greater success than the midwives they had displaced. By the early twentieth century, infertile patients and the practitioners who treated them oscillated from high hopes to regular disappointments. Surgical procedures, which had become dominant in the last half of the nineteenth century, rarely worked; doctors had little else. And as late as the 1920s, even in the practices of highly regarded infertility experts, pregnancy rates for couples having trouble conceiving hovered at 16 percent at best, and physicians almost never talked about how many of those pregnancies resulted in live births.[2]

The situation was about to change, however. The first new ideas about infertility in nearly fifty years were now beginning to make their way into clinical practice.[3] Important technological and scientific advances, which would become broadly accepted in the 1930s, were just emerging, the most important of which were the discovery of the sex hormones, research on male fertility, and the development of new nonsurgical methods of determining the patency (openness) of the fallopian tubes. The reopening of the MGH clinic and the creation of one at the Free Hospital suggest that their creators recognized that a new era in the field was about to begin.

In 1926, when Rock became director of the Free Hospital's sterility clinic, he resigned from the one at MGH. He could not, however, devote himself solely to this enterprise. Although Rock would make his career at the Free Hospital as a gynecologist and infertility specialist, in this period (and for a generation afterwards) it would be all but impossible for ambitious specialists to limit their practice to a single institution. In Rock's case, to make a living he had to practice obstetrics, and obstetrics was not part of the Free Hospital's mission. He delivered his patients' babies at the Boston Lying-In Hospital. And because not all of his private surgical patients wanted to come to the Free Hospital, he also needed his surgical privileges at MGH.[4]

Rock was fortunate in his senior colleagues at the Free Hospital. William Graves, the hospital's chief, and Frank Pemberton, his assistant chief and eventual successor, encouraged Rock's growing competence in the study and treatment of infertility. Graves's leadership was pivotal to both Rock's career and the hospital's overall transformation. From the time Graves arrived at the Free Hospital in 1902, and even more so after he became surgeon-in-chief in 1908, he emphasized research as much as he did patient care and teaching. He repeatedly exhorted the residents and young attending physicians who worked under him to "do all the surgery you can and publish the results of your clinical and research work often." The atmosphere at the Free Hospital encouraged its physicians to be productive researchers as well as effective practitioners.[5]

Rock was no exception. In assuming the directorship of the Free Hospital's sterility clinic, Rock had found his calling.[6] At the age of thirty-six, he arrived at the real beginning of his long, brilliant, and controversial career. From here on, his future would be tied to Harvard and the Free Hospital.

· · ·

The Free Hospital provided Rock with the opportunity to expand his professional expertise, teach, conduct research, and publish its results. His position was expected to pay off in experience and reputation. That's why physicians sought such posts. Appointments like this one paid little salary but conferred prestige, serving as springboards for the creation of a large and lucrative private practice. Elite medicine was a competitive world, and hospital positions were essential accessories for those who were ambitious. Rock wanted both professional recognition and financial success, and both goals had become more pressing. He had fallen in love and married. As 1926 opened, he had just become a father. He had a family to provide for now.

John had proposed to Anna "Nan" Thorndike, his close friend Sherman's sister, in 1924. He had known her family for more than a decade and vacationed with them at the family's summer home.[7] The young Thorndikes—Shermie, Martha, and Nan—were the children of General Sherman's youngest daughter, Rachel, and her husband, prominent Boston physician Paul Thorndike. The family lineages guaranteed their position among the city's elite, although they were a bit atypical in that Rachel and the children (although not Paul) were Roman Catholic.

Born on September 12, 1896, Nan grew up in Boston, where her father was chief of urology at Boston City Hospital. Educated locally as a young girl at Miss May's School, she enjoyed a year of German education in Munich at fourteen and another at a French convent school in Montreal at sixteen. She was a good student, taking courses in Latin, English (literature and grammar), French, algebra, German, physics, and logic. She also loved to have a good time. Her adolescent passions included sports as well as the music crazes of the era; letters to her sister ring with such popular slang terms of the period as "corking" and "crazy."[8] Like her sister, Martha, Nan came out as a debutante at the age of eighteen. ("Coming out" referred to the several months of parties and balls during which a wealthy and socially connected young woman was publicly presented to the social elite for the first time. It was a signal that she was now of an age for courting and marriage.) Unlike Martha, who had been debutante of the year during her coming out, Nan did not consider herself terribly suited to these trappings of society life. She was smart and fun loving, but she was a bit more than that. She had intellectual leanings, evident both in her decision to attend college and in her somewhat surprising choice.

In 1915, as she was about to turn nineteen, Nan entered Bryn Mawr, the most intellectually rigorous of the women's colleges. Headed by the formidable M. Carey Thomas, who had been its founding dean, Bryn Mawr had opened in the 1880s and was backed by the fortune of Quaker philanthropist Joseph Taylor.[9] It had been conceived as a female equivalent to Haverford College (the principal college for Quaker men, located in Haverford, Pennsylvania). Thomas, however, considered Haverford to be second rate. Her ambition was much higher—the creation of an institution where women could receive the kind of rigorous education available only to men at top-level colleges and universities.

Thomas, who constantly chafed at the educational restrictions placed on women, might have been disappointed at how lightly many upper-class young men wore their Harvard or Yale or Princeton educations. Certainly John Rock's Harvard was full of students whose social lives as undergraduates were far more important than their coursework. But Thomas would probably have insisted that such an attitude was beside the point—young men who valued learning at these institutions at least had access to it. Thomas had graduated from Cornell, having been thwarted by her first choice, the new Johns Hopkins University, when its president and board declined to admit women. She received her doctorate in linguistics at the University of Zurich, one of the few universities in the world that would allow women to earn the PhD.[10]

Thomas's vision for Bryn Mawr was shaped largely by her own desires and experiences. She wanted to provide for women—at least, for white, upper-class women—every opportunity enjoyed by their male counterparts. At Bryn Mawr she designed an education for women like herself and those from the even higher social backgrounds to which she aspired.[11] Under Thomas's leadership, Bryn Mawr offered graduate and undergraduate education; she insisted that the faculty be both researchers and teachers. The undergraduate program was modeled on what was called the "group system," pioneered at Johns Hopkins. A forerunner of the undergraduate major, the group system steered a middle course between the elective system that had been introduced by President Charles Eliot at Harvard (but would be discarded by his successor Lawrence Lowell) and the classical curriculum favored by most women's colleges.[12]

By the time Nan enrolled as one of ninety-five members of the class of 1919, Bryn Mawr's curriculum remained little changed from the previous decades. Nan's classmates were much like her; their families ranged from the well off to the truly wealthy. Nearly all were Protestants, although Nan's Catholicism (bleached as it was by social prominence) had been no obstacle to her acceptance. She selected mathematics and physics as her major areas of concentration, fields in which she would have excellent role models. In mathematics, both senior faculty positions were held by women with PhD degrees, and in physics, the two junior faculty members (who did not hold PhDs) were women. Thomas hired men as well as women, but she preferred to hire women whenever possible. As a result, Nan and her fellow students had ample evidence that women could excel in mathematics and the sciences. Besides courses in her area of concentration, Nan studied English, biology, economics, philosophy, and psychology. Having been well prepared in Greek as an adolescent, she was declared proficient by examination and studied only French and German in college. She passed the required examinations in both languages in her senior year. Nan also explored electives that suggested a broad curiosity about the world around her, taking courses in architecture and in the history of the Slavic peoples.[13]

Bryn Mawr also allowed Nan to indulge her passion for athletics and music. She played tennis, hockey, water polo, and basketball and was also on her class's swimming and track teams. She was the "song mistress" for the class of 1919.[14] And her interest in the world around her was profound. The Great War was raging, and Nan, who had traveled in Europe as a child, was deeply affected. M. Carey Thomas herself was an impassioned Allied supporter. Even before the war started, she refused to hire pro-German faculty members and was vociferously and publicly critical of those who did not support the French and the English.

As a student, Nan, influenced by her own experiences as well as the college's pro-Allied stance, joined a group of volunteer ambulance drivers who traveled to France to aid the war effort. Her service engendered a long-lasting compassion for the suffering and devastation wreaked on that nation by the war. She remained concerned for its people; after she graduated, she returned to France in the early 1920s as part of a humanitarian relief mission sponsored by the American Committee for Devastated France. She recorded this later trip in photographs—of her friends driving and fixing motor vehicles, carrying relief supplies, and posing amid French villagers, as well as the invariable tourist snaps of churches, landscapes, and picturesque village scenes. Grateful to Nan Thorndike and women like her, the French government presented her with the Medaille de la Reconnaissance for her service.[15]

Once she returned from her second trip to France, however, for the first time Nan seemed to settle into a conventional postdebutante life. According to her daughters, she worked for a while in an exclusive dress shop. There is no indication that she expressed any career aspirations, although if she had, her family would have discouraged her. She did not seem to repine, however, and in 1924 became engaged to John. They married on January 3, 1925. Because of Nan's mother's social standing, William Cardinal O'Connor himself performed the sacrament. Cardinal O'Connor rarely officiated at a wedding, and this was considered a great honor.[16]

John and Nan honeymooned for a month in Quebec. A snapshot shows them on ice skates, and they certainly were an eye-catching couple: She was nearly six feet tall, and although not conventionally beautiful, was strikingly attractive with an engaging smile (more Katharine Hepburn than Vivien Leigh—not so much pretty as handsome). He was about an inch taller, was quite handsome, and would become even more so as he got older.[17] Catholics who had waited until the ages of thirty-five and twenty-nine to marry, they made an early start on having their family. Rachel was born slightly less than a year after the wedding, in December 1925, and John Jr. was born eighteen months later. Nan and John would go on to have three more children: Ann Jane (called A. J.) arrived in 1929, Martha in 1930, and Ellen in 1932.

John was happy with Nan and proud to be a father, but he sometimes despaired when he considered the financial resources needed to raise a family in the kind of comfort he expected for them and for himself. Nan had been accustomed to servants all her life—she had even enjoyed domestic help at Bryn Mawr, since M. Carey Thomas, unlike the administrators of the other women's colleges, insisted that her students should not have to make their own beds or tidy their rooms. John, too, had grown up in a family with household help. In their generation, most upper-middle-class families employed domestic workers.[18] John and Nan, therefore, expected no less. The young Rock family generally had a cook and other daily domestic workers in their large West Roxbury home and, at least when Rachel and A. J. were small, had live-in help as well. John and Nan each had a car, perhaps not too great a luxury for the family of a doctor out delivering babies at all hours.[19]

The big house, the cars, the cook, the maid, the children, and their nursery maid—they all cost money, and money was often in short supply. John's clinical position at Harvard and the appointment to the Free brought prestige and recognition and opened the door to private practice possibilities, but they did not pay the bills. In 1927, with a child already and another on the way, Rock earned a total of $800 for the year (less than $9,000 today) from his job at the Free Hospital, of which he "spent $200 on . . . office and car and practice expense."[20] Nan's family had lived well and was socially prominent, but Nan herself had only $7,000 (around $80,000 today), an inheritance from an aunt. She had invested $5,500 of that, keeping the other $1,500 for family expenses.[21]

· · ·

Rock's new clinic responsibilities, private patients, and growing family kept him busy, and he heeded his chief's advice to put his name before the profession through publication. As a first step, he took on the occasional task of writing the "Progress in Obstetrics" articles for the *Boston Medical and Surgical Journal*, soon renamed the *New England Journal of Medicine*.[22] These "Progress in" articles, written by specialists in a particular field, were designed to appear approximately once a year. Their purpose was to provide general practitioners with summaries of current research. The articles on obstetrics were especially welcome, since most babies in this country delivered by doctors were delivered by general practitioners, not obstetrical specialists.

In his own early "Progress" pieces, Rock addressed such matters as how to diagnose a pregnancy, prenatal care, and pregnancy complications such as anemia, heart disease, placenta previa (a condition in which the placenta is covering the opening of the cervix, which can cause obstetric hemorrhage), and late toxemia (now called preeclampsia, which can result in high blood pressure, seizures, and fetal death).[23] He offered advice on managing patients with tuberculosis. He emphasized the importance of prenatal care in the prevention of some of the most serious complications, such as eclamptic seizures, and gave his opinion on what had by then become a staple of obstetrical discussion, the kinds of anesthesia to use in delivery.[24]

In these years, there was no simple way to determine in the first few weeks after a missed period whether a woman was pregnant or not. Researchers, naturally, were eager to find one. In the 1920s Rock dutifully wrote about reports of success with a simple albumin test. Unfortunately, in his next "Progress" article, he had to say that the reports were wrong: the "sugar tolerance" test was unreliable. In fact, he said, there was still only one way to be sure a

woman was pregnant—time. "Fortunately," he concluded in one of his typical dry asides, "the diagnosis of pregnancy is not always of immediate importance. Time is probably still the surest aid: indeed, for all practical purposes
it may be considered certain."[25]

The "Progress" articles provide a sampling of some of Rock's maverick
opinions, which would become more evident as the years unfolded. Much later in his career, Rock would tell an interviewer that he had never been a fierce
opponent of abortion because he believed the fetus was a *potential* person but
not yet a human being. He suggested as much in 1927 when he insisted that a
pregnant woman's health should take precedence over the life of her fetus. If
a woman's health would be endangered if her pregnancy were allowed to continue, he wrote decisively, "good obstetrics . . . demand[s] . . . prompt empty-
ing of the uterus." Physicians should also perform an abortion if they were
unable to treat uncontrolled "toxic" vomiting in early pregnancy. And abortion was indicated for women with certain types of heart conditions (a patient with "clear signs of congestive failure, [or with] complicating nephritis
or hypertension, . . . auricular fibrillation, absolute disorder of the heartbeat,
. . . [or] who has at present a rheumatic fever"). Women suffering from tuberculosis, he was pleased to note, were enjoying more successful pregnancies
with appropriate treatment, and hence abortion should not be necessary.[26]
Although Rock opposed elective abortion, he insisted there were sound medical indications for performing an abortion. He did not mind that his views did
not conform to the teachings of the Catholic Church, which as early as 1895
had ruled against abortion performed for medical reasons.[27]

Perhaps more interesting than Rock's stance on therapeutic abortion,
which may have been condemned by his church but conformed with progressive obstetrical opinion, was his explicit support of contraception.[28] Rock
did not shy away from expressing his views, even in this journal published
in Massachusetts, a state with a draconian anti-birth-control law. In his 1932
"Progress in Obstetrics" article, he boldly discussed the "Prevention of Pregnancy." Reviewing a new book on contraception for physicians, he praised
its discussion of "the best modern methods of prevention." Recommending
it as a source that would allow the "honest sincere obstetrician" to prescribe
contraception, he insisted that such a practice was essential for those patients
in whom pregnancy would result in "serious impairment or destruction of
health or reason." And he concluded with a direct slap at doctors who claimed
that their moral scruples would not allow them to dispense contraceptive devices. It was one thing, he said, for a doctor to oppose contraception as a pri-

vate person, but "it is wrong . . . for the doctor to make believe he is practicing medicine" when so doing.[29]

Rock used the occasion of these review articles both to articulate his own developing views about fertility, pregnancy, and contraception in the first decade of his career and to shore up the claims of obstetrical specialists over those of general practitioners. In these years most physicians in America's cities and towns were general practitioners, and a woman typically looked to the general practitioner for all family medical care, including her pregnancies. Specialists like Rock sought to persuade general practitioners to refer their patients to obstetricians, although Rock was careful not to offend his generalist colleagues. As he preached the gospel of full prenatal care, prompt and expert attention to any possible complications in pregnancy, and the superior knowledge of the best and most up-to-date kinds of anesthesia to use in childbirth for a successful outcome to the pregnancy, he suggested simply that these services were more likely to be provided by an obstetrical specialist.

In a presentation to the White House Conference Institute devoted explicitly to public policy issues surrounding pregnancy and childbirth, he argued the case of the superiority of specialists even more forcefully. American doctors were well aware that in the United States, the death rate in childbirth had climbed as births moved from the home to the hospital.[30] Unwilling to admit that control of childbirth by physicians might be part of the problem, he argued instead for systematic prenatal care: "If our pregnant women would go early and often to the doctors our maternal mortality would be halved."[31] And although he was not, he claimed, insisting that "all doctors . . . be specialists," he declared that "each doctor must know enough to recognize the patient whose condition surpasses his qualifications safely to deliver and care for." "Many" generalists, he believed, "would willingly be excused from maternity work, but are forced to do it to establish themselves in the community." Either medical schools and professional boards must do a better job of training and certifying general practitioners, he concluded, or the obstetrician should replace the general practitioner in the delivery room.[32]

Rock spoke passionately from experience about the superior claims of the specialist. He knew firsthand the difficulties of establishing a specialty practice and keeping it up in these early years of the Great Depression. Medicine was a highly competitive profession, with generalists and specialists vying for the same patients. But while he sincerely believed in the efficacy of prenatal care and in the importance of training medical students and interns to recognize potential complications of pregnancy, it would be surprising if he found much intellectual satisfaction in the routine practice of obstetrics. A normal pregnancy, thank goodness, is uneventful. Physicians who revel in solving complex problems, managing difficult pregnancies, and successfully bringing a tricky delivery to a close would be hard pressed to find much of a challenge in a routine pregnancy, labor, and delivery. But the practice of medicine was such during this era that even gynecologists—*especially* gynecologists—could not afford to do without obstetrics. It was at the heart of their day-to-day practice.

Unlike some of his colleagues, who justified the need for specialists by advocating increasing obstetrical intervention, ranging from routine induction of labor to the promotion of cesarean sections, Rock was a minimalist who, in the absence of complications, trusted nature to take its course. He did, however, believe strongly in pain relief during labor; to his mind, anesthesia and other analgesics were simply adjuncts to a natural labor.[33]

Rock would continue to publish in the field of obstetrics until 1939 and to deliver babies until the mid-1940s. Obstetrics remained his bread and butter in these early years. Increasingly, however, his passion lay in the study and treatment of fertility and infertility. The *New England Journal of Medicine* published his first article in this area, a review of the state of research and treatment of infertility, in 1928. Placing considerable emphasis on the concept of relative fertility and the importance of fertility testing for husband as well as wife, Rock reflected the common wisdom among his colleagues. He also incorporated several hints of what was to come—a mention of "endocrine factors" and a veiled curiosity as to how exactly a newly fertilized ova makes its way to the uterus.[34] Overall, however, this was not an article that dazzled with originality. In later years, he would omit it from his list of significant publications.

· · ·

By the end of the 1920s, Rock's life seemed to consist of an endless round of practicing, publishing, and trying to develop a research program that would build his reputation. Some days, he would operate for more than four hours straight in the morning, then see patients in the afternoon and evening. And after all that, his day might not be over; he could be called to a delivery in the middle of the night. The nonstop grind took its toll. He was constantly worried about money, and at times he wondered why he was pushing himself so hard. "It's about six at the end of another day of ceaseless detail," he wrote Nan in the summer of 1928, when she and Rachel had gone off for a vacation to Cranberry Island, Maine. "I don't know where all this work comes from," he puzzled, then added hopefully, "but it's probably leading somewhere."[35]

If nowhere else, it was leading to a breakdown. By early 1929 Rock had pushed himself beyond his endurance. He felt debilitated. Not wanting to have his health gossiped about among his Harvard colleagues, he turned for advice to Rusty McIntosh, one of his closest medical school friends. Rusty, now at Johns Hopkins Medical School, suggested that Rock come there for an evaluation. With Nan's encouragement, John spent a week at Hopkins in April under the medical scrutiny of the hospital's physician-in-chief, Warfield Longcope. As hospital stays go, Rock's was pretty pleasant. Although for part of each day he was poked, prodded, tested, and x-rayed, in the evenings he went out for drinks and dinner with Rusty and his friends. When not being examined, he dropped in to watch J. Whitridge Williams, the hospital's chief gynecologist, perform a cesarean section and visited the wards to see how they functioned. Sometimes he just sat in his room and read. He had always loved to read, and the enforced rest allowed him to read for pleasure. He had managed, he wrote Nan with considerable satisfaction, to finish the new Lytton Strachey biography of Queen Victoria.[36]

His week of rest and freedom from the demands of his work and family may have done him good all by themselves. Nan, indeed, had insisted that her "own diagnosis" was not overwork but "too much family." John disagreed with her, but still, in addition to his worry about his work, he and Nan now had three children under the age of four. Back in Brookline, Nan described a typical family evening: "Your son and eldest daughter are in the kitchen, . . . one probably eating coal off the floor and the other ironing her dollie's clothes—and little Ann Jane has been calling her ma but is now sleeping peacefully."[37] And before too long, Nan would be pregnant again. Even with regular household help, the children kept Nan, and often John as well, extremely busy these days.

According to his doctors, John's troubles seemed to have no discernible physical causes. The specialists at Hopkins had studied his heart, lungs, gall bladder, and digestive system; but in the end, all the examinations, tests, and x-rays uncovered no disease. And what did Warfield Longcope think? The great physician told Rock that he was "emotionally upset." And while John claimed to be relieved that he did not have any physical illness, he did not like the idea of a psychological diagnosis. He wrote not-quite-jokingly to Nan that she would "be pleased to know there's nothing mentally wrong—you're not married to an incipient madman or imbecile." Still, Longcope "suspects I have 'complexes,' though he did not term them that."[38]

Given his relationship with his family, especially his father, complexes would have come as no surprise. Even so, his well-founded professional and financial worries no doubt were major contributors to his unspecified physical symptoms. What he wanted to do in his career was to combine academic medicine, which privileged research and teaching, with a productive and profitable private practice. But this was a difficult goal to achieve. Even today, of course, most gynecologists also practice obstetrics, but nowadays we would not expect a doctor who specializes in reproductive endocrinology and engages in research to have a generalist practice in obstetrics and gynecology. That, however, was Rock's situation. During the 1930s, as he became an increasingly prominent practitioner and clinical researcher in a new field that would eventually be called reproductive medicine, he still would have found it extraordinarily difficult, perhaps impossible, to make an adequate living specializing in infertility research and treatment. After all, his hospital position paid little, which meant that a substantial private practice was necessary for him to make a living.[39] And because far more women were having babies than seeking medical care because they were having trouble having babies, Rock continued to perform deliveries. Not until nearly the end of World War II would he be able to give up obstetrics, which is both demanding and exhausting. It would not be until the late 1940s that Rock could devote himself almost entirely to problems of fertility. Even then, he would continue to perform gynecological surgery until his mid-sixties and practice some general gynecology for his entire professional life.

From the outset of his career, therefore, and for nearly two more decades, Rock was an obstetrician, gynecologist, infertility specialist, teacher of medical students and residents, and clinical researcher, all in one. By all accounts his patients loved him, and he enjoyed respect from many of his colleagues. He would become quite successful, except for one thing. He could never manage money. Although he eventually did get in the habit of billing his private patients, he would never allow himself to insist on collecting their fees. That he brought many of his financial problems on himself did not make him worry less. And he had reason to worry.

Rock's income in the late 1920s and the early 1930s might not seem meager by the standards of typical beginning young professionals, but it was not sufficient to enable him and Nan to move among Boston society, where membership for Nan in the Chilton Club (an exclusive women's club), for him in the Tavern Club, and for them both in the country club in Brookline, seemed de rigueur. From 1928 through the early 1930s, his gross annual income ranged from about $10,000 to $12,000 (about $110,000 to $140,000 today) before deducting the expenses of running his private practice—rent, phone, part-time secretarial assistance, supplies, and the like. (In 1928, the only year for which exact figures are available, his practice cost was just under $1,600.) In addition, he may have incurred other expenses connected with his research work at the Free Hospital. Money worries more than anything else probably fueled the symptoms that sent him into the hospital just after his thirty-ninth birthday. Fortunately for the Rock family, brother Charlie could almost always be counted on to step in as fairy godfather.[40]

Chronically short of money, throughout the 1930s John often turned to Charlie, now the wealthiest by far of the three Rock brothers. Charlie had parlayed his experience at various New England firms, and even more so his year in the Middle East and Asia, into his own business, founding a company called Media Records in 1928. An early clipping service with a twist, Media Records provided advice, data, and related services to companies attempting to figure out the best advertising strategies in the brave new world of national and international markets. The firm kept, for example, a national database of advertising campaigns. Its subscribing companies could receive a record—copies of advertisements in newspapers throughout the country—of their competitors' advertising strategies. The firm kept data on the activity of all advertisers in every newspaper published in cities and towns with populations of ten thousand and above, as well as on radio advertising.

As Charlie put it, his firm preserved "the records of what advertisers had done and were then doing, in order that each advertiser might study the program of any other advertiser whose success or failure could be followed or avoided, as the case might be." Based on data it gathered, the company also advised companies on how to distribute their advertising among various newspaper and radio outlets. This was one business that continued to thrive during the Depression; by the mid-1930s, Charlie's venture, headquartered in New York, had four "bureaus," as Charlie called them, located in different parts of the country, and a total of 350 employees.[41]

John could always count on Charlie to write a check when the taxes came due, make up shortfalls in the family budget, and provide loans or outright gifts whenever John was overwhelmed financially. Charlie also helped support their sister Nell, whose husband's income was often uncertain in these

Depression years, and whose own health was poor. The money came, for the most part, from the estate of Frank Rock, who had died in 1932. With the Marlborough theater income Frank had signed over to Charlie when Frank married Delia, Charlie had made sure his father received a comfortable retirement living; at the same time, he had assisted his two youngest siblings. When Frank died, his estate was worth a bit more than $88,000 (about $1.2 million today). Charlie, as Rock and Hayes trustee, kept control of the estate. Frank had chosen not to reassign the trust to Delia, instead providing for her by putting his other properties in her name before his death. Charlie treated the trust as a source of support for himself, John, and Nell. Harry, who made a very comfortable living working for Charlie, had never asked for a share, and Charlie apparently decided unilaterally that their sister Maisie didn't need any. Delia was furious that she did not get this money, too, although Charlie continued to support her after Frank's death.[42]

With Charlie's assistance, John fretted somewhat less about money. Charlie distributed about $2,300 to John and Nan from the income of his father's theater in 1932 and 1933 (a bit over $31,000 today). All told, between the time Frank Rock died and 1940, John and his family received about $10,400 (close to $150,000 today).[43] This financial cushion, and John's disciplined work habits made it possible, if never easy, for him to continue to juggle all aspects of his career.

Rock's career choices were, in some respects, costly to his family. The most practical decision would have been to make his private practice his priority, concentrating on treating those patients who could pay and making sure he collected their fees. That was certainly the option many of his colleagues at the Free Hospital chose. If he had done so, he would have made an excellent income and had many fewer monetary worries. He could have traded on both his position at a Harvard teaching hospital, which conferred professional cachet, and Nan's social connections. Those connections, including a listing in the Social Register, would have enabled him almost completely to overcome his Irish Catholic roots and would have virtually guaranteed financial success.

Rock needed his private practice, but his ambitions went far beyond it. His drive may not have been on display, but it was there nevertheless. He was simply not willing to take the obvious path. He wanted to combine practice and research, and he was committed to providing care to whoever needed it. Charlie supplemented the family income, and Nan worked too, teaching bridge for several months a year. For two years she also managed a summer resort. Their support—financial as well as moral—allowed John to do what he wanted.

. . .

John Rock's research, built on nearly a half-century of scientific and clinical discoveries and developments, was pivotal to the creation of the field of reproductive medicine.[44] He came to the study of human fertility at a propitious time. As Rock was composing his first article on infertility for the *New England Journal*, ideas about the nature of fertility and infertility had begun to take a new and exciting turn.

Advances in the ability to diagnose male sterility and female tubal occlusion (blockage) were two of the most important new discoveries. In the 1920s Gerald Moench made pioneering discoveries about the structure of sperm in humans; for the first time, doctors were able to determine what "normal" male fertility was in terms of sperm quantity, motility, and morphology. It became much easier to diagnose male infertility, even if it remained generally untreatable.[45] And I. C. Rubin's announcement in 1921 that he had developed a nonsurgical test to determine the patency of the fallopian tubes addressed one of the most common causes of infertility in women.

Tubal blockage was then, and remains today, a significant cause of infertility. During the 1920s and 1930s, clinicians attributed the condition to gonorrhea, infections during a prior childbirth, appendicitis, and other pelvic disorders. Before Rubin, only major surgery via laparotomy, in which the abdomen was opened to reveal the uterus, tubes, and ovaries, could diagnose this condition. Rubin created a relatively simple apparatus that could be set up in a doctor's office. The physician would insufflate the tubes using carbon dioxide, which traveled through the cervix and uterus, then into the tubes. If the tubes were open, then the gas would pass through them easily and enter the abdominal cavity. If the gas passed, the patient experienced pain in the shoulder region. The doctor judged the degree of patency by how much pressure was needed to force the gas through the tubes. By the end of the decade, both the Rubin test and a similar procedure known as hysterosalpingogram, in which an oil-based solution was used while the physician watched the progress of the procedure under x-ray guidance, became common diagnostic procedures. Both could dislodge tiny bits of debris in the tubes and open those with minor blockages. Severe damage remained almost impossible to treat.[46]

Both advances made it easier to diagnose infertility but not necessarily to treat it. The recent discoveries of female hormones in the 1920s, however, seemed to promise to do both. The so-called sex hormones of estrogen and progesterone would soon be isolated and synthesized, and they promised to reveal the complex biology of human reproduction and offer treatment when this function failed. The fact that in the late 1930s Rock would change the name of his sterility clinic to the Fertility and Endocrine Clinic would be just one manifestation of the importance of the new field of endocrinology to fertility and infertility.

It would be hard to overestimate the impact of the hormones on the development of the field of reproductive medicine.[47] Scientists had known about their existence since the late nineteenth century, even if they had not been able to isolate many of them yet. (And the hormones couldn't be synthesized—that is, created in a laboratory—until they had been successfully isolated.) However, estrogen and progesterone were mysterious entities until just about the time Rock began serious work on infertility.[48] It was still unclear in the 1930s—and even beyond—what exact role these hormones, and the gonadotropic hormones that controlled them, played in the workings of the human female reproductive cycle.

Today we know that estrogen and progesterone, with two hormones from the pituitary gland called follicle stimulating hormone (FSH) and luteinizing hormone (LH), control a woman's reproductive cycle. Follicles within the ovary produce estrogen, and the increased production of estrogen causes the lining of the uterus to thicken and develop. The follicles contain the ova. Ovulation occurs somewhere around the fourteenth day of an average menstrual cycle, after which the estrogen-producing follicle, having released an ovum, becomes the corpus luteum, which then produces progesterone. If the ovum is not fertilized, then the production of both estrogen and progesterone drops sharply, and menstruation occurs.

The discovery and isolation of estrogen and progesterone in the 1920s and 1930s had been preceded by nearly three-quarters of a century of speculation and experimentation in pursuit of understanding what were then referred to as the "ductless glands." In 1849, Thomas Addison presented his first paper on the adrenal disease that would later be named after him. That same year, Arnold Adolph Berthold performed his famous experiment in which he castrated roosters, then implanted their testicles back in their abdominal cavities to see whether the roosters' secondary sex characteristics would reemerge. They did.[49]

One scientist who confirmed Addison's theory was Charles Brown-Sequard, who became even more famous in later life for injecting himself with animal testicular extracts in an effort to restore his sexual powers at the age of seventy-two. It didn't work, but Brown-Sequard was one of the earliest medical researchers to argue that both the testicle and the ovary produced "internal secretions," defying the skepticism of many of his colleagues, who did not believe that these reproductive organs demonstrated properties similar to the adrenal, thyroid, and pituitary glands on which research was then concentrated.[50]

Brown-Sequard, however, was proved correct. By the early twentieth century, researchers knew that these "glands of internal secretion," including the ovaries and testicles, produced something, but they didn't know exactly what. Only one hormone had been isolated, the adrenal hormone epinephrine. And the only hormonal extract of proven therapeutic value was thyroid extract, which at the time was processed from sheep thyroid. Until the early twentieth century, there was not even agreement on what to call these substances. In 1905, however, British scientist Ernest Henry Starling began to call all of them "hormones," a term derived from the Greek by way of a classicist friend of his. The name soon found favor and came into common use.[51]

Once researchers were persuaded that the ovary, like the thyroid and adrenal gland, produced hormones, laboratory scientists around the world foraged in abattoirs for the unwanted organs of animals destined for the dinner table, collected the urine of mares and stallions, and killed many a little mammal—mostly rabbits but also guinea pigs and rats—in attempts to isolate these substances. Success eluded them, but they persevered, seeking to understand, explain, and create artificially these fascinating substances. Meanwhile, clinicians grew impatient and took matters into their own hands. After all, they had their patients' immediate needs and demands to consider.

Physicians who treated the always importunate infertility patients seemed ready to try almost anything to bring about a pregnancy. Knowing that scientists were attempting to isolate the substances secreted by the ovaries, and having already seen the effectiveness of animal thyroid extracts on myxedema (the edema and dry skin seen in primary hypothyroidism), by the early twentieth century clinicians took matters into their own hands. Not willing to wait for the pure crystalline forms that still eluded laboratory scientists, they began to prescribe animal extracts to women who sought infertility treatment.

By the 1910s and 1920s, American and European physicians who treated infertility (and other suspected hormonal imbalances) became swept up in a rage for glandular preparations. Pharmaceutical companies prepared manuals for physicians. Many practitioners, including some who were less than scrupulous, rushed to provide their patients with what one advocate called "practical hormone therapy." Extracts of animal ovaries, pituitaries, and testicles were given almost whimsically. In the 1910s, Henry R. Harrower, the driving force behind the creation of what eventually became the respectable Endocrine Society, published tables of available preparations and advised physicians to use the trial-and-error method. If one preparation didn't work, he wrote blithely, try something else. There were scores of products, the risk as he saw it was minimal, and there was a possibility of significant benefit.[52]

This was a medical craze, where it was almost impossible to distinguish between respectable practitioners and the lunatic fringe. Like Harrower, physicians busily prescribed extracts manufactured from desiccated animal organs by pharmaceutical houses in Europe and the United States for numerous couples who had failed to conceive. Even self-described "moderates" prescribed wild hormonal and herbal combinations with little justification. One well-respected authority, whenever he was faced with an unexplained case of infertility in which he suspected a hormonal imbalance, prescribed a preparation called thelyglan, which was a combination of "ovarian, thyroid, and pituitary" animal extracts, plus calcium and the "vegetable extract" yohimbin, long considered an aphrodisiac.[53]

These preparations were widely available more than a decade before any of the hormones that regulate the reproductive process had been isolated, let alone synthesized. Clinicians were unwilling to wait for an understanding of these hormones' functions, not to mention the successful synthesis of the hormones themselves or any proof of efficacy, before attempting to make practical use of the information that had been filtering out from research laboratories.

Such a rush to prescribe before any verifiable reason to do so existed shows the desperation of both patient and practitioner. It also shows that practitioners were well primed for hormonal therapies long before successful ones were available. But even as they used such preparations, clinicians knew they didn't yet have the science. This was a problem for them, since by the 1920s the blessing of laboratory science had become critical to the legitimacy of medical decision making. Given their increasing sense of the medical profession as a science-based discipline, clinicians and clinical researchers wanted to know exactly how these substances worked.[54]

So while the clinicians were handing out compounds of dried animal organs, vitamins, and aphrodisiacs, bench scientists continued to toil away in their laboratories on the rats and rabbits. And if all we had to go on were their accounts, we'd be sure that the history of hormones began and ended with an orderly sequence of discoveries and isolations. When a laboratory scientist looks backwards, this history looks systematic and precise, with a new discovery flowing from each previous one, with milestones clearly demarcated and credit given to a particular person or groups for each successful discovery.

In reality, the story was messy and even chaotic, marked by individual and national rivalries, fueled not only by scientific curiosity but also by the profit motive of pharmaceutical houses and the ambitions of funding organizations. But not until scientists were able to isolate the hormones, truly understand their properties, and synthesize them would it be possible for clinical researchers to understand how the hormones worked in women and how the use of these hormones might affect both our understanding of the human reproductive process and the treatment of menstrual and ovulatory disorders in women.[55]

Estrogen was the first of the hormones to give up its secrets. In 1923, Edgar Allen and Edward Doisy, of Washington University in St. Louis, produced estrogen, what they called at first "the ovarian hormone." It then took until 1929 for Doisy to isolate it in a pure crystalline form. Estrogen products derived from animal sources were available by the mid-1930s; Russell Marker at Pennsylvania State University synthesized estrone (one of the estrogens) from plant sources in 1936, and the first synthetic estrogen, initially called stilbestrol and then diethylstilbestrol (DES), became available in 1938. Rock's colleagues at the Free Hospital, Olive Watkins Smith and George Smith, soon began experimenting with this one as a treatment for miscarriage.[56]

Estrogen was not the only ovarian hormone, however. As early as 1915, scientists understood that the corpus luteum (the ovarian follicle after ovulation) secreted a hormonal substance. In 1929 George Corner, then of the University of Rochester, led the team that produced the first "corpus luteum extract."[57] Corner wanted to call it progestin, but his name did not win out. In 1932, several teams working separately managed to obtain this hormone in an "almost pure" crystalline form, although they could not yet determine its structure. Four of those research teams, again working independently, isolated the substance in 1934. An international conference was called to give it a name, and it became progesterone.[58]

With a clearer understanding of the properties of both estrogen and progesterone, medical researchers could try to understand specifically how these hormones affected a woman's (rather than a rat's or a rabbit's) reproductive cycle. The animals on which scientists experimented in laboratories did not have the equivalent of a woman's menstrual cycle. Because physicians were so used to animal analogies, however, they at one time did equate animal estrus with women's menstruation, which is why in the nineteenth century they often told women, wrongly, that the fertile period was just before or after menstruation. But now, clinicians expected that the isolation of estrogen and progesterone would result in a better understanding of a woman's reproductive cycle.

. . .

It was just when the science was reaching this point that John Rock made his first major contribution to the newly emerging field. Researchers understood, more or less, the significance of estrogen and progesterone to a woman's reproductive cycle. Now they could try to answer one of the most important questions: When did ovulation occur in relation to menstruation and how could that time be accurately determined, preferably in advance? This was a bedrock question. Without an answer, it would be impossible to imagine the creation of the field of reproductive medicine. By the 1930s several researchers had weighed in on the subject, and there was enough information available to describe roughly a four-day window in which ovulation was likely.[59] But Rock sought a much more precise answer. Along with his young colleagues Marshall Bartlett and James Snodgrass, Rock worked on this problem during the 1930s. The Free Hospital for Women was the perfect place to do so.

Journalist Loretta McLaughlin referred to the Free Hospital as "a private research preserve for its principal staffers," who enjoyed "almost absolute research freedom."[60] That is a bit of an exaggeration, but not much of one. Harvard Medical School seemed to exercise little oversight at any of its clinical outposts, whether the small Free Hospital or the sprawling Massachusetts General Hospital. Researchers faced few constraints as they decided how to conduct their studies. Nevertheless, the hospitals did not exist in an ethical vacuum. Historian Susan Lederer, a leading expert on the history of medical research ethics in the United States, observed that "ethical guidelines," even though they lacked "enforcement policies and [were] far from perfect," did indeed influence "the conduct of [human subject] research . . . in the decades before World War II. At no time were American investigators free to do whatever they pleased."[61] However, given the clear and sometimes shocking abuses of those standards, it would be hard not to conclude that following them was voluntary.

As a relatively small institution dedicated to treating women's reproductive problems, the Free Hospital offered Rock and others a particularly hospitable environment. Its medical staff had broadly congruent research and clinical interests, which provided circumstances conducive to meaningful collaboration. Medical students, residents, and research fellows enjoyed opportunities for practical surgical experience as well as research. And of course, many of the patients who came to the Free Hospital were receiving "charity" care. Indeed, some of the physicians who treated these women hardly appeared to have seen them as individual human beings. George Smith, who would become chief surgeon in 1947, used the unfortunate and chillingly impersonal term "teaching material" when referring in his memoirs to the clinic patients he served.[62] Smith was not alone. Among this group of mostly Protestant, Harvard-trained, and typically upper-middle-class physicians, the temptation always lurked for them to depersonalize the working-class and often Catholic patients whom they treated.

Rock was not cast in that mold, even though outside the hospital setting and among his friends and club mates, he would openly display the casual racism, anti-Semitism, and misogyny characteristic of his gender, era, and social milieu. Throughout his life, he could be callous and insensitive toward *groups* and carelessly employ racial and ethnic slurs, yet he never viewed his patients in such stereotypical ways. To him, each was an individual deserving of courtesy and kindness.

We can see precursors of this behavior in the empathic qualities toward individuals he developed in his youth. He had demonstrated courage in Guatemala, where despite his own racial assumptions, he had defied his superiors and defended the striking banana cutters. He treated his patients as rational human beings and by so doing earned their trust. Perhaps more unusually, Rock did not limit himself to clinic patients when he conducted a study—his research volunteers included private patients and even the nurses and secretaries who worked at the hospital.

Rock's first major research project addressed fundamental questions about a woman's reproductive system: What triggers ovulation? What is the relationship between ovulation and menstruation? How can it be determined if a woman has ovulated? And is it possible to predict in advance when ovulation will occur? Rock began by asking, How can a woman's menstrual cycle be charted? What signs indicate that she is about to ovulate, or that she has ovulated? Rock collaborated in this research with Marshall Bartlett, who had graduated from Harvard Medical School in 1926 and would go on to have a successful career as a general surgeon and clinical professor of surgery at Harvard. Rock and Bartlett looked at tissue from the endometrium (the lining of the uterus) and correlated it with each day in the menstrual cycle. This enabled clinicians to determine after the fact, with fair accuracy, the timing of ovulation. By "dating" the endometrium, as this technique was called, physicians would know whether a woman had ovulated in a particular cycle, but they still could not predict precisely when ovulation would occur.

Rock was disappointed that his and Bartlett's techniques could not determine when a woman would ovulate, but they had been unable to make day-to-day classifications of the first half of the menstrual cycle, what Rock called the "estrogen phase." Once a woman had ovulated, however, it was possible to detect daily changes in the endometrium. By using this technique, they noted, "one can determine whether and when a patient ovulates, and, if she is anovulatory, whether any of the gonadotropic substances either from the pituitary gland or from pregnancy urine is effective. One may perhaps determine also the integrity of the corpus luteum."[63] To have this information would enable a physician to know at least whether a patient could not conceive because she didn't ovulate, or if the couple failed to have intercourse during the woman's most fertile time. And if a physician was treating anovulation (failure to ovulate) with gonadotropins, he or she could take a sample of the endometrium to determine month by month if ovulation had been restored.

This study launched Rock's research career, and its importance for further research became even more evident as the decade wore on. George Smith, then the Free Hospital's research director, hailed him as a "pioneer" for this work. Rock was invited to give several presentations elaborating on the study to various audiences, including one at the New York Academy of Medicine in 1936. In 1937 the Journal of the American Medical Association published the study with Rock as lead author.[64]

The ability to date the endometrium, even if only in the postovulatory phase, was an important medical advance, but what physicians really wanted was a technique to determine the exact time of ovulation. Researchers had discovered, using rats and rabbits, that electrodes measured differences in what were called "ovulation potentials" in both kinds of animals during estrus. Rock attempted to discover whether the same thing happened in women.

His first step was to recruit volunteers among patients scheduled for laparotomy near the expected time of ovulation. These women agreed to have a probe either inserted into their vaginas or attached externally to the abdomen for several days before their scheduled operations. This would mean a few extra days in the hospital, the inconvenience of being hooked up to a device, and the chore of keeping a log of their activities. The idea was to begin the monitoring close to, but before, the time of ovulation, in the hope that some signal could be recorded indicating ovulation and that confirmation of this would be made at the time of laparotomy.

Twenty-two-year-old Mrs. L. B. was one of the willing volunteers. An infertility patient in Rock's clinic, Mrs. L. B. suffered from severe menstrual pain that sometimes kept her in bed for days. She agreed to participate in the electrode study just before her diagnostic laparotomy. Arriving at the hospital four days before her scheduled surgery, she kept a log of her daily activities, from connecting and disconnecting the electrodes when she rose from bed and returned to it, to inserting her own vaginal thermometer, to drinking water, eating, reading, filing her nails, and kissing her husband. She took her role in the experiment seriously and seemed proud of her potential contribution to medical research.[65]

But Mrs. L. B. and the other dozen or so women who joined her took their notes in vain. Rock's experiment was not working. Getting nowhere and ready to give up, Rock read about some new findings from researchers who claimed that electrode readings of index fingers could indicate ovulation. Rock abandoned the vaginal and abdominal probes and directed his young colleague, physiologist James Snodgrass, to set up an electrode-equipped table outside the lunchroom of the Free Hospital.[66]

Every day for two months in 1939, Snodgrass waylaid a group of thirty nurses and twenty-three miscellaneous employees to have their electrical measurements taken just before lunch. One group included regularly menstruating women with cycles generally considered within the normal range. In the other group were women who only in the loosest sense of the term could be deemed controls—"one surgical castrate, one woman in natural menopause, one pregnant individual, and two women who, on the basis of their clinical history, doubtless had anovulatory cycles." All the women dutifully proffered their index fingers, and the investigator was not informed about which women belonged to which group or about the menstrual cycles of any of the women. Entrusted with the secret of which women were the subjects and which the controls was Millie, the switchboard operator. Millie kept the menstrual data in "careful, secret custody" until the end of the experiment because she, according to research assistant Miriam Menkin, "was . . . a holy terror [who] . . . would even bawl out the chief surgeon . . . It was generally agreed that this secret information would be safe with her."[67]

What a picture! We can just see the study participants revealing the details of their menstrual cycles only to Millie the switchboard operator. Then we look for young James Snodgrass sitting outside the lunchroom, his graph paper within reach, snagging the women on their way to lunch. The table at which he sits holds his electrical equipment and beakers of saline solution for the nurses, secretaries, lab technicians, and sundry other women to immerse their fingers. The whole scene provides an amusing and fairly accurate picture of the ad hoc quality of some of the activities that came under the rubric of research.

Rock, based on his and J. Reboul's earlier findings about the general use-lessness of the vaginal probes and surface electrodes, was not optimistic that this would lead to anything. One might wonder why he even kept up with this idea, given that none of the techniques he employed thus far showed any in-dication of working. But researchers in other institutions had claimed posi-tive results, leading him to believe that the only way to determine who was right and who was wrong was to give it one more try. And besides, as every-one working in this field well knew, "the establishment of a clearly defined criterion of ovulation time" was critical to progress in infertility research, and if such a simple mechanism could indeed determine ovulation, it seemed worth this one last effort. Endometrial biopsy was uncomfortable for the pa-tient—sometimes acutely so—and only indicated ovulation after the fact. An electrode applied to the index finger was nonintrusive and nearly effortless for the patient. But it simply did not work. Claims of previous experiment-ers notwithstanding, these researchers concluded that "the electric methods hitherto proposed are unsuitable for the detection of ovulation."[68]

Rock was disappointed but hardly surprised. He and his associates under-took numerous investigations in these and later years. Not all of them worked out, but both of these particular studies, the successful endometrial dating study and the spectacularly unsuccessful electric "potentiator" project, illus-trated Rock's typical manner of conducting an investigation and the pattern of clinical research more generally.

First, the studies were collaborative. Collaboration would become routine for investigators in these decades. Clinical research often required several different sets of skills and generally called for a number of pairs of trained hands. Rock's own accomplishments, he always recognized, would never have been possible without the assistance of young colleagues, residents, medical students, research fellows, laboratory technicians, and secretaries, not to mention the occasional switchboard operator. Rock was not then, and would never become, the kind of researcher who could spend hours engaged in the actual day-to-day minutiae that experiments require. Throughout his career, Rock posed questions, devised protocols (sometimes alone, sometimes with others), often personally recruited patients to participate in studies, and closely monitored the results. The painstaking detail work was carried out by his collaborators and assistants.

Creativity and intuition were Rock's hallmark intellectual qualities. He could drive colleagues who had better scientific training to distraction by his blithe willingness to change a protocol for an experiment in midstream if he thought he might get what he believed were "truer" results. Fellow gynecologist George Smith, who collaborated with his wife, biochemist Olive Smith, years later complained that he and Olive simply could not do any work with Rock, because "he refused to run control observations and frequently ruined a case-study by changing the protocol in mid-stream."[69]

No doubt, but we can just imagine Rock asking why in the world he should keep going in a certain direction if it looked like he was treading the wrong path and another one seemed more promising. This was both his strength and his weakness. Rock's focus was always less on the study itself and more on the likely medical knowledge gained by a particular line of inquiry. He was a specialist in reproduction, and he wanted to advance knowledge in that field. If advancing that knowledge meant he changed a protocol in the middle of a study, so be it. For such a consummate scientist as Olive Smith, this attitude smacked of sacrilege.

. . .

Clinicians think differently from bench scientists. It would have been almost impossible for Rock not to think in practical terms, since he spent so much of his time as a practicing physician. In the mid-1930s, while his assistants were busy in the laboratory, he kept up an extraordinarily busy schedule of patient care. He left his house for the hospital every morning at 6:30 or so. Once he arrived at the Free Hospital, he would spend two hours on his research projects. Next, he might be headed for the operating room, where two hours were generally allotted for each procedure, though one or more might take longer. After performing surgery, on some days he met his scheduled appointments with private patients. The clinic patients came in one afternoon a week. In between, he made follow-up phone calls to patients, visited his hospital inpatients, prepared his correspondence, consulted with colleagues, and met with his assistants and staff. He was also still delivering babies, who arrive when they arrive, so that part of his job could never be scheduled.

Of Rock's collaborators and assistants, the young doctors and medical students were almost all men, and the secretaries, nurses, technicians, and occasional volunteers were all women. Many of this latter group worked with him for years, but no one's loyalty or dedication surpassed that of Miriam Menkin, who first came to work for Rock as a secretarial assistant and technician in the late 1930s. She would spend nearly her entire career with Rock.

Miriam Menkin's story is unique in some respects but in many others was all too common for women with scientific ambitions who came of age in this period. Born Miriam Friedman in 1901, she earned a bachelor's degree from Cornell in 1922, with concentrations in histology and comparative anatomy. The following year she earned a master's degree from Columbia in genetics, then briefly taught biology and physiology in New York. Like scores of other science-minded young women born at the turn of the twentieth century, Miriam Friedman wanted to be a physician. But unfortunately, she came of age at a time when medical education for women was becoming less available and increasingly beyond their ability to afford.[70] Instead of becoming a doctor, she married one—to be more precise, she married a medical student, Valy Menkin, in 1924.

Although she abandoned the idea of becoming a physician, she still hoped, once her husband had finished his own training, that she could eventually earn a PhD in biology from Harvard. But first, to have a practical and marketable skill to support herself and her husband while he completed his medical education, she acquired another bachelor's degree, this one in secretarial studies from Simmons College. In the late 1920s she undertook further coursework at Harvard and spent a summer studying histology in Berlin, but she never did manage to complete a PhD. Tight finances were a major factor, and she and her husband were having marital difficulties. She apparently decided to keep working rather than complete her PhD, even after he began earning an income, so that she could save up enough money for a divorce.[71]

In the mid-1930s she worked as a laboratory technician at Harvard, a member of that legion of well-educated women who, with job titles such as technician or secretary, were indispensable to medical research in the first two-thirds of the twentieth century.[72] Working behind the scenes, often barely acknowledged, many of them with PhDs themselves, these women took the only jobs they could get, typing the papers of male researchers or performing tedious laboratory experiments. Many of the women who made critical contributions to the work of the men whose names were so prominently displayed on the title pages of major journal articles remained anonymous.

Menkin seemed destined to vanish into that stream. Perhaps as a young woman, since she and her husband had no children, she considered such positions as only a temporary holding pattern for her, until she could afford to leave him and begin a career of her own. But her life took a fateful turn when she unexpectedly conceived. She believed that having a child meant that she would never end her marriage. Since forsaking science was as unthinkable as leaving her marriage had become, she seems to have resigned herself to going on indefinitely as a technician and secretary.

From 1930 to 1935, Menkin served as a research fellow in pathology at Harvard Medical School. She went from there to work at Harvard College for Gregory Pincus, who would soon become famous—perhaps "notorious" would be a better word—for the creation of "fatherless rabbits."[73] When she worked for him, her title was secretary and technician in the biology laboratory. Among her tasks was the preparation of extracts of the gonadotropins FSH and LH in order to "superovulate" the rabbits.[74]

Pincus left Harvard in 1937 when he was denied tenure, and Menkin may have lost her job because he lost his, or she may have decided to stay at home for a while with her infant son. She applied for a job with Rock in 1938, having heard about the opening from an acquaintance who was about to vacate it. Rock hired her immediately. Menkin's experience was all with animals, but her technical skills were superb, and she had been educated in the relevant scientific disciplines. She had the patience for detailed and painstaking work that Rock lacked.

Menkin came to the Free Hospital just as Rock was beginning work on the two studies that would make his career. The first would bring Rock great distinction within his profession and help propel him into prominence as one of eighteen leading figures who transformed our understanding of human reproduction in the twentieth century, ushering him into the Gynecological Hall of Fame of the American College of Obstetricians and Gynecologists. The second would make his name familiar to the press and public. Both studies would have been impossible without the groundwork laid by others as well as his own research on the dating of the endometrium. Both would take him into uncharted territory.

When Menkin arrived, Rock and pathologist Arthur Hertig were just embarking on the first of the two research studies. They intended to discover precisely how a newly fertilized egg became implanted in the uterus and went on to become an embryo. And Rock had a second project simmering as well. If rabbits could be fertilized without sexual intercourse, he mused, if egg and sperm could unite in a "watch glass" rather than in the rabbit's fallopian tube, then why not in humans too?

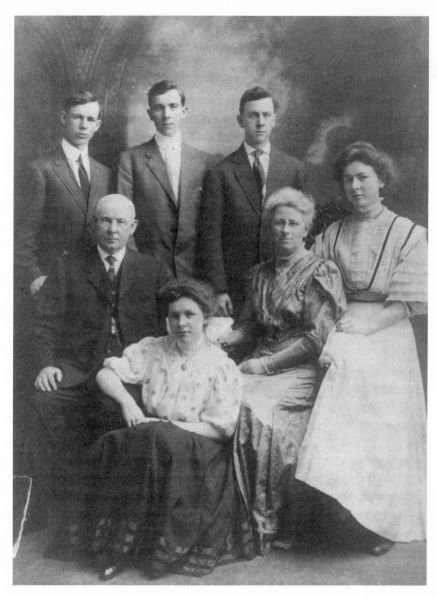

The Rock family has its picture taken just before John leaves for Guatemala in 1909. From left to right: (seated) Frank, Nell, Annie, and Maisie; (standing) Charlie, John, and Harry.
Courtesy of Rachel Achenbach.

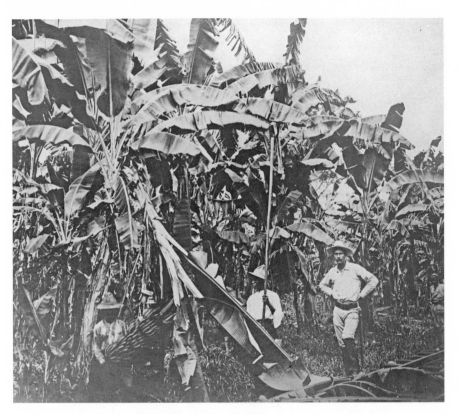

Victor Cutter, John's boss in Guatemala. This photograph was taken in the banana fields in 1908, the year before John arrived. At the time Cutter was superintendent of the Guatemala division of the United Fruit Company. He later became its president.
Courtesy of Dartmouth College Library.

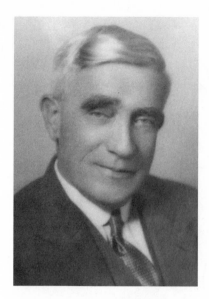

Neil MacPhail, the doctor who befriended John in Guatemala, in an undated photograph. When he and John met in 1909, MacPhail was twenty-seven years old. Courtesy of Rachel Achenbach.

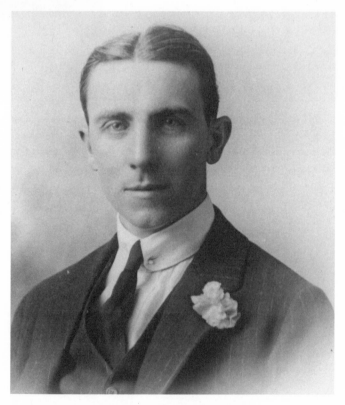

John Rock in the early 1920s. Courtesy of Rachel Achenbach.

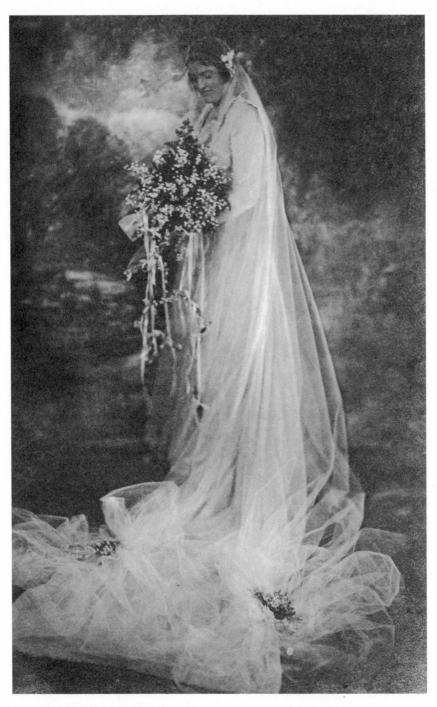

Anna (Nan) Rock in her wedding dress, January 1925. Courtesy of Rachel Achenbach.

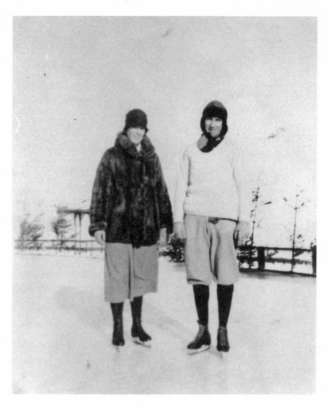

Nan and John Rock in Quebec on their honeymoon, January 1925.
Courtesy of Rachel Achenbach.

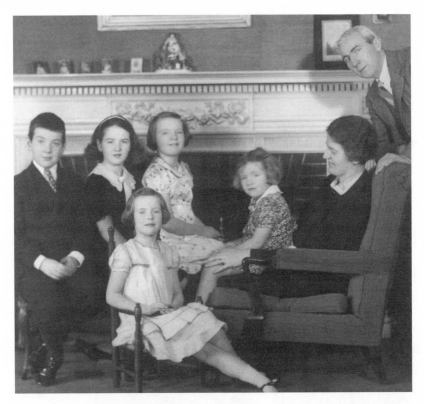

Nan and John Rock and their five children (left to right): Jack, Rachel, Martha (in child's chair in front), Ann Jane, and Ellen, around 1937. Courtesy of Rachel Achenbach.

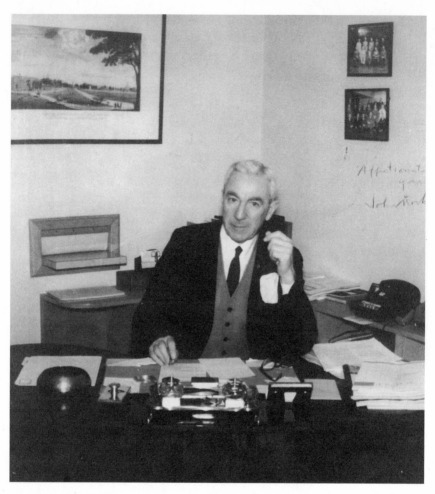

John Rock in his office in the 1940s. Courtesy of Rachel Achenbach.

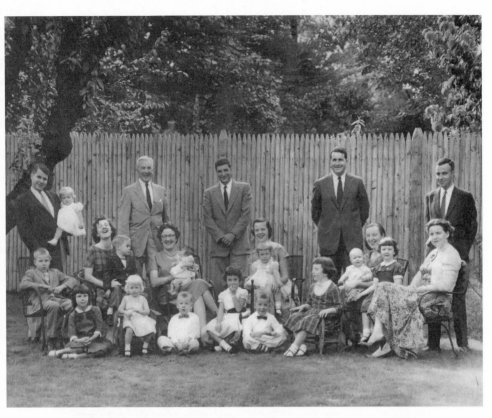

John and Nan Rock, their four daughters and sons-in-law, and thirteen grandchildren, in the 1950s. John Rock's grandchildren would eventually number nineteen. Adults left to right: Hart Achenbach, Rachel Achenbach, John Rock, Nan Rock, Eugene LeFevre, Martha LeFevre, Hank Levinson, A. J. Levinson, Ellen Phillips, and Jerry Phillips. Courtesy of Rachel Achenbach.

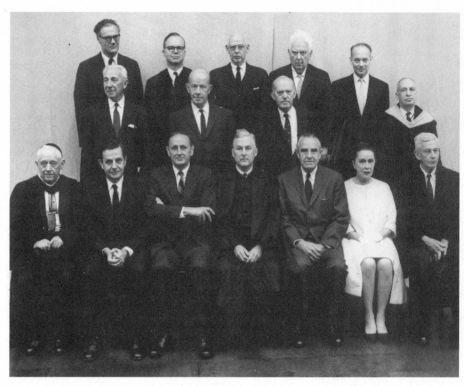

John Rock and his fellow recipients of honorary degrees from Harvard University in 1966. The only woman in the photograph is choreographer Martha Graham. Rock is in the second row, far left. Courtesy of Rachel Achenbach.

Chapter 4

FIRING THE FIRST SHOT IN THE
REPRODUCTIVE REVOLUTION

Boston, 1937. An unsigned editorial in the *New England Journal of Medicine* hints at the possibility of creating human embryos outside the uterus by means of in vitro fertilization.

Brookline, Massachusetts, 1938. John Rock and Arthur Hertig set forth on a fifteen-year quest to trace the path of the fertilized egg from fallopian tube to uterus, providing the first visual record of the early days of human conception.

Science magazine, 1944. Rock and his technician Miriam Menkin electrify the scientific world with the announcement of the successful fertilization of four human ova outside the womb, firing the first shot in the twentieth century's reproductive revolution.

In January 1938, John Rock, nearly forty-eight years old, was in his twelfth year as director of the Fertility and Endocrine Clinic at the Free Hospital for Women. He had become a prominent Boston obstetrician and gynecologist and had developed a respectable reputation in research. He could take pride in a satisfying, if not stellar, career.

Fast forward a decade, to 1948, when Rock would enjoy an international reputation as an infertility expert, receive one of his profession's most coveted honors, and astonish the nation with an announcement of the first successful fertilization of a human ova outside the uterus. His name was not yet a household word, but women from around the globe could nevertheless come to any Boston hospital, ask for the "fertility doctor," and be directed to Rock. Articles about his work appeared regularly in national magazines. Men and women from across the nation and the world sought his advice about their difficulties in having a child, and young physicians from everywhere vied for a chance to work with him.

John Rock's metamorphosis from prominent local gynecologist to internationally recognized fertility expert was the result of determination, hard

work, and good fortune. People who had known him only socially were sometimes caught off guard by his ambition. His bonhomie, self-mocking sense of
humor, and obvious pleasure in society life could deceive the casual observer.
His cultivated modesty and genuine grace were among his notable public characteristics. But beneath that charming exterior dwelt a driven temperament.[1]

Two studies formed the twin centerpieces of a large and ambitious research
program that Rock directed and that helped to lay much of the groundwork
for the development of reproductive medicine in the second half of the twentieth century—the first was on the process by which a fertilized ovum becomes
an embryo and the second, on the fertilization of ova outside a woman's body
(what came to be called in vitro fertilization). In these studies, he and his
collaborators, including Arthur Hertig for the embryo project and Miriam
Menkin for what was called the ova study, sought answers to what had been
insoluble mysteries of human fertility.

By the time Rock embarked on these two studies in 1938, his personal situation had become more stable. He had learned to pace himself; he no longer,
even privately, agonized so much about his ability to manage his myriad responsibilities. His brother Charlie, in spite of a health scare three years before, remained at the helm of the family and provided financial assistance
whenever John needed it. John and Nan had completed their family; their
youngest child, Ellen, was nearly five. It was now easier for him to focus on
his research interests.

John was lucky in his wife. Nan was both a supportive spouse and a woman
of independent interests who had a life of her own. As a couple, they often
entertained and had friends to stay with them. She would accompany him to
professional meetings, but she would also travel without him, either alone or
with one or more of the children, to visit her friends or her family. She seemed
in general the more self-reliant of the two—she, after all, could take apart
and reassemble an automobile engine; he couldn't be bothered even to put in
a quart of oil. She also relished her times away more than he did. He did not
like to travel without her.[2]

Rock worked hard, but he and his wife both liked to socialize; he had a
close circle of friends and a broader one of friendly acquaintances, many of
them physicians. Thanks to Nan's social connections, the Rocks belonged to
the exclusive country club in Brookline (always referred to in Boston simply as
the country club) for a time, and they had a listing in the Social Register. John
and Nan were of a generation, and a social class, in which same-sex social
activities made up much of a person's life. The Chilton Club Nan belonged to

was a women's club for the social elite, and John's Tavern Club was an exclusive, almost entirely Protestant, Boston men's club to which his father-in-law Paul Thorndike had introduced him.

In later years Rock recalled that Dr. Thorndike successfully proposed both his son, Sherman, and his new son-in-law for membership in 1927, but the Tavern Club's list shows Rock as a member a few years earlier than that, probably during his and Nan's courting days. The Tavern Club, as Loretta McLaughlin noted, "catered to the wealthy and well-positioned." Bigelows, Cabots, Lowells, and Shattucks punctuate the roster of members, but the club's venerable history includes figures in medicine, law, literature, diplomacy, politics, and science. Among its officers had been the novelist William Dean Howells and Supreme Court Justice Oliver Wendell Holmes, Jr. Members over the years would include politicians and diplomats such as John F. Kennedy, Christian A. Herter, Jr., and Leverett Saltonstall; novelists Henry James, Owen Wister, and John Marquand; and artists, among them sculptor Augustus St. Gaudens and poet Archibald MacLeish. The physicians are too numerous to mention but in Rock's day included many of his colleagues at the Harvard Medical School.[3] Rock took enormous pleasure in acting in the club's theatrical productions, of which there were three a year, often written by the members themselves. Particularly when Nan was away, he often ate at the club, either alone or with friends.[4]

The Great Depression still cast a pall over the nation in the late 1930s, but a reader of Rock's correspondence for these years would scarcely have known. His patients' husbands were often out of work, and they and their families struggled with economic hardship. The nation still staggered under the weight of the most devastating and longest-lasting economic setback in its history, but Rock and his family seemed relatively untouched. Right now his finances were in as good an order as could be expected for a physician reluctant to remind patients to pay their bills in the best of times. He worried about money, of course, but he *always* worried about money. For now, he was content; he went to work every day and hoped for the best.

• • •

In developing his ambitious research program, Rock's overarching goal was nothing less than to understand the entire process of conception and fertilization, from the ripening of the Graafian follicle, through the meeting of sperm and egg and the fertilized egg's trip through the fallopian tube, to implantation in the uterus and growth of the tiny embryo. With Arthur Hertig,

Miriam Menkin, and a host of medical fellows and technicians, Rock studied ova taken directly from the ovary before ovulation, ova in the fallopian tube, and the embryo after fertilization. Sperm from medical students and from his artificial insemination patients found their way into the IVF experiments. He continued, without success, to try to find a simple way to determine when ovulation was just about to occur.[5]

All in all, for about a decade and a half, more than a thousand women, from hysterectomy patients to women undergoing various surgical procedures for infertility and pelvic disorders—such as diagnostic laparotomy, lysis of adhesions, and ovarian resections—participated in one or another of these studies, conducted concurrently from the late 1930s into the early 1950s. This work would establish Rock as one of the leading fertility researchers in the United States by the end of the 1940s, and without question the leading clinician in the field of infertility treatment. The authors of the official history of the American Society for Reproductive Medicine would call Rock one of the field's most important early figures, an "extraordinary man, . . . a revolutionary."[6] He was so well known by the mid-1940s, one story goes, that when "a famous movie actress"—Merle Oberon, we suspect—arrived in Boston to see "the fertility doctor" and didn't know his name, she was sent directly to Rock. When she told him how she found him, he told her not to feel embarrassed. After all, he said, "Before we met, I'd never heard of you, either."[7]

Rock's embryo study was referred to in the medical literature as either the Rock-Hertig or Hertig-Rock study and the ova study is known also as the in vitro fertilization experiments.[8] Because the terminology can bewilder, here is a brief primer: An *ovum* (*ova* in the plural) is an unfertilized human egg. When a woman's reproductive system is working properly (in other words, when she ovulates regularly) an ovum is released from the ovary at mid-cycle and travels through the fallopian tube, where fertilization occurs. A *fertilized egg* is the ovum after it has had contact with the sperm. A *blastocyst* is the term for the fertilized egg in its early stages of cell division. Rock and Hertig used the term *conceptus* to refer to a recently fertilized egg until implantation, and *embryo* to refer to the fertilized egg once it was implanted in the uterus.[9]

In the embryo study, Rock and Hertig broke new ground in the scientific and medical understanding of human fertility. Their work addressed a series of fundamental questions, beginning with the most basic: How is a pregnancy established? Rock and Hertig wanted to find out whether it was true, as many clinicians and scientists believed, that ovulation occurred fourteen days before menstruation; to determine the interval between ovulation and fertilization; to understand the length of time it takes for a newly fertilized ovum to implant in the uterus and the location of that implantation; and to learn how frequently a woman is likely to produce an abnormal embryo that would be destined for miscarriage. Rock also hoped to learn something about how long it generally takes for a fertile woman to conceive. And finally, Hertig and Rock wanted to create a visual record of the process of conception—from ovulation, through fertilization, to the attachment of the new embryo to the uterine wall and the establishment of a pregnancy.[10]

The IVF study was intended to capture the process of fertilization at its earliest stages, including the initial cell division of the newly fertilized ovum. This stage was beyond the technological capabilities of the Rock-Hertig study—surgery could not be timed in such a way that a two- or three-cell fertilized ovum would be found. And in practical terms, Rock also knew that if physicians could fertilize an egg "in glass" and then implant it, they would eventually be able to circumvent damaged fallopian tubes, a widespread and at the time mostly untreatable cause of female infertility. In both studies Rock had a clinical as well as a research outcome in view. A clear understanding of the process of conception and fertilization would lead to more effective infertility treatment, and in vitro fertilization would make it possible for women with blocked or absent fallopian tubes to become pregnant.[11]

Nowadays, we take reproductive technology for granted. With a simple test available at any drugstore, a woman can learn early on whether she has conceived. Within several weeks of conception, she can see her tiny embryo on a screen as a technician performs an ultrasound, and she can take home a picture of her fetus to post on the refrigerator to show to family and friends. Advances in assisted reproduction have rendered IVF almost routine for several kinds of infertility problems. Women with premature ovarian failure or those beyond their reproductive years can avail themselves of donor eggs and even donor embryos.

But in the 1930s clinicians were able merely to estimate the time of ovulation in advance. They had no data to help them determine for what period a newly released egg might be fertilizable. They did not know how long it took for the fertilized egg to travel to the uterus, attach itself to the uterine lining, and develop its amniotic sac. They were uncertain of the ratio of abnormal embryos to normal ones, or what proportion of normal embryos would successfully implant. This research, designed to provide answers to these critical questions, was not just of great interest to researchers and clinicians. It was of truly monumental significance.

Like his colleagues in the now growing area of infertility treatment, Rock was hopeful that at least some of the intractable difficulties facing infertile couples could be treated, or at least diagnosed more accurately so that treatments could be developed. The 1930s had witnessed important progress, particularly in diagnosis. Thanks to Gerald Moench, whose studies of sperm motility and morphology enabled clinicians to analyze the semen of the male partner for its potential fertility, male factors in infertility received more serious study than heretofore. And thanks to Rock and Bartlett's success in dating the endometrium, clinicians could determine (at least after the fact) if and when ovulation had occurred. This was useful information. If a woman was menstruating regularly but was failing to ovulate, she could not conceive. Endometrial dating, greater precision in semen analysis, and the new nonsurgical methods of determining the patency of the fallopian tubes were genuine advances. However, the earliest stages of conception and implantation remained an enigma.[12]

· · ·

Arthur Hertig was thirty-four years old and just eight years out of Harvard Medical School when he began working with Rock on the embryo study. He had first met Rock in 1930 when he was a fourth-year medical student at Harvard on an obstetrical rotation at the Boston Lying-In Hospital. Rock had given a lecture to the students on birth control. In 1931, as a resident at Boston Lying-In, Hertig founded its pathology laboratory. He was well on the way to becoming one of a small number of young pathologists to specialize in obstetrical pathology. In 1933 he won a fellowship to work at the Carnegie Institution of Washington with George Streeter, the preeminent human embryologist of the era and director of the Carnegie's Department of Embryology.

This fellowship shaped the next two decades of Hertig's career. The Carnegie laboratory possessed an extensive collection of human embryos as well as a colony of rhesus monkeys, whose reproductive systems are analogous to humans'. Hertig worked with Streeter and embryologist Chester Heuser in their development of a graded series of embryos from that species. Heuser, by all accounts a "technical wizard," taught the young pathologist how to search for tubal and intrauterine fertilized primate ova. Carl Hartman, considered the nation's leading expert on the reproductive life of the rhesus monkey, was at the Carnegie during those years as well.[13]

Hertig and Rock first worked together in 1934, just after Hertig returned from the Carnegie. Foreshadowing their later studies, this one consisted of "preliminary studies in which [they] attempted to recover segmenting ova from human fallopian tubes." They did not succeed at that time, but when Hertig was named pathologist at the Free Hospital in 1938, they went back to the drawing board. Their collaboration would last fifteen years.[14] Hertig never became quite so public a figure as his older colleague, but he went on to have a long and distinguished career, all of it at Harvard. Besides this embryo study, for which he was long remembered, he conducted important research on spontaneous abortion and on abnormalities of the placenta. He also served for more than two decades as chair of the Pathology Department.[15]

A remarkable feat of clinical research, the Rock-Hertig study enabled scientists and clinicians for the first time to visualize the process of human conception. Creating a photographic record of the earliest stages of pregnancy, Hertig and Rock documented a continuum of the early development of the human embryo, from the travels of the ovum through the fallopian tube to the implantation of the fertilized egg in the uterus and the beginning stages of embryonic life. In the course of the study, they recovered thirty-four fertilized ova and embryos, representing, as one journalist later put it, "the first seventeen days of life."[16]

Before the results of their research appeared, there were only two ways for researchers to learn about human embryology. They could analogize from the studies on the rhesus monkey, the most important of which were being conducted at the Carnegie. (And indeed, Rock and Hertig made use of those studies even as they sought to recover human eggs and embryos.) But the only way to study humans, until this point, had been to rely on embryos and fetuses that had been discovered accidentally. Not coincidentally, George Streeter at the Carnegie already presided over the largest scientific collection of these embryos as well. The Carnegie's human embryos had been acquired by happenstance—during autopsies, surgeries for ectopic pregnancies, emergency hysterectomies, and on occasion during a dilatation and curettage. But they did not represent a continuum.

No one had ever attempted to trace the origins of human embryonic development from fertilization through implantation and beyond. Indeed, without reliable knowledge about the timing of ovulation, such an attempt would have been extremely unlikely to succeed.[17] As to which one of them came up with the idea, as Hertig later remembered it, both of them did, maybe even independently. Hertig recalled numerous discussions he and his colleagues had during his fellowship at the Carnegie about the absence of "material" for the first two weeks of human development, and Rock's interest in the relationship between "ripe ova" and the menstrual cycle had already begun.

They may have been thinking along parallel tracks, but neither could accomplish the research alone. Rock had access to potential research volunteers among his own patients and the patients of other surgeons at the Free Hospital. Hertig had the unique training and expertise needed to find the ova and embryos. Both had skilled technical assistance: Rock, the indefatigable Miriam Menkin, and Hertig, the accomplished Eleanor Colby Adams.[18]

Their collaboration was emblematic of Rock's style of working. Later, an envious and frustrated George Smith, Rock's longtime colleague at the Free Hospital, would bitterly characterize Rock, who had been a friend, as someone who rode the coattails of more technically accomplished researchers.[19] Rock might have seen Smith's point; he always had a pretty good idea of his limitations as well as his strengths. He recognized that he lacked advanced scientific and technical training. But he did have imagination, exceptional intuitiveness, and the good sense to gather around him those who possessed technical expertise and intellectual tenacity. When he lavishly credited the accomplishments of those with whom he worked as making possible his own, he was speaking the literal truth. To say that Rock was skilled in selecting his collaborators, however, neither denies his originality nor diminishes his accomplishments.

All in all, 211 women participated in the Rock-Hertig study.[20] The protocol for the study, although it underwent a few changes over time, is relatively simple to describe, but it was not simple to execute. First, the researchers had to find women of known fertility who needed a hysterectomy but not necessarily immediately. Then, the women had to agree to have unprotected intercourse at the time they were most likely to conceive. The participants were recruited from two groups, those seen in the gynecological outpatient clinic and women from the "rhythm clinic" begun by Rock and run by social worker Elizabeth Snedeker since 1936.[21]

One of the goals of the rhythm clinic was to assist the Free Hospital's many Catholic patients to limit their pregnancies without violating the strictures of their religion (not to mention the laws of Massachusetts). It was an excellent source for recruitment. These women were clearly fertile. (Otherwise, why would they be there?) And their many pregnancies sometimes wreaked havoc on their reproductive organs, making them candidates for hysterectomy. In addition, many of these women, who waited for their appointments just down the hall from the infertile women who sought help from the Fertility and Endocrine Clinic, were familiar with and sympathetic to those who could not conceive. When the study's purposes were explained to them as a way to understand conception so that women like the infertile women down the hall might be able to bear children, many were pleased that they could help.[22]

Rock later declared that he did not personally recommend the hysterectomies, but patient records do not back him up. And Hertig remembered the recruitment process with a bit of sophistry, writing years afterwards that "patients destined for a hysterectomy were selected by the staff, not by Dr. Rock [emphasis in original], and then placed on the operative list." Only after they had agreed to participate, he continued, were they "transferred to Dr. Rock's clinic and treated as his private patients." Given the way the hospital operated, however, "selected by staff" might mean that they were selected by one of Rock's residents or fellows, or even by Elizabeth Snedeker or Miriam Menkin.[23]

In the stiff language of the scientific article, the participants were women of proven fertility whose "symptoms[,] caused either by gross uterine displacement or minor uterine pathology[, . . .would] be best relieved by hysterectomy," according to the best medical judgment of the time, but who did not require immediate surgery.[24] They were then put on a waiting list for an elective procedure and called in accordingly. The women agreed to track their menstrual cycles for one to several months (and the later participants also had their urine tested for hormonal activity) so that the nurses could determine, when the time came, participants' likely dates of highest fertility. In the month before they were scheduled for surgery, either Miriam Menkin or one of the staff nurses then asked each woman to have unprotected intercourse during that time.[25]

The women in the study ranged in age from twenty-five to their middle forties, and most of them came from the clinic population, although there were enough private patients both in this and the related IVF study—around 10 percent of the total—to suggest that one's status as a clinic or private patient was not absolutely determinative of participation.[26] In addition to the requirement that volunteers be married and living with their husbands, they needed to be "intelligent," have had at least three full-term deliveries, and be "willing to record menstrual cycles and coitus without contraception." Many of the women in the Rock-Hertig study had experienced more than three full-term pregnancies, and several had been pregnant a dozen times or more.[27]

The participants' gynecological complaints ran the gamut from prolonged and profuse menstrual flows to incapacitating menstrual cramping, from constant pelvic pain to "falling of the womb." Some of the women had endured their problems for several years—one had suffered for more than a decade and a half—before attempting to seek a remedy. Others had recently experienced a worsening of their conditions.

Highly fertile women maximized researchers' chances of finding a fertilized egg. Some of them had a dozen or more children. All had real gynecological problems.[28] They typically waited for their operation about one and a half to six months, although a few women experienced delays of a year or longer. (Any patient with an immediate need for surgery received it. If she was a participant in the study and her condition became acute, she was simply operated on and taken off the research list.)

While they waited, the women sent in prepaid postcards noting the dates of their periods and sometimes came in for additional examinations. For nearly all the women whose surgery occurred more than six months after their initial visit, the delay appeared to have been by choice. Some had trouble deciding if they wanted the surgery. Others had child-care problems. Occasionally a husband lost his job and the wife had to take one. Or a woman needed to schedule surgery during the summer when older children were available to take care of the younger ones. And still others had additional health problems for which they required more immediate medical attention.[29]

Many of these women had experienced numerous pregnancies in a relatively short time and were hard pressed at home with the care of their children. Often they had little assistance and were poor or nearly poor. Others had teeth that needed to be pulled, or varicose veins requiring surgery. Still others suffered from constant exhaustion and seemed prone to undefined illnesses.[30] Some of them had suffered for a long time. One complained of pain "of 17 years duration," another of "falling of the womb" accompanied by backaches and "weakness, fatigue, and nervousness." Others spoke of constant "soreness," or "pulling pain[s]," or "profuse flow[s]" lasting for up to six weeks and sometimes longer.[31]

At their initial visits, as a part of their general workup, all patients provided a menstrual history. At that point, some of them were noted as possible volunteers for one of the research series—embryo, early tubal ova (one component of the Rock-Hertig study), or ova. Either Rock or one his assistants, usually Miriam Menkin but sometimes one of the nurses, explained the purpose of the research, generally describing the studies as a way to learn more about how to help infertile women conceive.

Probably in part so that Hertig could perfect his proficiency at finding specimens, in the first few years Rock operated on the participants close to the next expected date of menstruation, because the later the surgery, the larger the fertilized egg. Rock never wanted to schedule a surgery any later than the date of the next expected menstruation. Missing a period, in those days before early pregnancy tests, was generally considered the first indication of a possible pregnancy. Hertig later recalled that every patient was operated on before the next expected menstruation. However, Rock miscalculated at least once, operating two weeks later than he had intended.[32]

Since the "embryo" patients, it was hoped, would conceive during the cycle in which the surgery was planned, the researchers did not want them conceiving before that time. The patient records do not indicate in all cases the advice the doctor or nurses gave them for preventing conception between the time of their initial visit and the menstrual period preceding their surgery. A few charts indicate that the patient was advised to continue using rhythm; others noted a woman's ongoing contraceptive practice. During the month in which her surgery was scheduled, when each woman was instructed to have unprotected intercourse during her expected fertile period, the instructions were oral and simply noted as such on the chart in the early years of the study. But by the late 1940s, the staff began to follow up with a letter containing explicit written instructions, as Jean Nauss, one of the office nurses, wrote to Mrs. W.: "About the other matter which you discussed with Dr. Mulligan [one of Rock's assistants]—we would like you to have intercourse on the following dates without using a douche or any other precaution: December 26, 28, and 30, and January 1 and 3. Since you will be coming here on the 3rd, it will mean having intercourse in the morning if you can possibly arrange to do so."[33]

Several days before a participant's surgery, Rock's staff alerted Hertig's laboratory and provided him with the patient's history, estimated time of ovulation, and the likely age of the fertilized egg, should one be found. Once the organs were excised, they were rushed from the operating room to the lab, where Hertig stood by, ready to examine, dissect, and fix the specimen with Bouin's fluid. In the earliest stage of fertilization, the egg became visible only after being fixed; older ones could be viewed even before fixation. The process, recalled Hertig, took an entire day "by the time one carefully dissected the tissue, flushed tubes, pipetted uterine fluid, examined fluid in which the uterine sac was opened, and described the procedures and everything that goes into a specimen in a pathology laboratory." If the organs contained an ovum, fertilized egg, blastocyst, conceptus, or embryo, that was cause for celebration.

Given that a human ovum is much, much smaller than the period at the end of this sentence, great skill and perseverance were necessary. If Hertig found what he was looking for, he packed up the specimen and personally took it by train to Baltimore and the Carnegie Institution, where the specimens were prepared and photographed.[34]

Rock and Hertig were profoundly indebted to the scientists and technicians at the Carnegie. Streeter and Heuser participated in the interpretation of the data. In 1940, when Streeter retired as director, the equally illustrious George Corner (the first to discover progesterone) succeeded him. Also important to this enterprise was Hertig's devoted technician at Harvard Medical School, Eleanor Colby Adams, who worked with Carnegie technician O. O. Heard to reconstruct the specimens from serial sections. The fertilized eggs, blastocysts, conceptuses, and embryos then joined the collection at the Carnegie.[35]

This study began long before the federal government provided support for scientific and clinical research. In later years, Hertig would state proudly that "the original, full study did not cost the taxpayer one cent," being financed principally "from Dr. Rock's private practice and my hospital salary and small grants—small even in those days." Outside grants came from the Milton Fund at Harvard, the Carnegie Corporation, the National Research Council, and the American Cancer Society. The Carnegie Institution paid the salary of the indispensable Eleanor Adams.[36]

Hertig and Rock began presenting their results as soon as they had their first findings. By June 1942, when they traveled to Sky Top, Pennsylvania, for the annual meeting of the American Gynecological Society, sixty-one surgeries had been performed as part of the study. Hertig had discovered, as Rock informed the audience, one "perfect unfertilized tubal ovum," two follicular ova "in the first maturation division," and "twelve very young human conceptuses." Two of them, reported for the first time at Sky Top, were aged seven to eight and nine to ten days old, the youngest human embryos ever seen.[37]

From these specimens, Rock and Hertig sought to learn the probable time of ovulation and the number of days that elapse between ovulation and fertilization. The data confirmed Rock's belief that the timing of ovulation could not be calculated in advance, from the most recent menstruation, but only after the fact. He used two cases as examples, instances in which the women had only a single coitus during the relevant cycle. In one case, endometrial dating for the woman in whose uterus the seven-to-eight-day-old embryo was found indicated that there were still six days to go before menstruation, on the thirtieth day of her cycle. Ovulation had probably taken place on the sixteenth day, and intercourse occurred within a few hours. As Rock declared, "the post-ovulatory phase approaches a constant; the pre-ovulatory phase is of variable length."[38]

The first full report on the study appeared in 1941 in *Contributions to Embryology*.[39] Later results appeared in the *American Journal of Obstetrics and Gynecology*, and other fruits of the study continued to appear in scientific and medical journals throughout the 1950s. Annual reports of the Free Hospital described the status of the study and the number of embryos found. Occasionally the press reported on it; one article mentioned the "very fertile women . . . who cooperated before the surgery by trying to get pregnant."[40] The study came to an official end in 1954. In 1989, the year before he died at the age of eighty-six, Hertig remarked proudly, "I have been told by experts in in vitro fertilization that this series of naturally occurring human ova laid the foundation for their pioneering work in solving developmental aspects of human infertility."[41]

. . .

The Rock-Hertig study was what we call "nontherapeutic" medical research. Although the patients were having a therapeutic procedure, and a review of their preoperative and postoperative diagnoses suggests that a hysterectomy was legitimately indicated according to the diagnostic guidelines of the time, the *research* performed did not directly benefit them as individual patients.[42] What did that mean for the women involved?

Early twenty-first-century readers may think immediately about the ethics of encouraging women to have unprotected intercourse in the hopes of finding evidence of conception. Although Arthur Hertig would insist several decades later that "the patients were *not* instructed when to have coitus, but [only that] if they did so without precaution they were to record this fact on a postal card," his recollection does not jibe with the records.[43] Indeed, more specific directives than those given by the office staff can hardly be imagined.

The best way, everyone knew, to increase the chances of finding an embryo was to ask the patients to have intercourse when conception was most likely. It is possible that some patients failed to understand the connection between having sex and getting pregnant, but most of them appear to have gotten the point quite clearly. Some, perhaps many, of these women were poor. They were not stupid. Not only would women who had been attending the rhythm clinic have a good idea of their fertile period, but there is also evidence in the patient charts that before women agreed to participate, they wanted absolute guarantees that the surgery would occur as planned.

None of them wanted an unplanned pregnancy. "Suppose something happens and they change their minds about operating?" one woman worried. Another patient, fully confident that her doctors would not let her down, was unable to persuade her husband to equal confidence. He became so nervous that the surgery might be canceled that he was unable to cooperate after the first scheduled date for intercourse. He need not have worried; she had her surgery as scheduled. Indeed, the records suggest that they all had their surgeries.[44]

One woman did wonder, after the surgery, whether she had conceived. "I . . . would like to know . . . what Dr. Rock found—if conception had occurred—and if it helped him any—I'm just sort of curious." She hadn't, the record shows. One of the staff wrote back that Hertig had at first thought she might have, but "when your womb was examined a very interesting condition of its lining was found, but apparently conception had not taken place."[45] The tone of the woman's letter seems anxious, although the overall tenor of her correspondence with the staff suggests that her ambivalence was not about participation in the study but about having had the surgery itself. She had put off her operation for several months until Rock convinced her that she needed it.

If Rock believed that a woman truly needed a hysterectomy, he would tell her so; if there were other options, he offered those. Rock's relationship with his patients was complicated. It does not conform to a stereotype of physician-as-authority-figure imposing his will on women-without-power. As Luigi Mastroianni, one of Rock's fellows from the 1950s, recalled, Rock never misled patients, keeping them fully informed of the reasons he was asking for their participation in a study and the purpose of the research.[46] These women were decidedly not passive creatures blindly accepting whatever an authority figure told them.

To the contrary, at least some of the clinic patients who participated in this study were surprisingly well-informed consumers of medical services. One woman scheduled for surgery wrote to the staff in 1948 that she decided against an operation Rock recommended because she had "read up on the subject," and she believed that she could put off the operation for a while, particularly since her husband was out of work and she could not "go to the hospital and have peace of mind." This patient was not asked to participate in the study because after examining her, Rock had concluded that she did not need a hysterectomy but needed a myomectomy (removal of only the fibroid tumor). In another case, Rock had informed a patient that he could alleviate her condition, which according to her chart included a lacerated perineum, a cystocele, a hypertrophic cervix, and cervical erosions, either with or without performing a hysterectomy. The choice, he said, should be hers; he could cure her either way. After consulting with her husband, she wrote to say that she wanted the hysterectomy rather than the repair. Rock did as she requested.[47]

Rock never encouraged women to have unnecessary surgery so that he could increase the number of cases in the study, and there is nothing to suggest that any of them were pressured to participate in the study if they did require a hysterectomy. This is not to say that many were not *flattered* into participating either by Rock or the staff, who told them that they would be helping to make an important contribution to the medical understanding of fertility and the alleviation of infertility. There was no coercion, but could the women have felt a more subtle pressure? It's hard to tell. Rock was a well-loved doctor whose patients were devoted to him. Both clinic and private patients often expressed a personal gratitude for his care that went beyond appreciation of his medical skills. Some, perhaps many, of his patients might have wanted to do as he asked, particularly when agreeing to participate assured them of a more personalized level of care and attention from the staff as well as the doctors.[48]

The Rock-Hertig study relied on the willingness of mostly clinic and some private patients to attempt to conceive with the understanding that they would have a hysterectomy before a pregnancy, in their view, could be established. A majority of these women were probably Catholics, who nevertheless agreed to participate in research that would allow Rock and Hertig to use their embryos to enhance medical knowledge about, in Rock's own words, "the earliest stages of human development." The women were told that they were expected to try to conceive, and they in turn expected assurances that their hysterectomies would occur as planned. They did not consider these early embryos to be life, notwithstanding the Catholic Church's contention even then that life begins at conception. Historian Leslie Reagan has documented that as late as the 1920s, women generally did not believe a fetus was alive until it could be felt to move. "Quickening continued to have real moral meaning for women," Reagan says for that period, and the fact that Rock's patients did not think of themselves as possibly pregnant suggests that the idea may have had considerable staying power into the next couple of decades.[49]

Neither Rock nor Hertig ever doubted that this was a responsible, ethical study. Although Hertig remembered that they had thought "long and hard about the ethical implications" of this research, the record contradicts him. Neither they nor their patients seem to have been troubled in the least by ethical difficulties.

Should they have been? Given the context of the times, we don't think so, although it is true that during this period, other nontherapeutic research studies were doing harm to their subjects. The Tuskegee experiment, conducted by the National Public Health Service, is perhaps the most infamous example. For twenty years, beginning in 1932, black men suffering from syphilis in impoverished rural Alabama were recruited for yearly tests that would track the progress of the disease. The researchers deliberately withheld treatment that had been proved to cure this disease (effective antibiotic treatment was available by the 1930s) and even refused to provide simple information to the men. They did provide "free medicines" for other diseases, "hot meals" when the men came to the hospital for tests, and free transportation to and from the hospital, including a stop in town to shop and hang out. And their families were guaranteed fifty dollars in burial assistance if, once an afflicted man died, they would agree to an autopsy.[50]

It is impossible to read about the Tuskegee experiment without feeling the chill of revulsion—here we have a group of impoverished African American men, denied treatment for a disease for which a cure was available, observed and studied until they died and even afterwards. Not all nontherapeutic studies were this egregious, and some were neutral or benign, but Tuskegee was not an isolated instance. The exploitation of mental patients and children in orphanages in research that sometimes caused physical pain and even permanent damage was the subject of public outcries. During the Great Depression, state employment bureaus sent jobless men to laboratories that paid them to be research subjects, which was coercive if not always physically harmful to the participants. For example, eighty unemployed men, sent to the Department of Pathology at the University of Illinois College of Medicine, participated in a study of human response to "various forms of stimuli" designed to study the influence of weather.[51]

Although some elite physicians had urged the American Medical Association (AMA) to adopt formal rules regarding human experimentation as early as 1916, and although campaigns against such experimentation—called in the parlance of the time "human vivisection"—were active in the 1930s, it was not until 1946 that the AMA Code of Ethics included any reference to the obligations of a researcher to a subject.[52]

But just because some medical researchers could get away with doing harm

to patients or other research subjects doesn't mean that all clinical researchers did so. Rock and Hertig were among those who did not. As far as Rock
was concerned (and as the patient records confirm), the patients were genuine
candidates for surgery and were given the opportunity to consider whether
they wanted to have an operation. After that, they were then asked if they were
willing to participate in a study that would not harm them and would contrib-
ute to medical knowledge.

Later critics notwithstanding, Rock and his collaborators did not subject
poor women, with little power to say no to authority figures, to what the wom-
en would have considered a possible abortion in order to obtain "research
material."[53] Nor did they force women to wait months for urgently needed
operations to satisfy their research designs, or deliberately use their positions as figures of authority to coerce patients into cooperating and to mislead them about their possible condition. These criticisms would come later,
of course, both from opponents of abortion and from some feminists. Among
the former was physician Herbert Ratner, who in 1963 denounced this study
as "lethal human experimentation" and branded Rock as a renegade Catholic
who displayed a longstanding "intransigence to the teaching of his church."[54]
On the other side of the political divide, a group of feminists opposed to reproductive technology in the 1980s saw the Rock-Hertig study as a harbinger
of everything they deplored in modern reproductive medicine, which they
viewed as "a form of medical violence against women." Or, as Gena Corea
put it in The Mother Machine, "women in [the Rock-Hertig study] belonged to
a lower economic, social, and gender class than the doctors who asked them
to participate . . . Did they truly understand the nature of the experiment?
. . . Were they confident that if they did refuse to do what the doctor asked of
them, they could still receive health care and be treated decently?" The answer, for Corea, was a resounding no.[55]

Even journalist Loretta McLaughlin, who wrote a flattering biography
of Rock in the early 1980s that highlighted his struggles with the Catholic
Church over birth control, expressed serious reservations about the propriety
of the Rock-Hertig study, describing the "delicate ethical maneuver" required
of the two researchers before they could justify the research. In an interview
with Hertig around 1980, McLaughlin said, she pressed him: If a patient was
pregnant at the time of the surgery, "wouldn't [she] have considered the result
an abortion?" Hertig, she continued, recoiled from such an notion. "No! How
could it be?" he shot back. "There was no way in God's world at that time of
knowing whether they were pregnant or not. There were literally no tests."

But then again, he recalled, he never actually talked to the patients. Forced to justify himself in ways that would never have occurred to him in the 1930s or even the 1950s, Hertig's "vehement" response to McLaughlin's questioning reflected the influence of the charged contemporary political climate in which questions about reproduction were asked and answered.[56] He was responding to the issues of the 1980s, not to those of an earlier era.

. . .

The Rock-Hertig research raised no controversy in its day; neither the patients nor the researchers considered these embryos to be babies-in-waiting.[57] And except for the occasional mention in a Boston newspaper, the study received little attention from the media. Not so for Rock's companion project on human in vitro fertilization. This one would receive national attention and make Rock a media celebrity. The in vitro project had as its immediate goal the understanding of human fertilization, the initial event leading to the formation of an embryo. Like the embryo study, which had as one of its immediate purposes obtaining information about the timing and process of ovulation, the in vitro project was aimed at finding knowledge applicable to overcoming female infertility.

Rock began this project at the same time he and Hertig embarked on the embryo study. It was preceded by an anonymous editorial in the *New England Journal of Medicine* in 1937, which suggested that if fertilization could be accomplished outside the uterus in humans, as Gregory Pincus had already shown was possible with rabbits, "what a boon for the barren woman with closed tubes!" The editorial's author, as he later admitted, was Rock himself.[58] Just six years after beginning the IVF study, he and Miriam Menkin would electrify the readers of *Science* magazine with their announcement of the successful fertilization in vitro of four human ova. Although a few scientists would later raise questions about whether Rock and Menkin had achieved true in vitro fertilization, the two are generally credited as the first in this research.[59]

Closed fallopian tubes, which could be caused by endometriosis, scarring arising from complications of abdominal surgery or appendicitis, or sexually transmitted diseases such as gonorrhea, were responsible for about 20 percent of the infertility cases in Rock's practice. At the time, a woman's only hope for conception was to have the tubes surgically reconstructed and opened, a procedure requiring extraordinary skill and delicacy. Success rates were low, with the best surgeons reporting around 7 percent. Gynecologists were frustrated by their inability to help women with this condition.

Eventually, in vitro fertilization, with the embryo implanted in the uterus, would enable women with occluded (or absent) fallopian tubes to bear children. Today it is the first line of treatment for infertility caused by tubal disease. But in the 1930s the idea of human "conception in a watch glass," as it was sometimes called then, seemed far fetched, even frightening, raising the Orwellian specter of babies fertilized in test tubes, then spending their prenatal life in artificial wombs, fatherless and motherless. Gregory Pincus, who would later recruit Rock as his chief clinical collaborator in the development of the oral contraceptive, had been denied tenure at Harvard only a year before Rock and Menkin began their experiments, and the notoriety of his in vitro fertilization and related experiments on rabbits has been viewed as a contributing factor. (A Collier's magazine article on his work talked about Pincus as the creator of "fatherless" rabbits and suggested that such experiments could mean that if women no longer depended on men to bear children, they might not need them for anything else, either![60]) But by the time Rock and Menkin announced they had succeeded, the climate of opinion had changed, and the public was more excited than dismayed.

Pincus's successful rabbit experiments were much on Rock's mind when he decided to undertake experiments in human IVF. Menkin later recollected, only half-jokingly, that when she interviewed for a position with Rock in 1938, the only thing that impressed him was that she had worked for Pincus on his rabbit studies. "In my interview," she told a group of fellow scientists at Cold Spring Harbor in 1949, she tried to impress Rock with her "interest in cytology . . . Many years before that, I had had the great privilege of taking Dr. Wilson's course in cytology at Columbia. I was trying very hard to make a good impression . . . I was dying to get the job . . . but that didn't seem to cut much ice with Dr. Rock . . . about cytology and the great E. B. Wilson. What did impress him, however, was when I told him that I had once worked for Dr. Gregory Pincus, though in a very minor capacity. I used to prepare those pituitary extracts: FSH and LH, for Dr. Pincus's experiments on rabbit eggs. SUPEROVULATION! that one word did it . . . I was hired."[61] And so in March 1938, Menkin began her career as an "egg chaser." She was a dream hire for this project. Smart, tenacious, meticulous in her technique, and a perfectionist (perhaps even obsessive) about documentation, she devoted her considerable talents to this project for the next six years.

The cool, analytical, scientific language that Rock and Menkin would use in 1944 to announce the success of their research did nothing to capture those tumultuous six years of trying out different research protocols, changing them often in midstream. When they began, all they had to go on were the earlier animal studies. In humans, after all, no one had ever done this before. The researchers had no idea of the optimum time in the ovulatory cycle for an egg to be fertilized, although it was believed that the best time was just after ovulation. Should they try to find ova that had just ripened? Should they wait until the ovum was in the fallopian tube, where fertilization appeared to take place in nature? Or should the eggs be taken directly from the ovary and then be "developed" a bit further in a culture medium before the insemination was attempted? How were they to know? And just how helpful were those animal studies anyway?

Among our animal relatives, only primates menstruate. IVF researchers had worked with mice, rats, and—most successfully—rabbits. All of these animals experience estrus, not menstruation. That meant it was possible to control an animal's ovulation—mate the female rabbit, for example, with a sterilized male, and she ovulates. Afterwards, the rabbits lost their lives at various stages of the process.[62]

Although it was hard to know how much of practical value could be learned from the rabbits, Menkin and others, with the cooperation of the Fearing Laboratory at the Free Hospital, studied rabbit eggs and embryos, conducting several IVF experiments concurrently with those on the patients. The Fearing, directed by biochemist Olive Smith, was the hospital's center for basic research. Olive Smith was well known for her work on the estrogens, particularly diethylstilbestrol (the later infamous DES). Rock was her obstetrician as well as a friend and colleague, and she allowed Rock's researchers to conduct these experiments, although she was not a collaborator on them.[63]

Unlike the embryo study, the human ova study called only for participants to keep track of their menstrual cycles. In the first years of the study, when Rock believed that the ova most likely to be fertilized would be those that were, in Menkin's words, "just ready to pop," the staff attempted to schedule surgeries when it seemed most likely that the patient had just ovulated. In these early days, he had been hopeful that one could predict the exact time of ovulation using the electric "potentiator," but after a brief period in the late 1930s, when Rock admitted the women into the hospital a few days before their anticipated surgery and hooked them up to the device, rushing them into the operating room just after the potentiator indicated that ovulation had occurred, the sheer fruitlessness of it soon became obvious. And besides, the staff found the scheduling to be a logistical nightmare; it was simply impossible for them to do the clerical work required to keep track of all the cycles.[64]

Once it had proved impossible to figure out when a particular woman was about to ovulate, Rock decided that perhaps they should look for an ovum already in the fallopian tube, since this procedure had worked with Pincus's rabbits. Scheduling the surgery was a bit easier; these women were operated on between days sixteen and eighteen of their menstrual cycles. But this didn't work either. In the first place, only women who required complete hysterectomies could be asked to participate, since an ovary and tube would have to be removed, and unless there was severe pathology of the ovary (which could be a bad indicator for the health of the tubal egg), an ovary was not removed except in hysterectomy. Tubal eggs were, therefore, hard to find: only two were found over the course of the entire study. Finally, in early 1942 Rock approved a protocol in which the participating women were scheduled for surgery about a week after the onset of their menstrual periods. This was easier on the women and provided Miriam Menkin with more ova.[65]

A total of 947 women agreed to have parts of their reproductive organs used for the study. They were a much more varied group, in terms of their diagnoses, than those who participated in the embryo study. All the surgical procedures they were having involved laparotomy. Some of the women were scheduled for hysterectomies; others were infertility patients undergoing ovarian resection, which was at the time performed not only for polycystic ovaries but also for unexplained infertility; still others were having diagnostic laparotomies, mostly for infertility.

Out of the 947 women, 359 of them had their cases, in Menkin's words, "discarded." Of these, some were found during the surgery to be treatable without the removal of any ovarian tissue. Others became pregnant. Some dropped out, and still another group had menstrual irregularities that precluded their participation. In another 200 or so cases, the ovaries were too damaged to be of any use, or the laparotomy was not performed because more minor procedures were sufficient. When all was said and done, the researchers had obtained "research specimens"—that is, ova—from just under 300 patients. Of those patients, 47 had their eggs inseminated. In all, Menkin attempted to fertilize 138 eggs from these 47 women.[66]

After the operation, the ovarian tissue was "minced with fine scissors" and "flushed" with a mixture of blood serum and Locke's solution, which contains albumin, later considered to be the substance that triggers sperm "capacitation," or its ability to fertilize the egg. In the early stages, the serum came from the patient. Later, Menkin used serum from postmenopausal women to avoid potential hormonal variations. After several changes of the sterile serum, the ovum was incubated overnight. Spermatozoa were added the next day. The sperm Menkin used came from "leftover" semen that had been used for artificial insemination, either from husbands of infertility patients or from donors.[67]

Week in and week out, for six years—except for a brief maternity leave to have her second child—Menkin waited outside the operating room for the specimens, then literally ran upstairs to the laboratory to begin the process, occasionally varying the length of culture or the concentration of sperm. She was dogged and careful, and seemed rarely to become discouraged, although six years without any progress could have seemed an eternity. Then, between February and April 1944, Menkin managed to fertilize four ova from three women.

Why did the experiment work after so many years of failure? According to Menkin, success resulted from a combination of accident and exhaustion. Until now, she had washed each sperm suspension three times in Locke's solution before beginning the insemination attempt. But that day, worn out from having been kept awake two nights running by her teething baby, she washed it once and then used a more concentrated suspension. She also used a longer contact time, which may have made a difference. Previously, because it had worked with the rabbits (although one would think the researchers would have known better by now than to keep relying on animal analogies), she had allowed only a twenty-minute contact time. Now, "I was so exhausted . . . that I couldn't get up, so I just sat there, watching this remarkable sight, . . . which never fails to fascinate me—the human egg, with a mass of spermatozoa on its surface . . . So great is the force of their combined efforts that the egg is made to rotate around and around." She sat for at least an hour, transfixed.[68]

The first success, however, was not an unrelieved triumph. Everyone became so excited that an argument ensued about the best way to preserve the newly fertilized ovum. After making a quick sketch, Menkin wanted to use her normal half-hour procedure, but Arthur Hertig held out for the more elaborate process used by Chester Heuser at the Carnegie Institution. In the heat of the discussion, they forgot to photograph the egg, and when the argument was over, and Hertig had prevailed, Menkin went back to the microscope and couldn't find the egg! Rock told her not to worry, that now at least they knew it could be done, and although she endured a considerable amount of teasing for her "miscarriage in vitro," she at least thought she would be able to repeat the fertilization. Because she was unsure which of the accidental new factors had made the difference, she incorporated all three into her next experiments and was successful again—with three ova from two women. These specimens were carefully photographed before being preserved.[69]

To her enormous disappointment, Menkin was forced to leave the project just at this point because her husband lost his job in Boston. Although Rock tried to find him another position in the region, he was unable to do so, and the Menkins moved first to Duke University and then to Temple Medical School in Philadelphia. She was unable to continue the experiments in either place. The physicians and researchers at Duke were scandalized (one of the doctors called her research "rape in vitro" behind her back), and in Philadelphia they were uninterested. Meanwhile, back at the Free Hospital, her successors apparently did not have her technical proficiency. In 1949, Rock wrote her, "Weep. This P.M. Dr. Finkel [sic] lost a beautiful 3 cell in vitro fertilized egg, fortunately after photography. A 2 cell one was lost only a few months ago just before photography. We need you badly."[70] (Before too long, Menkin would be back working for Rock, but by then he had become interested in other things.)

The announcement that human ova had been fertilized outside the womb brought Rock a great deal of journalistic attention. Menkin had done almost all the detail work on the project, but it had been Rock's idea. He had designed the protocols and overseen the study. He had the MD and the clinical reputation. The first report appeared in 1944 in *Science*—a brief communication with the description of the fertilized ova, but no illustrations. The full report would not appear until 1948, and Rock would insist that Menkin be the lead author. In part because her name was going first, but also because of her perfectionism, it took so long before publication because Menkin insisted on investigating every hint of a reference to previous animal studies. She also understood that this would be—literally—a seminal article if there ever was one, and she wanted it to be as perfect as possible.[71] But the press would never have waited for the full explanation anyway.

Almost immediately after the *Science* article appeared, newspapers across the United States and around the world picked up the story. As journalists converged on Rock, he tried to temper their (and his) excitement. He was convinced that what he and Menkin had achieved would have a major impact. Pregnancy through in vitro fertilization, he told more than one journalist, was "not beyond the realm of imagination, and it seems to offer about the only hope for women whose tubes have been destroyed."[72] Nevertheless, as he would often remind people over the next several years, a great deal of research would be needed to make the leap from a two- or three-cell fertilized ovum to an embryo that could be placed into a woman's uterus and grow into a baby.

Rock and Menkin's IVF research garnered more praise than criticism, in part because it was viewed as a potential means of aiding infertile couples to have children, and in part because this was an era that celebrated scientific discoveries. *Time* magazine even recalled the Pincus rabbit experiments, noting that Rock and Menkin's research was "a development from similar work on rabbits by Biologist Gregory Pincus." *Time* remembered—correctly—that in the case of the rabbit, Pincus had "planted [sic] the resulting cells in [her] uterus and she bore normal, healthy bunnies."[73] But a few critics there definitely were, including one Missouri woman who wrote indignantly to the president of Harvard, telling him that "when you interfere with the laws of Nature, you interfere with the laws of God, and when you interfere with the laws of God, you insult the intelligence of the Christian people."[74]

In later years, some doubts would surface about whether Rock and Menkin had actually achieved in vitro fertilization. Carl Hartman, a leading zoologist and former scientist at the Carnegie Institution, was a skeptic, telling Rock in 1954, "I don't believe you ever got *in vitro* fertilization."[75] But most of Rock's contemporaries were believers. George Streeter, the most distinguished embryologist of his day, told Rock that "Dr. Corner, Heuser, and I are convinced that it is the real thing."[76] Rock and Menkin would not be the last of the IVF researchers to face the skeptics. Even Robert Edwards and Patrick Steptoe, the two men responsible for the birth of the world's first acknowledged IVF baby, faced disbelief when Louise Brown was born in 1978.

. . .

In the mid-1940s, Rock's research career had reached new heights. He and Arthur Hertig were on the receiving end of professional accolades for their embryo study, a major breakthrough in fertility research. (In the 1980s, it would be this study, rather than the IVF companion research, that was viewed as having laid the foundation for successful human in vitro fertilization.) The American Gynecological Society—the oldest and most prestigious gynecological organization in the United States—would award its 1949 Research Prize to Hertig and Rock, and embryology textbooks until around 1980 would continue to use their images. When he had begun both studies, he had been a prominent Boston specialist with an excellent reputation as a skilled and compassionate physician. Now he had become a nationally recognized expert

in fertility, and once the war came to an end, his reputation spread internationally, and he received letters asking for advice from women and men in
infertile marriages from around the world.

His growing fame, however, was accompanied by personal heartbreak, ill
health, and tragedy. The first blow was the loss of his eldest brother in 1940.
Charlie was just fifty-five. John and Charlie had become quite close as adults.
And while Charlie continued to provide financial support when needed to
his younger brother, the relationship became one more of equals, with John
providing both medical and family advice to Charlie. The two Rock brothers
turned out to be more alike in some ways than they ever might have expected.
Late bloomers both, once they found their respective callings, they shared a
powerful work ethic. Like John, Charlie threw himself into his work. Both
thrived on their seven-day commitments, although it would be a mistake to
call either of them by the contemporary term "workaholic," because they
knew how to enjoy themselves as well.

Unfortunately, Charlie, like John and Nell, suffered from hypertension—
in his case, quite severe. He had a "sudden cerebral vascular disturbance" (a
mild stroke) in the summer of 1935, which caused John considerable worry.
Charlie, however, once he began feeling better, was resistant to medical advice. John persuaded him to see his internist friend Paul White at Massachusetts General, but Charlie did not like White's advice, which was to limit his
activity, take regular vacations, and watch his weight. White had told Charlie not to drive for six months and advised an experimental operation, called
splanchnic resection, if diet and behavior changes failed to work.[77]

Charlie, who had expected to receive some medication and be sent on his
way, was furious. Obstinate as ever, he claimed that White, considered one
of the best internists in Boston, was little better than an "interne." Charlie
refused, he said angrily, to be some "white rat or a guinea pig or some other
kind of animal" for experimentation. Furthermore, he ranted, "The thing I
want to do most in the world is drive my car and it is the thing I must not do.
If I told White I was staying up late at night reading then he would tell me to
stop reading . . . If I told him that I was rushing for a train, running down the
platform, hopping on as the gates closed, he would tell me to get in a car and
ride." And just to make sure that John understood that he was going to ignore
as completely as possible all this medical advice, he concluded, "I don't have
any headaches and I don't have any pains and I don't have anything but a desire to work and drive my car. And I'll do both these things either in small or
big doses until I find out what the effect is and I will stay away from all profes-

sional counsel until I am in a mental attitude to accept it. And I don't know when that will be."[78]

John knew, and tried to make Charlie understand, that hypertension is a silent disease. People often have no symptoms until it is too late. But Charlie was a stubborn man and refused his brother's advice. As his health deteriorated in 1939, he described how he felt as "something falling out of the system." Still, he kept busy with Media Records, with his attempts to motivate a less-than-ambitious son either to do well in school so he could go to college or to decide to go to work, and with the ongoing saga of dealing with the fallout from their father's financial affairs.[79]

Frank Rock had died in 1932 at the age of seventy-five. His widow, Delia, with whom apparently only Maisie had a good relationship, was only in her fifties when he died. All the property they had owned together, or that he had deeded to her during his lifetime, came to her at his death. But Frank died without a will, already having tied up his most profitable property—the theater and its related real estate in Marlborough—by making Charlie the trustee. He had done so for several reasons. Family lore attributes that decision to Frank's guilt over not following Charlie's instructions to sell a substantial amount of Gillette stock Charlie had owned while he was working for that company.[80]

But there was more to the story. The theater property was linked in Frank's and his children's minds with their mother, Annie, who had nurtured it along. Then, too, Frank cared about his children as well as about Delia, and he had long counted on Charlie to use the revenue from the theater to take care of the whole family. So Charlie did. He made sure that Delia got regular checks, as did his sister Nell, in poor health and with a disabled husband unable to provide for his family sufficiently. John, as we've seen, periodically called on Charlie to be bailed out of one financial hole or another. It isn't clear whether Maisie ever benefited; although she often complained about her family's finances, Charlie seemed to think she was well off enough. Harry, still employed by Charlie, may not have asked for anything more. Certainly, Harry seems to have been satisfied with what he had. Charlie had powerful family feelings, he had money, and he cheerfully shared his and his father's wealth with at least the siblings he thought needed help.

Charlie certainly did not expect to die in the prime of his life. But as his health failed, he and John discussed whether Charlie should divide what he considered the Frank Rock legacy among Delia and the siblings. Apparently, Charlie planned to provide the most to Nell and the next biggest chunk to

John, with everyone getting something, but the others receiving considerably less. John, in his desire to "save" Charlie "from possibly bad family reaction" while he was in poor health, advised him to put it off. As John later told Charlie's widow, Kathryn, "I figured if he could arrange to have it done after his death, no reaction could hurt him, and indeed, disapproval from anyone was less likely after his death than before." But then Charlie died before he was able to "give the final directions," leaving Kathryn to handle the details.[81] Unfortunately, John was completely wrong about the reaction from Maisie and Delia, who sued Kathryn and Harry (Charlie's executors) for control of Frank Rock's estate after Charlie's death, leaving the family bitterly at odds.[82]

According to Nell, Maisie may even have been the instigator of the suit, although Delia surely had no love for Nell or John. Several years later, Maisie, without apologizing for her actions, wrote Nell about seeing each other again, asking, "Do you think we could rely on our sense of humor to help us?" Maisie's action had deprived Nell of a monthly income that had made the difference between poverty and comfort, Nell responded bitterly. How dare she want to be sisters again after joining with Delia to try "to prove before the world that . . . Charlie was an embezzler and that my and your father had softening of the brain because he didn't leave his affairs to your and Ed [Maisie's husband] and Delia's liking." Indeed, Nell's husband was often unable to work; John and Nan would help her financially once the income from their father's Marlborough property had been redistributed to Maisie and Delia.[83]

From then on, John had nothing to do with either Maisie or Delia. Only Harry seemed to keep up any sort of relationship with either. John had lost the brother to whom he had been the closest, and the fight over the will resulted in a break from his elder sister. He remained close to Nell, his twin, but she was already in poor health, which would bedevil her for the rest of her life. He and Harry retained their cordial relationship, but it was not an intimate one.[84]

His brother's death and the family estrangement took a toll on Rock, although his friends and patients may not have noticed it. Rock cultivated a cheerful, calm, and steady demeanor, but his public face belied the periods of worry and unrest, and sometimes outright depression, which tended to manifest themselves in physical symptoms such as severe stomach and intestinal pains. Although he was relatively attentive to his physical health, he shared some of Charlie's and Nell's physical problems. In 1944, at the age of fifty-four, he suffered what would be the first of six heart attacks. In fact, he was in the hospital recovering when the first IVF report came out. At the time, enforced inactivity was part of the recovery process for a heart attack, which meant that Rock's income from private practice was greatly curtailed while he remained in the hospital. He gradually recovered and returned to all his activities except delivering babies, which he gave up entirely. He restricted his travel for a bit longer but soon returned to that as well.

Rock's heart attack made him anxious for Nan and the children. Rachel had graduated from Milton Academy, decided against college, and would soon come to work for the Free Hospital, where she became proficient in cytology. The younger girls were still in school. Jack was in the Marines. During Jack's adolescence, John fretted over what he viewed as his son's lack of ambition and unwillingness to apply himself in school or to think of his future. Father and son were often in conflict.

Could John have forgotten how long it took him to find himself as a young man? If he had remembered, perhaps he would have been less worried about Jack. But the situation had begun to turn around. By the time Jack joined the Marines, John had developed more confidence in him. This would be the most charitable interpretation of Rock's decision to unburden himself to Jack about the family's difficult finances. Less charitably put, John's letters eerily recall his own father's letters to him about the family's 1909 financial set-backs. Rock seemed completely oblivious that he was acting like his own not-very-beloved father. Of course, his heart attack must have made him feel how vulnerable Nan and the younger girls would be if he died, and the passage of time had no doubt obliterated the pain of his youthful experiences.

Jack, however, did not seem to resent his father's confidences, and by then he had grown closer to John. As John confided in him, he came to confide in his father, even feeling comfortable enough to write from his base about his sexual temptations away from home and his confusion about how to handle himself. John, while cautioning Jack that mere physical release was not by itself a good reason to have sex, expressed his faith that Jack could depend on his own judgment and sense of right and wrong. Or, as he put it, don't feel you necessarily have to use the condoms when the military hands them out, but take them anyway![85]

His brother's death, his sister's failing health, his estrangement from Maisie, and his own heart attack—these were difficult enough, but in 1946 he and Nan faced the worst experience any parent could have, the death of a child. Jack died from injuries he sustained in a car accident in the summer of 1946. He had never been sent to Europe or the Pacific theater and would soon have been discharged. He and John had been talking about the future, with

John steadily urging him to go to college rather than take a job right away. Jack had been home on leave and was headed back to the Portsmouth Naval Base. It was raining heavily, he was tired, and his car went off the road. He was alive when they took him to the hospital but died soon afterwards. John blamed himself for Jack's death because he had urged Jack to stop at a party for disabled servicemen to help Rachel entertain by playing the piano while she sang.[86]

Publicly stoic, John kept his feelings from showing to the world. Even his staff had no sense of the depth of his feelings—not just of grief, but of self-blame. One of Rock's secretaries, writing to Miriam Menkin just two weeks after Jack's death, remarked, "It has been a tremendous loss to the whole family and . . . a great shock but Dr. R. seemed rested and serene when I saw him last week."[87] He wasn't serene; he was shattered. One of his famous patients invited him and Nan to spend a couple of months at her Hollywood mansion so that they could grieve away from the glare of his public life. When they returned, he tried to take up the threads of his life, but he never ceased to grieve, to blame himself, and to feel that his life had been irretrievably altered.

Rock's personal tragedy seems not to have affected his professional life at all. His career soared. As the nation entered the postwar period, the start of the baby boom fueled the development of reproductive medicine even more than Rock's and others' research achievements, most of which had no immediate practical application. But Rock was famous because of them, and infertile couples from around the nation and the world beat a path to his door.

Chapter 5

THE WORLD OF THE PATIENTS

Baltimore, Maryland, 1934. Samuel Meaker's *Human Sterility: Causation, Diagnosis, and Treatment: A Practical Manual of Clinical Procedure* is published, setting a new standard of practice for the diagnosis and treatment of infertility in both men and women.

Brookline, Massachusetts, 1936. John Rock opens the rhythm clinic at the Free Hospital, which becomes the state's first free clinic for providing contraceptive advice, offering the only contraceptive practice that is legal in Massachusetts.

Brookline, Massachusetts, 1949. Rock finally persuades the Free Hospital to establish a male infertility clinic and to hire Dr. Fletcher Colby as its director.

In 1948 John Rock told one of his colleagues, "I am not a research man nor have I a research mind. All I know are some of the problems I want answered."[1] This statement is surprising given his research accomplishments during the 1930s and 1940s. But Rock was not just being modest; he was also describing his priorities in a way that made sense to him. For him, research was a means to an end, not an end in itself. He wanted to find solutions for the problems of reproduction that beset his patients and the millions of men and women around the world who joined them in suffering either from infertility or repetitive childbirth. Although he started out in 1926 to direct a sterility clinic, his experiences over the next two decades changed him. By the 1940s his interests encompassed fertility matters in all their complexity—infertility, what he called overfertility, and marital sexuality.

This chapter explores Rock's medical practice in the 1930s and 1940s through the lens of his patients' experiences. In many ways, Rock's own beliefs and behavior evolved through his patients' influence. His interactions with them helped to shape his ideas about infertility, contraception, and broader issues of sexuality and reproduction. They started him down new lines of inquiry, led him to develop new treatment protocols, and changed his attitudes toward reproductive questions and problems over the years.

Rock built his professional life around "the problems I want answered." He cared little for abstract scientific questions; he sought practical clinical solutions. How can we determine the time of ovulation in *women*, not just in rats or rabbits? How exactly is a *human* ovum fertilized, and what happens to that fertilized ovum as it travels from the fallopian tube to the uterus? Are some embryos destined to abort, either because of their own abnormalities or because they fail to implant and develop in the uterus? Can we make it possible for women with blocked or absent fallopian tubes to become pregnant? How exactly do hormones function in a woman's body—on a daily basis, during pregnancy, or during menopause—and can artificial versions of them be used to treat such conditions as menstrual disorders or infertility?

When he first took up these questions in the early 1930s, there really had been no answers. Scientists who did possess "a research mind," as Rock called it, had hypotheses and conjectures about human reproduction based on laboratory or agricultural research.[2] Basic science had come to serve as the underpinning for all reputable medical education. Insights from the laboratory infused the practice of medicine, and Rock never minimized the significance of these landmark laboratory discoveries and achievements of others. He followed their work with great interest. He found the discoveries that came from the laboratory of Gregory Pincus particularly useful, and he was deeply indebted to the scientific research staff at the Carnegie Institution for their expertise in embryology.

But Rock did not do that kind of laboratory work himself, had a tendency to express a good-humored but decided skepticism toward any literal reliance on animal analogies to explain the problems of human reproduction, and always declared that any interest he had in basic science lay in its application to clinical conditions.[3] More than once he laughingly recounted a discussion he had with the great biochemist Otto Folin, his former medical school professor and now a colleague at Harvard. Rock was telling Folin about his plans for a new study. Folin listened for a while, then finally, exasperated by Rock's casual attitude toward accepted research protocols, shot back, "I think you have a good idea, but I would have no confidence in your results."[4]

Rock was impervious to Folin's retort, since as far as he was concerned, laboratory results by themselves offered little immediate benefit to the women who turned to him for alleviation of their diseases and conditions.[5] Whenever

Rock asked a research question, at its heart was his desire to address the needs of the human beings who came to him with their problems day after day.

Rock saw his patients as individuals, never as their diseases. Their conditions, needs, and longings drove his clinical and research agendas. Some might find that surprising; after all, our image of American medicine in Rock's era is a reductionist one. We think of the twentieth century as one in which patients became their diseases, and physicians treated disorders, not people. Gynecology and obstetrics were particularly suspect specialties, ones with a long history of reducing women patients to objects. The record of the past century and a half is full of examples of powerful men using the authority of science to establish an interpretation of reproductive health and illness that valorized medical expertise and disparaged women's own understanding of their body's functions and needs.[6]

Rock was different, although it would be too bad if he were unique. Luigi Mastroianni, one of Rock's research fellows who went on to have an illustrious career of his own, recalled that Rock was not like most other male doctors. "Back then," he said, "the practice of medicine was—the unpopular name for it was paternalistic—not John Rock! . . . The way this man communicated with patients was something I'll never forget." Rock treated all his patients, whoever they were, with courtesy, Mastroianni remembered, explaining procedures in detail and telling them who would be involved in their care.[7]

We do know, from the records he left behind, that throughout his career Rock cared about his patients as well as the thousands of men and women from around the world who poured out their hearts to him in anguished letters.[8] They, in turn, respected him. Perhaps equally important, they had considerable impact on the way he practiced his profession.

When John Rock became director of the sterility clinic, the Free Hospital for Women was one of three hospitals in the Boston area dedicated to women's medical problems. The two others were the New England Hospital for Women and Children and the Boston Lying-In Hospital. The former was an independent institution founded in 1862 and staffed in the late nineteenth century by New England's leading women physicians. In the 1930s and 1940s, it continued to treat women and children whatever their medical complaints. The latter was a maternity hospital, founded to care for the poor in 1832. It was connected with Harvard Medical School, but it did not take gynecological cases, making the Free Hospital the only Harvard-affiliated hospital devoted solely to gynecology. As a result, although the Free Hospital had been founded to care for the poor, women who could afford to pay for care had increasingly sought its services.

To meet the demands of women with means, the hospital had a separate facility, the Parkway wing, which had been completed in 1922. Five stories tall, it had a separate entrance, laboratories, offices, a lecture hall, and forty rooms that provided more luxurious accommodations for the many private patients who wanted to have the advantage of being treated by the distinguished physicians at the Free Hospital. The basement was reserved for "the X-ray room," radium vault, and the outpatient clinics. The hospital was now set up to treat the wealthy and the poor. Those with incomes somewhere in between were sent to the free wards and asked to pay whatever they could for the hospital's services.[9]

Rock's private office was on the third floor of the Parkway wing. There he saw his private patients and managed his research projects. The clinics were held in the basement, where the outpatient department was also located. By 1936 Rock oversaw two clinics—the sterility and endocrine clinic for those unable to conceive, and the rhythm clinic for those who couldn't stop conceiving. Elizabeth Snedeker, a social worker married to a prominent Harvard physician, managed the rhythm clinic and was a valued addition to the core group of men and women who worked with Rock over the years.[10]

On clinic days, he and his staff would take their charts and head down to the basement, where at one end of the hall were the patients looking for ways to keep from getting pregnant. At the other end were the infertile women trying desperately to conceive. There were also, along with the infertility patients, women with a range of disorders of the reproductive system who also waited to be seen by the doctors, either Rock or one of the young fellows or residents.

In the 1930s and 1940s, Rock continued to deliver many a baby among the wives of his colleagues and of at least one of his colleagues herself, Olive Smith. His private patients, in those years before the ritual of an annual gynecological exam had become established, mostly saw Rock for obstetrical care or a range of gynecological problems, including infertility.

Rock's clinic was created initially to treat infertility only, but it evolved over the years into the sterility and endocrine clinic by the mid-1930s and the Fertility and Endocrine Clinic shortly thereafter, for women with infertility and other kinds of gynecological disorders. Rock treated women with ectopic pregnancies; cancers of the cervix, uterus, and ovaries; pelvic inflammatory disease; endometriosis; and a range of other conditions.[11] In the 1930s, he had only about two hundred or so infertility patients per year in the clinic, and the numbers in his private practice were also relatively small. After all, during the Great Depression more couples were concerned with limiting the size of their families than with adding to them. But if the demand for fertility services in these years was limited, interest in the problem among gynecologists was growing. During the 1930s Rock was part of a small but increasingly influential cohort of practitioners redefining clinical practice in the area of the diagnosis and treatment of infertility.

One of the milestones marking this redefinition was the publication in 1934 of *Human Sterility*. An up-to-date guide for practitioners treating the problem of infertility, the book was underwritten by the National Committee on Maternal Health (NCMH), a birth-control advocacy group founded and headed by physician Robert Latou Dickinson. In the 1930s, the NCMH became involved in the development of standardized protocols for infertility treatment. It encouraged systematic data gathering in infertility practices and supported research on male fertility.[12] The committee's hand was visible everywhere, from the design of a widely used form on which physicians would record a couple's medical history to the classification of the steps in a diagnostic evaluation. Not every doctor followed the new standards, but clinics run by elite practitioners in major cities were indeed coming to agreement on certain key protocols.[13]

In the early 1930s, when Dickinson proposed that the NCMH fund a new study of sterility treatment, he first planned to fund a research project. It soon became clear to him, however, that what practitioners really needed was a treatment guide. Samuel Meaker, a professor at the medical school at Boston University, took on the task.[14] In *Human Sterility*, Meaker attempted to assess the extent to which Americans experienced infertility, codified the current state of knowledge about human reproduction, and provided a step-by-step guide for practitioners who wanted to develop expertise in infertility treatment.

We say "attempted to assess" the rate of infertility because precision on this matter was impossible at the time (and remains elusive even now). Race suicide alarmists in the early twentieth century had dramatically inflated the infertility rate among native-born white Protestants for their own purposes, and Meaker had to counteract this information. His own data suggested that infertility rates were relatively constant, at between 10 and 13 percent of married couples.[15] As for its causes, Meaker highlighted disturbances of the endocrine system; in his view, more than half of infertile couples suffered from hormonal imbalances.

Although he emphasized the importance of testing the husband, Meaker was not persuaded that male sterility was a major problem. In this he was much like his predecessors in the field. From the 1870s on, many physicians ignored the advice of leading practitioners, who had urged their colleagues to test a man's semen before subjecting his wife to treatment. Even those who tried to act on this advice found husbands reluctant to accept that the problem could be theirs, either in whole or in part. Regardless of economic, educational, and social status, men equated manliness with the ability to father children. Since most of the doctors who treated infertility were men, they had no difficulty identifying with the severe dejection of a man who learned he was sterile. Meaker was so sensitive to the masculine ego that he insisted men were absolutely responsible for a couple's infertility "only in rare instances."[16] He was also much more optimistic that male infertility could be treated than the evidence warranted.

Perhaps his most important practical finding was that infertility usually resulted from several predisposing factors rather than a single cause. He argued that successful treatment of most infertility required a team of specialists rather than a single practitioner, and he encouraged the development of group infertility practices, combining the services of a gynecologist, urologist, endocrinologist, and pathologist.[17]

Human Sterility provides us with a snapshot of what physicians associated with medical schools considered effective measures to treat infertility in the mid-1930s. Rock did not formally adopt the team approach, but he had access to specialists among his colleagues whenever he needed it. Also, his own training in urology gave him a familiarity with the disorders of the male reproductive system that was not a part of the typical gynecologist's expertise. In the late 1940s, Rock would finally succeed in getting the hospital to establish a separate clinic for the diagnosis and treatment of male infertility.

• • •

A woman seeking infertility treatment in the 1930s at Rock's clinic would, at her first appointment, provide her medical history and undergo a complete physical examination. If she was not menstruating at all, or she menstruated irregularly, the doctors would suspect an ovulatory disorder and order an endometrial biopsy. If it turned out that she was not ovulating, then Rock would prescribe various hormonal treatments, including equine gonadotropins and other hormones.[18] She would also be tested for tubal patency, by insufflation with carbon dioxide (the Rubin test), or by a hysterosalpingogram. Either of these tests might also clear a minor tubal occlusion.[19]

Before proceeding, Rock always asked the husband to have his semen tested. He was one of the few specialists who consistently argued that men were responsible for a larger share of infertility than the medical profession believed. Today we know that in about 40 percent of infertile couples, the male is either the sole cause or a contributing cause of infertility. Some infertility specialists, mostly women physicians such as Sophia Kleegman, refused to treat a woman unless her husband agreed to be tested. Rock was not among them. He did not turn women away if, despite all efforts, a husband would not cooperate.[20]

If after all these tests there was still no clear diagnosis, Rock would recommend a diagnostic laparotomy. Some conditions were impossible to diagnose definitively without opening the abdomen. Endometriosis was one of them. An often painful condition in which tissue from the uterine lining migrates to other sites in the pelvis, causing ovarian cysts and the formation of adhesions and scarring, endometriosis remains a significant factor even today in female infertility. In Rock's era the only treatment was surgical—lysis of adhesions and removal of the ovarian cysts. Another diagnosis that could only be confirmed by laparotomy was polycystic ovarian syndrome, which impairs ovulation and causes multiple cysts to develop in the ovary.

At the other end of the hall from the infertility patients sat the women who couldn't stop having babies. The rhythm clinic, which was the first free clinic in Massachusetts to offer any form of birth-control advice, provided the only kind that was legal in Massachusetts, which prohibited the prescription and use of contraceptive devices. The rhythm method required a couple to avoid intercourse during a woman's likely fertile period.[21] But since a woman's fertile period could only be determined after the fact, the method actually required a woman to abstain from sex for about a ten-day period during the middle of her menstrual cycle. Rock was not being naive when he began to provide this service. He knew there were Massachusetts couples who used diaphragms, condoms, and douches to prevent pregnancy. He was even surreptitiously teaching a course on birth control to Harvard Medical School students. But he could not legally open a clinic that would provide such devices. And besides, many of his patients were Catholics who would not agree to a diaphragm and whose husbands would not use condoms.

After a patient at the rhythm clinic provided her medical and obstetrical histories and underwent a complete physical exam, she was asked to chart, for the next three months, the date on which her menstrual period began. The nurses also asked her to make a note each time she and her husband had intercourse. To have any chance of success with the rhythm method, it was important to have a regular cycle and to know when to abstain. Those women who were lucky enough to have regular cycles were then taught how to determine when it would be safe to have sex. During the next four years, 225 women came to the clinic seeking help, nearly 90 percent of them Catholic. The size of their families ranged from one to fourteen children. Some of them simply wanted to figure out how better to space the births of their children. Others wanted to end childbearing completely.[22]

From these two clinics, from other gynecological patients in the Free Hospital, from Rock's private practice, and from among the thousands of men and women who asked for his help in other ways, come the stories in the following pages. Many of the women participated in one of the research studies, and others were his correspondents. Because the field of reproductive medicine was in its infancy, and human fertility so little understood, it comes as no surprise that Rock's education in understanding reproductive disorders and the women who suffered them was in part provided by the women themselves.

Although most of the women in these pages were clinic patients, they are probably not fully representative of that group of women as a whole. For several of the research projects, especially the embryo study, women had to be both willing and able to cooperate with a set of complex instructions that included keeping track of their menstrual cycles and remembering to notify the hospital, following a schedule for intercourse, having a level of understanding that would enable them to explain what they were doing to their husbands, and sometimes providing additional information. Less active involvement was required for the IVF studies and some of the others, but the patients nevertheless had to keep track of their cycles and notify the hospital of their menstrual dates.

But even if they did not represent the entire universe of his patients, the overwhelming majority of these women were nevertheless clinic patients. Not all of them came from truly impoverished households, but almost all were from working-class families with relatively low incomes. They represented most of the ethnic groups in Boston. Nearly all were housewives. Their husbands were laborers, laundry workers, bakers, elevator operators, machinists, and steel workers. A few were married to clerks or salesmen. In the 1930s some of the husbands had been employed by the New Deal's Works Progress

Administration.[23] Irish and Italian surnames abounded here, but there were Polish and German, as well as typically Anglo-Saxon and Scots names. Some were Protestant and Jewish, and many were Catholic. A few were African American, but it is difficult to tell how many. Our guess, based on Boston's geography with its pronounced racial segregation, is that African American patients would have been more numerous in the clinics of Boston City Hospital than in these clinics, although only in a tiny number of cases was a notation about race listed on a chart. The few instances in which a patient was listed as either "colored" or "white" give no basis for even a guess about how many African American women were treated at the clinic.[24]

. . .

By the early 1940s, Rock's interests were evolving from an emphasis on the treatment of infertility to the treatment of reproductive disorders more broadly. Among the problems faced by these women were chronic severe pelvic pain, incapacitating menstrual periods, and what they called "falling of the womb." Some of them had suffered from their conditions for a dozen years or more, while the conditions of others were of more recent origin.

Women sometimes came to the hospital for the specific purpose of obtaining a hysterectomy, which would provide them with both a cure for their medical problems and an end to their childbearing. But others had no fixed idea about what might help them. They simply wanted relief. Rock's handling of their situations reflected his own commitment to involving his patients in decisions about their medical care. Whenever feasible, he offered them more than one choice of procedure to relieve their gynecological disorders.

If a woman insisted on a hysterectomy, as long as the procedure was medically justifiable, Rock seemed generally to accede to her wishes. When thirty-six-year-old Mrs. J. H. appeared in the clinic, she was the mother of five children and had been married for fifteen years. Her youngest child was just a toddler, the oldest a teenager. She immediately announced to Rock and the nurses that she and her husband did "not wish any more children." Her "periods [were] too troublesome," she said, and she felt "extremely tired all the time." She got her wish, receiving a hysterectomy for what was diagnosed postoperatively as chronic cervicitis, chronic salpingitis, and chronic oophoritis.[25]

There were also women who had so many children that they felt overwhelmed. Mrs. L.A. at thirty-two had already been married for fourteen years. She had borne eleven living children, most recently a set of twins, and had miscarried once. Her last five deliveries had been by cesarean section. She never used birth control, she said, and had intercourse about twice a month. Her husband, she said, was trying to be "careful" since the birth of their twins six months ago. She was exhausted and in pain.[26]

Given her childbearing history, imagine her surprise when a scheduling blunder sent her to the fertility clinic! Relieved at last to find the proper end of the hall, she said that she was exhausted, weak, and that she occasionally blacked out. Her periods had become painful and profuse. "P[atien]t desires hysterectomy," the file read. "Does not want to have any more children."

Her symptoms were not just severe; they were alarming. The doctors not only agreed that she should have a hysterectomy but also wanted to operate immediately. Rock, concerned that she might have endometrial cancer, urged her to have the surgery as soon as possible. But it was just before Christmas, and she balked. "With eleven children in the house?" She exclaimed, I'm expected to be in the hospital over the holiday? So they compromised. She came in a week before Christmas for a dilatation and curettage and agreed that if Rock found cancer, he would perform the hysterectomy. If not, she would have her hysterectomy after the holidays. She was lucky to have escaped a malignancy and in January had the hysterectomy.[27]

Other women were in a position to choose. Mrs. M. V., a thirty-nine-year-old mother of three, listened as Rock explained that he could perform a hysterectomy if that was her wish, but that less drastic surgery would also alleviate her pain. He suggested that she explain her options to her husband and then decide. Soon afterwards, she wrote the nursing staff that she and her husband had decided "it would be best if Dr. Rock went ahead and removed the womb and leave one ovie [sic] in for the change as he explained."[28]

Leaving "one ovie in for the change," as this patient called it, was the preferred practice both for Rock and those whom he trained, including William Mulligan, who would later succeed him as director of the clinic. They removed only one ovary, unless both were diseased, because Rock wanted the patient to continue to have the benefit of natural estrogen production until menopause. This was not, however, the universal practice at the hospital. Hysterectomies performed by Surgeon-in-Chief George V. Smith, for example, almost always involved the removal of both ovaries. Since we do not have cases for all the senior physicians, it is impossible to say how many followed Rock's practice and how many Smith's.

The women just described had good relationships with their husbands. Other women were not so fortunate, and some of them had terrible problems. Mrs. M. B. had been married for eleven years. She regularly used contraceptives, she said, but nevertheless she'd had six children and one miscarriage before her thirtieth birthday. When she first came to the clinic, she had been referred by the Boston Lying-In Hospital, where she had been treated after a bungled abortion. Her "difficult socio-economic and psychological situation at home," as one nurse called it, or her "domestic and mental problem," as another one put it more bluntly, had caused her doctors enough concern that they sent her for a psychiatric evaluation. Both the medical staff and the two psychiatrists at the Lying-In recommended a hysterectomy, clearly for sterilization purposes. But Rock did not think a hysterectomy was medically indicated and refused to allow one. Instead, he "discharged [her] to be fitted for a diaphragm."

Soon, she was pregnant again. Frantic, she tried unsuccessfully to abort herself, then sought medical help for her botched attempt. "Combined efforts of herself and shots from doctor aborted her," the chart reads. Three days later Mrs. B. went back to the Free Hospital, but not to Rock. The doctor she saw diagnosed her condition as a lacerated perineum and enlarged and prolapsed uterus. Consulting with two other colleagues, he decided that her physical and mental condition warranted a hysterectomy. This time Rock gave in. Perhaps the most recent abortion had worsened her medical condition. Or maybe he now believed that her mental state would drive her to keep on having abortions. He agreed to perform the hysterectomy.[29]

Mrs. M. B. was not Rock's only patient with a difficult life. Mrs. G. O., married at twenty, had borne thirteen children in twenty-three years, ranging in age from twenty-two years old to eleven months.[30] She and her husband had intercourse about once or twice a week, and like many of the other couples, they had never used contraceptives. Her husband, she says, was "careful sometimes," but if he was careful in this, he was careful in little else. He paid little attention to the children, and Mrs. O. fretted in the hospital when a cold delayed her surgery. She told the staff that her older children had been sent "elsewhere" and that her sister had moved in to care for several of the youngest ones. Even though her husband was once again out of work—he appeared to be more often out of work than in—he was no more help at home when he was unemployed, since he "doesn't know how to diaper a baby" and "refuses to care" for the children. Her sister became so angry over his laziness that she up and left.[31]

The situation of the O. family was in fact even more difficult than anyone at the hospital had initially realized. Their house was so dirty and disorganized that members of Rock's staff, who had taken on the task of trying to get her children cared for once her sister refused to keep doing it, were unable to find any housekeeper willing to go inside. They then got in touch with Mrs. O's minister. He tried to help but wasn't sure what could be done, now that the family was once again about to "go to welfare" because the husband had been so long out of work. Five of Mrs. O's older children, the minister said, had been removed from the family and were now in foster homes. The couple, "afraid that if they get in touch with Welfare, the other 4 children will be taken from them," were in a desperate situation.

In the end, the staff was able to arrange for the younger children to be cared for by the Home for Little Wanderers, a private charity that would provide temporary shelter. Finally, Mrs. O had her operation, her husband got a job, the danger of losing the other four children lessened, and the staff was able to get "Welfare" to provide her with home assistance for three weeks after the operation. Mrs. O's case was more dire than most, but many of the clinic patients faced hardships of one sort or another every day.[32]

These women represent a group of patients who chose—and sometimes demanded—their hysterectomies. Others were more reluctant, like one forty-year-old mother of two children who was a favorite among the medical staff because of her "extremely pleasant" manner. She had always wanted more children and had not yet given up hope, even though after two miscarriages and a stillbirth she knew there was little likelihood of having her wish granted. When Rock told her that her condition called for the hysterectomy, she agreed only reluctantly.[33]

. . .

As a result of his experiences with so many couples whose problems arose at least in part from having families that were much larger than they either wanted or could afford, by the 1940s Rock was becoming bolder in his advocacy of birth control. He had long been sympathetic to their plight. As a resident at the Boston Lying-In Hospital, he had witnessed many sad situations among the impoverished women in the North and East Ends of Boston when he delivered their babies in shabby tenement apartments. Even then, he believed that both his church and the state of Massachusetts were wrong in opposing birth control.

Still, in the 1920s he had remained aloof from the birth-control movement, even though he had written openly and favorably about contraception for a medical audience toward the end of that decade. He inched closer to the movement in the early 1930s. In 1931, in spite of a papal encyclical the year before that affirmed the opposition of the Roman Catholic Church to "artificial" birth control, he had taken a stand as one of only fifteen Boston physicians (and the sole Catholic) to sign a petition in favor of repealing the Massachusetts law prohibiting contraception.[34]

When he first opened the rhythm clinic at the Free Hospital, Rock asked his brother Charlie to have Media Records keep track of newspaper articles on birth control. That same year he began, somewhat reluctantly, to make common cause with the birth-control forces, accepting an invitation to a conference sponsored by Dickinson's NCMH.[35] Rock was still not sure he wanted to be associated with the birth controllers, however. As an elite Harvard-affiliated physician who moved in the most exalted circles of the medical profession—at least that's how Harvard physicians in Boston viewed themselves—he was not sure about the tone of the new company he was keeping. Returning from the NCMH-sponsored conference, he confided to his diary that some of the participants were "not quite first raters."[36]

For the next decade he kept some distance from the NCMH, even as his medical practice led him to become an ever-stronger proponent of a couple's right to limit their family size. But at the end of the 1940s, in a funny twist of fate, he would find himself for a couple of years at the helm of the NCMH, trying to keep it afloat as it promoted scientific and medical research on the pressing reproductive issues of the day.

In the 1940s Rock also became more interested in the reproductive context of the lives of the women he treated. For example, he began including a question about his patients' contraceptive and sexual habits on the form each woman filled out on her first visit.[37] Among the clinic patients, withdrawal (known formally as coitus interruptus or euphemistically as "being careful") was the most widely used method, followed by condoms and rhythm. Almost none of these patients used a diaphragm, which required a doctor's prescription that in Massachusetts would have been legal only for serious medical reasons. And whether his patients employed contraceptive measures or not, their sexual habits were remarkably similar. Most women had intercourse once or twice a week (commonly twice); about 20 percent, only one to three times a month. And not a single patient admitted to having sex regularly more often than three or four times a week.[38]

Contraception and sexuality were of increasing interest to Rock in the 1940s. His own experiences as well as those of his patients had contributed to the transformation of his thinking since he was a newly married husband and newly minted practitioner. He and Nan, after all, having brought five children into the world in the first eight years of their marriage, avoided childbirth thereafter. Although we know little of the Rocks' sex life, it seems unlikely that Nan became immediately infertile after Ellen's birth in 1932, or that the couple foreswore sex. Rock was interested in sexual questions. He was unembarrassed enough to have designed and taught a course in human sexuality to the medical students at Harvard (his daughter Rachel said it was "disguised" under the rubric of "primate behavior"), and he wrote openly about sex to his adolescent son, who had recently joined the Marines.

In 1945 Rock decided to investigate the impact of having had a hysterectomy on a woman's later health. Writing to one hundred women who had participated in the Rock-Hertig study, he asked them a series of questions about the aftermath of their surgery and about their subsequent lives, including their overall physical health, their sense of psychological well-being, their relationships with their husbands, and the quality of their sexual experiences. He then invited them in for a follow-up examination. Sixty-four of the hundred wrote back, sixty made appointments to see him, and fifty-two actually had the follow-up examination. Some of the others wrote friendly letters, saying that they would really love to see him, but they no longer lived in the area. Several promised to get in touch if they came back into the vicinity. Some had moved, leaving no forwarding addresses. One unfortunate woman wrote back saying that she was pleased to hear from him and would be happy to come in once she recovered from throat surgery. She never did; she died unexpectedly from complications of that surgery soon afterward.

Doing research by asking the patients about their experiences had not yet been superseded by broad statistical studies, and Rock would use what he learned from these patients to understand the varieties of ways in which women and their spouses responded to hysterectomy. All these women had undergone the operation well before they would have expected to experience menopause; most were in their early forties or younger at the time of the follow-up study.[39]

Nearly all the women declared that they had fully recovered physically from their surgery, some within weeks, others not for several months. Several had developed unrelated health problems, others were experiencing the hot flashes and night sweats that heralded menopause, and a few had become overweight. Just half of the fifty-two women who came in for an appointment reported that their sex lives were no different from before, but it is not so easy to know what that meant. Did "no different" mean that sex was always pleasurable and remained so, or that it was never pleasurable and hadn't gotten any better? Although most of the women did not elaborate, four of the twenty-six said that it was "no different" because they had never had sexual desire or satisfaction before their operations and had none now.

Among the other twenty-six, women who declared that they had experienced a change in their sexual responsiveness, five found their sexual experiences to be worse. Either they no longer had orgasms or their orgasms were more difficult to reach. Eleven women reported improved sex lives. One was having a better experience, however, because she had jettisoned her marriage and now had a much better sexual relationship with her new fiancé. Several others, whose physical conditions before their hysterectomies had caused intercourse to be painful, enjoyed sex now that the pain was gone.

There were three very sad stories from women whose husbands had rejected them sexually. One woman cried when she told Rock that although her physical health was much better since her hysterectomy, her husband refused to have sex with her because, he said, she had lost her "nature." Another woman said simply that her husband "won't come near her." But then again, she recalled, he never had much interest in sex before the operation. The third woman told Rock that after her surgery, she began to enjoy sex much more, but because of this, her "husband doesn't want her" any more.[40] In the entire group, all but three women said that they were glad they had the surgery. Two expressed ambivalence—"glad in one way, not glad in another," said one. And only one, the woman whose husband taunted her with having lost her "nature," regretted the hysterectomy. All in all, about forty of the fifty-two women who came in for the follow-up examinations found their sex lives either unchanged or changed for the better. Twelve had worse experiences for various reasons.

These patients helped Rock to understand how women experienced the aftermath of a hysterectomy. And by taking a detailed sexual history, he also gained information about the length of time a normally fertile woman might take to conceive, a subject on which little research had been done at the time. Rock asked each how long it had taken them to become pregnant once they began having intercourse. In making this query, he was trying to assess how long a woman needed to be "exposed" (as doctors say) to the possibility of pregnancy before she actually became pregnant, in order to advise his own infertility patients. Of the fifty-two women, forty became pregnant within six months and another seven within a year. Of the five who took longer, one became pregnant within fourteen months despite her husband's using withdrawal; another said it took her a long time to become pregnant because she had an intact hymen; a third became pregnant after eight years of marriage once she had surgery to remove an ovarian cyst, whereupon she then had a child every two years; and yet another took seven years to achieve her first pregnancy and then bore five children. While these women did not constitute a large cohort, knowing how long it took them to conceive might have brought Rock closer to understanding how long he should wait before intervening medically when a patient came to consult him on her possible infertility.

...

During the first half of the 1940s, although most of Rock's patients came from Boston and the surrounding region, he was also developing a national reputation as a result of his and Hertig's embryo studies. But he did not become well known to the public until the IVF experiments. Once his fame spread, some of the women who wrote him hoped that test tube babies would become a medical reality within their own reproductive lifetimes.

Rock was interested in IVF for several reasons, one of them his desire to find a way around one of the most intractable causes of infertility, occluded or damaged fallopian tubes.[41] As word of his IVF experiments spread, he began to receive letters not only from women whose tubes had been damaged by disease, but also from anguished women whose tubes had been surgically removed. Many of the letters came from rural America, and the writers were often quite young. Several of the women knew the reason for their surgeries—ectopic pregnancies or complications from appendicitis, for example—but others had no idea what had happened. Their doctors might or might not have informed them of the nature of the surgery. Some women didn't know they were sterile until they attempted to become pregnant. "[My doctor] said [my] tubes were dried up so he removed them" during an appendectomy, said one. Another said that when she was nineteen, a doctor removed one of her ovaries and both tubes because, he said, she had adhesions. Another said her doctor had sterilized her without her knowledge immediately after the birth of her first child.[42]

As he began trying to figure out ways of helping at least some of these women, he acquired a famous patient, actress Merle Oberon, who had suffered the same fate. Famed for her exotic beauty and her sultry on-screen persona, Oberon was about thirty-five when she came to Boston to consult Rock. A star in the grand tradition of movie stars of that era, she had created an air of mystery about herself that obscured her difficult early life. Her mother, Charlotte, had been born in poverty and at times led a precarious existence, bearing her first child at fourteen and sometimes living dangerously on the fringes of the commercial sex trade in her native India.[43]

Merle was Charlotte's second child, so strikingly beautiful even as a teenager that her mother determined she should seek a career as an actress. Charlotte had little money and grand ambitions for her daughter, and she understood that Merle's beauty was her principal currency. Encouraging Merle to offer her favors to the powerful men who were drawn to her and to keep watch for things they might do for her, Charlotte did not want her daughter's life—not to mention her own hopes—destroyed by a pregnancy.[44] And so, without telling Merle what was about to happen to her, Charlotte had her sterilized at the age of sixteen or seventeen.[45]

Merle Oberon became Rock's patient just at the time he was hearing from other young women who had been sterilized. What was going on? As it turns out, he was learning about a troubling practice that was far more common than he had imagined. Beginning in the early twentieth century and continuing well into the 1940s and 1950s, involuntary sterilization was practiced in at least seventeen states. Poor white women, very young African American women, adolescent girls, and others—some but not all institutionalized for one reason or another, including expressing their sexuality outside marriage—were victimized by either overt or covert sterilization programs. Although it is not possible to document the true extent of such practices, historian Elaine Tyler May estimated in the 1990s that "tens of thousands of Americans" had been sterilized involuntarily by the middle of the twentieth century.[46]

Like Merle Oberon, the women who wrote Rock after having experienced the destruction of their fallopian tubes and subsequent sterility wanted children. And Rock wanted to help them. In the heady aftermath of his conviction that he and Menkin had taken a major if early step toward the goal of making in vitro fertilization a clinical reality, he was so caught up in the excitement that he told a reporter that pregnancy through IVF was "not beyond the realm of imagination and it seems to offer about the only hope for women whose tubes have been destroyed."[47]

Rock believed at the time that progress would be relatively rapid. In spite of his cautionary words—"There is still a tremendous amount of laboratory work to be done before the work can be applied on patients"—he sometimes could not help but convey what turned out to be unwarranted optimism. He expected success within a decade, or two at most. He even suggested to a few women in their early twenties that they might still be young enough to benefit from the procedure. In spite of his obligatory bow to caution in responding to one young woman, telling her that "our research work has not progressed to the point where it is of any clinical value," he couldn't help but add, "Fortunately you are young yet so don't give up hope."[48]

Whether human in vitro fertilization was one, two, or three decades away would not make a difference to most of the women whose tubes had been damaged by disease or removed by surgery. Their anguish continued to speak to him. He and Nan had become quite close to Merle Oberon. It was her California house where they spent two months after their son was killed so that they could take their grief away from the demands of his too-public life. Rock would remain in touch with her at least for another decade. He cared about her loss, and he sympathized deeply with the ordinary women who, like her, had been forcibly deprived of the opportunity to bear children. His inability to help them, or to treat other cases of sterility caused by absent, blocked, or otherwise dysfunctional fallopian tubes, caused him great frustration.

A letter in 1951 from a young wife in rural Kentucky seems to have struck a particular chord. Mrs. R. T. told Rock that she had been sterilized without her knowledge shortly after giving birth for the first time; she only learned the truth when her child died as a toddler and she wanted to have another baby. In an uncertain hand, writing with a formality that was both touching and dignified, she asked for his help. He responded, with barely suppressed rage that she had been sterilized without her knowledge and with enormous sympathy for her suffering, that if he could, he would try to help her. First, however, he said that he needed to be assured that her health could bear another pregnancy. He asked her to provide him with some additional details about her physical condition. She wrote back that since childhood, she had suffered from a serious heart condition, but she said that she felt much better now. Rock in turn said that he was sorry, but he thought her health was too poor for her to risk another pregnancy.[49]

When this exchange took place, he had become reconciled to the fact that in vitro pregnancies were a lot further off than he had hoped in 1944, so how was he planning to help her if she had been in good health? He was contemplating reviving and improving on a surgical procedure that had been abandoned in the earlier part of the century, often called the Estes operation. The surgery was named after a little-known gynecologist in Bethlehem, Pennsylvania, who was himself reviving an earlier procedure called ovarian transplantation.

Ovarian transplantation was a procedure developed by Robert Tuttle Morris, a highly respected abdominal surgeon, in 1895. He was reacting to a nineteenth-century gynecological outrage, the wholesale destruction of women's reproductive capacities by an operation called an ovariotomy. Physicians removed women's ovaries for a host of physical and mental symptoms that often had little relation to the reproductive organs. A number of Morris's patients, who had been victimized by this surgery, wanted to bear children, and he thought he could help them.[50] Engaging in a remarkable decade-long course of experimental surgery, Morris implanted sections of the ovaries of fertile women into other women who had lost their own ovaries through surgery, or sections of their own ovaries in cases where, for medical reasons, they faced removal of their ovaries and fallopian tubes.

One of his patients was a twenty-six-year-old woman with severe pelvic adhesions and diseased fallopian tubes. She needed surgery, but she did not want to be sterile. Morris removed her ovaries and most of the fallopian tubes; in hopes of retaining her ability to bear children, he left a stump of her right oviduct, to the interior of which he transferred "a small piece of the patient's diseased ovary." After returning home from a month-long stay in the hospital, the patient soon became pregnant, he reported; however, she miscarried after about three months. The cause, according to Morris, was "persistent pelvic adhesions."

In 1906 Morris claimed his only success, reporting that a woman into whose uterus he had implanted a section of another woman's ovary in 1901 succeeded in conceiving and carrying the pregnancy to term. Childless wives who had been subject to removal of their ovaries, on hearing of this successful outcome, beseeched Morris to operate on them as well. He agreed. His technique involved simultaneous surgery on donor and recipient, and the removal from the donor of a section of ovary about the size of a pea. Keeping the excised segment in saline solution, he either divided the uterus of the recipient and implanted the new ovarian tissue into it, or sutured the section of ovary to the fallopian tube. In the beginning, he was so excited about the potential success of this procedure that he urged his colleagues to "hunt up some of [their] old patients whose adnexa [i.e., tube and ovary] have been removed, and give them the benefit of a graft of new ovary, in the possibility of relieving them from the condition of barrenness." But as time passed, and no other patient conceived, Morris abandoned the operation.

William Estes revived it almost two decades later, using a slightly different technique. He implanted either the entire ovary, or a portion of it, in the uterine wall at the point where the fallopian tube would normally connect to the uterus. In 1924 his son, also a physician, reported that he and his father had performed ninety-five such surgeries, from which four pregnancies resulted.

Others tried but could not replicate their success, and the operation had pretty much fallen into disuse, although not entirely. The gynecologist that Merle Oberon consulted before she saw Rock had performed this operation on her, "only making conditions worse" in Rock's view.[51] But Rock, who attempted to reconstruct her fallopian tubes, also failed.

And then, in 1951 a Scandinavian physician who had revived the Estes procedure reported that out of twenty-three cases, four pregnancies had resulted. If true, this was a significant improvement over the earlier results. Nevertheless, it seems that after Rock's exchange with Mrs. R. T., he chose not to pursue the idea further. Whether he had concluded that the Scandinavian report was flawed, or had simply succumbed to the press of other interests, is not clear. But he continued to try to think of solutions to the problem of absent fallopian tubes for a while, even consulting with a plastics company about the feasibility of creating artificial tubes. He soon concluded that the current state of technology made that an impractical idea as well. In his surgical practice, he decided to concentrate, with William Mulligan, on improving surgical techniques for damaged and occluded fallopian tubes instead. With his ambitions for IVF postponed, and these other options seemingly foreclosed, for the present he was unable to think of any ways to help a woman to conceive if her tubes had been removed.[52]

. . .

Male infertility was at least as resistant to treatment as a woman's blocked fallopian tubes. True azoospermia, or the complete absence of sperm, is relatively rare and completely incurable, except in the infrequent instances when adequate sperm is produced but their passage is blocked. Oligospermia (inadequate sperm count) was (and still is) much more common. Little was known about how to treat it, but practitioners in the 1930s and 1940s eagerly embraced anything that was likely to help. Mostly they offered advice that could do no harm and might be helpful. Physicians advised infertile men to change their eating habits, get more exercise, work less, relax more, avoid excessive exposure to x-rays and automobile emissions, and have sex only a few times a week.

Possibly a bit less benign were the hormonal treatments. Men, like women, received thyroid hormone—just in case it might do some good. And just as women were sometimes given extracts of animal ovaries for infertility, men were given injections of bull testicle extracts. In truth, unless a man's inadequate sperm count really had resulted from a thyroid disorder, correctable dietary deficiencies, or an infection that responded well to treatment—an infected tooth that could be pulled, for example—all the bulls' testicles in the world would not make him fertile. Not until the 1990s would significant progress be made in the treatment of male infertility.[53]

By the time he wrote Rock, poor Mr. M. H. had been through it all. He had changed his eating habits, lost weight, and received "many types of injections" over several years. He was willing to keep taking them if it would help, he said, but not if he was wasting his time. "If it is hopeless I would stop," he wrote. Rock was pleased to hear from a man who was willing to undergo treatment, given his own not-always-successful battle to involve the husbands of his infertility patients. Rock's treatment options for men, however, were as limited as everyone else's. But recently, he had developed a new technique for concentrating semen for use in artificial insemination, to be used in men who possessed some level of fertility but lacked the sufficient quantity of sperm to make fertilization likely.

As Rock explained to Mr. M. H., he had tried his new technique on only twelve men, but he had met with some success. "In two out of twelve cases such as yours," he explained, "I have obtained pregnancies by laboratory treatment of the ejaculate before placing a concentrated portion of it high in the uterus." Don't become overly optimistic, he cautioned, because the procedure "was still definitely in the experimental stage." Nevertheless, he suggested that Mr. M. H. see William Carey, an infertility specialist in New York to whom Rock often referred that city's residents. And if Dr. Carey "would like to try this method with you," he wrote, "I shall of course be very glad to give him the details of the laboratory technique."[54]

Rock believed that one of the things that discouraged men from dealing with infertility was feeling uncomfortable in a gynecological clinic waiting room surrounded by women. For years he sought separate facilities. Finally, in 1949, he persuaded the Free Hospital to hire Fletcher Colby to establish a separate clinic for men. Rock's records indicate that in the postwar period, the numbers of men receiving infertility treatments did increase, but it is hard to know the extent to which that increase reflects the existence of the new male facilities rather than simply the dramatic overall interest in infertility treatment during the baby boom. The increase was certainly not a result of new treatment successes, with the possible exception of the use of concentrated ejaculate with targeted placement—the treatment he described to Mr. M. H.

. . .

At the end of the 1940s, John Rock was the most prominent infertility specialist of his era. New patients crowded into his clinic. Journalists, medical poli-
cymakers, physicians, and ordinary men and women from around the nation
and abroad sought his opinions. He treated African royalty and American film
stars, Boston socialites and the wives of elevator operators and mechanics.
His and Hertig's embryo research was bringing him professional acclaim, including one of gynecology's major awards. Harvard promoted him to clinical
professor. He was a public figure, nationally and internationally, as a result of
his and Menkin's work on in vitro fertilization. More and more, young physicians from around the country and abroad begged to be invited to the Free
Hospital to observe his methods and to work on his research projects.

At his age, many of his colleagues were looking back on their achievements
and considering resting on their laurels. There is no indication that resting
occurred to him, despite his professional success remaining shadowed by the
sudden death of Charlie, then the irrevocable breach with Maisie. Nell was
suffering from a range of chronic and sometimes nearly incapacitating illnesses, which would leave her partially paralyzed by the end of the decade.[55]
His own debilitating heart attack in 1944 was followed in 1946 by the tragic
car accident that killed his son, Jack. His personal life had been marked by
one terrible event after another for much of the 1940s, and yet he managed,
not to put them behind him, but to achieve in spite of them.

Nearing sixty, he had not slowed down. He continued to take on new projects and a growing number of patients. Now nationally recognized as an infertility specialist, he would soon take a turn to the opposite direction. He
had long sympathized with the all-too-fertile women he saw in the clinic and
the hospital, suffering from a host of conditions brought on by too many children and too little money. The more he saw, the more convinced he became
that every couple should be able to choose freely the number of children they
could afford—materially and emotionally—to bring into the world.

The ideas that consumed John Rock—in his words, the "problems I want
answered"—involved central questions about human reproduction, whether
the issue was infertility treatment or fertility control. To a casual observer
it might have seemed contrarian for him to choose a career dominated by
the treatment of infertility during the Great Depression, when most people
wanted to have as few children as possible, and then to become interested in
birth control during the baby boom, when everyone seemed to want, if not
as many children as possible, at least more than the previous generation. In
later years, most of the stories about the development of "the pill" consider

it a delicious irony that one of the nation's most prominent physicians in the treatment of infertility would end up being most remembered for his work on the oral contraceptive. Rock saw it differently. There was little contradiction in his mind between his work to enhance fertility and his work to control it. And so, within two decades he would move from being seen as one of the leading figures among his generation in the understanding and treatment of infertility to becoming a household name as the chief advocate of the birth-control pill.

Chapter 6

THE FERTILITY DOCTOR MEETS THE PILL

Shrewsbury, Massachusetts, 1944. Biologists Hudson Hoagland and Gregory Pincus establish the Worcester Foundation for Experimental Biology, one of the nation's first independent research organizations. Among its clients is a Chicago pharmaceutical company called Searle.

Santa Barbara, California, 1952. Wealthy feminist Katharine Dexter McCormick seeks introduction to Gregory Pincus with an eye to funding the development of a birth-control pill.

Brookline, Massachusetts, 1953. John Rock joins forces with Pincus to develop an oral contraceptive.

John Rock's seventh decade—he turned sixty in March 1950—would turn out to be one of the most challenging, and fulfilling, of his professional life. Changes in the way medicine was practiced in the postwar period, combined with the childbearing frenzy of the baby boom era, helped to make his infertility clinic the most prominent in the nation, as young couples filled its waiting rooms. In growing numbers, Rock's colleagues from around the country invited themselves to observe the clinic's operation with an eye to replicating its success in their own cities. And young doctors from across the nation and around the world sought positions as fellows to advance their careers. Just as his fertility clinic was bursting at the seams, Rock launched his now-famous collaboration with biologist Gregory Pincus on the development of the oral contraceptive. His work on what became known simply as "the pill" brought him international attention as well as new allies and opponents.

In retrospect, John Rock and Gregory Pincus seemed to be such an odd couple that those who told the story of the pill in later years believed their collaboration had to have been an accident. Much has been made of the seeming incongruity of Rock and Pincus using the same hormone for opposite purposes and not even realizing it until they met—by fate or by chance—at just the right moment. Almost everyone who has written about the two men tell one or another version of the happenstance story. As one writer put it, their coming together was "one of those haphazard, inscrutable accidents that spangle the history of science." And a 2002 television series on science and sexuality based an entire program on what the show's writers called the "serendipity" of this encounter.[1]

The general outlines of the fateful meeting story go like this. In the early 1950s, Gregory Pincus began work on the birth-control pill, but he was in a quandary about exactly how to proceed. Then, as luck would have it, he happened to run into John Rock at a conference, not having seen him for decades. To their mutual amazement, they discovered that Pincus in Worcester was engaged in animal research on progesterone as a potential contraceptive, just as Rock in Brookline, using the very same substance for cases of infertility, had accidentally discovered that the hormone prevented ovulation. What a shock! Rock was finding in women what Pincus believed he had achieved in rabbits, and the world would never be the same. It's a great story. It's just not true. Rock and Pincus, although they were not close friends, were professional acquaintances of long standing who were very familiar with each other's work. Rock had made his first appearance in Pincus's correspondence in 1937.[2] A year after that, when Miriam Menkin interviewed with Rock, he hired her principally because she had worked for Pincus on superovulation in rabbits. And Rock's embryo and ova studies were inspired by Pincus's animal studies on ovulation, in vitro fertilization, the manipulation of ova, and embryo implantation. The men had, in short, followed each other's work for years. Once Pincus began work on the pill, it would have been much more surprising, given the convergence of their interests, if the two men hadn't gotten together than that they did.

So, how did the story get started? Its genesis may lie in the many ways Pincus and Rock were polar opposites—in their personalities, upbringing, and career paths. Rock was Catholic; Pincus, Jewish. Rock was socially ambitious and had married into Boston's upper crust; Pincus took pride in his immigrant heritage. Rock was smooth; Pincus had a decided edge to him. Rock was part of the establishment; Pincus was something of an antiestablishment scientific entrepreneur.

Pincus would become the driving force behind the pill's development. Without his organizational brilliance, scientific acumen, and entrepreneurial persistence, the pill never would have made it from lab bench to the physician's drug closet. But Rock, who in later years would call himself the "stepfather" of the pill, would in the end become nearly as important to the project as Pincus.

Gregory Pincus, born in 1903, grew up in Woodbine, New Jersey, an immigrant Jewish farming community in the southern part of the state.[3] He attended Cornell's agriculture school intending to follow the footsteps of an uncle into agronomy, but in college he became more interested in other areas of biology. He earned his PhD at Harvard in 1927, after which he took a postdoctoral research position in England at Cambridge University. In 1930, Harvard offered him an assistant professorship in biology. Brilliant and original, with a dazzling research agenda, he was also viewed by some of his colleagues as a publicity hound. In the mid-1930s, after reporting that he had succeeded in producing "immaculate conception" (parthenogenesis) in female rabbits, he allowed himself to be profiled in *Collier's,* a popular national magazine. The author of the article, J. D. Ratcliff, was the one who speculated that the eventual outcome of Pincus's work would be a reproductive future for humans in which men were no longer necessary, maybe not even desirable. Ratcliff predicted a future in which "the mythical . . . Amazons . . . [would come] to life" and create a "world where woman would be self-sufficient; man's value [would become] precisely zero."[4]

This article sounded the death knell of Pincus's Harvard career. In those days, Harvard preferred its researchers to be notable, not notorious. Its leading professors may have personified old-family New England arrogance, but they wished to seem, if not to be, modest about their professional triumphs. To engage in media self-promotion was a cardinal sin. Brilliance was not enough. Harvard did not grant him tenure, which meant he lost his job.

He was shocked, but maybe he shouldn't have been. Even some of his admirers wondered, in historian James Reed's words, whether his "experiments were too complex to be carefully controlled or easily reproduced." University politics and anti-Semitism also came into play. William Crozier, Pincus's department chair and mentor, had troubles of his own at Harvard and could not help his young protégé. Harvard's new president, James Conant, viewed Crozier as an "empire builder" and saw to it that Crozier's department was cut out from under him and his power in the university destroyed. Crozier and his supporters believed that the university's action against Pincus was aimed at them just as much as at Pincus. And Harvard was not immune to the virulent Ivy League anti-Semitism of the era. In Reed's words, the whole sad saga reflected "prejudice against [Pincus] as a student of Crozier and as a self-advertising Jew who published too soon and talked too much."[5] Maybe he would have been denied tenure anyway, and the fatherless rabbits only sealed his doom.

Harvard gave Pincus a paid research leave at Cambridge University for the academic year of 1937–1938, but after that he was out of a job. To his dismay, despite the best efforts of both Crozier and the influential William Castle at the University of California at Berkeley, another of the young scientist's supporters, Pincus received no offer of a position in the United States. War in Europe loomed, and Pincus was eager to get home, but he needed a job. His very career as a scientist imperiled, he was rescued by Hudson Hoagland at Clark University in Worcester, Massachusetts. Hoagland offered him a position as a visiting professor in his laboratory and provided the desperate scientist with a research base. Unfortunately, Hoagland had little else to give—no salary and no faculty perquisites. Luckily for Pincus, a wealthy benefactor, fellow scientist Lord Nathaniel Rothschild, stepped in to provide two years' salary.

This was not the career that Pincus had envisioned, but in the end, it gave him the freedom he craved. Together, he and Hoagland moved on to create an entirely new scientific enterprise. Hoagland, like Pincus, was an entrepreneur at heart whose ambition was to build his own research empire at Clark. Clashing regularly and rancorously with the university administration, he became fed up, so he and Pincus decided to strike out on their own in the late 1930s. They founded the Worcester Foundation for Experimental Biology (WFEB), an independent research laboratory, locating it in Shrewsbury and incorporating in 1944.[6]

At the time, theirs was a daring undertaking. This was more than a decade before the federal government, under the aegis of the National Institutes of Health and the National Science Foundation, would become the principal funding source for science in the United States. The two scientists had no safety net. Although some of their research was conducted under grants from foundations, their most profitable relationships were with the burgeoning pharmaceutical industry, for which they developed new processes to produce compounds and performed animal testing on existing ones.[7]

As it happened, their timing was excellent; they caught the first wave of the new era of antibiotic and steroid therapy. Pharmaceutical companies, in fierce competition for patents and profits, were developing scores of new chemical compounds and seeking advice on how to synthesize others. The WFEB was prepared to provide biological expertise in both these arenas. One of these companies was G. D. Searle and Company, still a family-owned and operated business. Pincus began regularly performing scientific studies for them as early as 1939. However, by the early 1950s, his relationship with the company had become rocky at best. In fact, Searle and Pincus in 1951 nearly had a fatal break. Having invested a half-million dollars in various Pincus enterprises, Searle—in the person of research director Al Raymond—came close to pulling the plug permanently on Pincus and the Worcester Foundation.

The crisis came over the synthesis of cortisone, which had recently been shown to treat severe rheumatoid arthritis. Cortisone was a treatment, not a cure, and its side effects would soon become evident, but the fact that men and women who had not been able to lift their arms without pain were now able to move freely and go about their daily lives was indeed a medical miracle. But it was a miracle available only to a few at first, because it was difficult and expensive to synthesize the drug.

If a way could be found to synthesize cortisone cheaply and simply, enormous profits would follow. In the late 1940s, Searle and other American pharmaceutical companies raced to see who could figure out how to produce large quantities of hydrocortisone at a moderate cost. Pincus, under contract to Searle, had figured out a synthesizing process based on perfusion. On the plus side, he could produce large quantities. On the minus side, this was a very expensive way to manufacture the product. But almost as soon as they had purchased, at Pincus's urging, this expensive equipment, Searle was beaten out by a rival pharmaceutical company. Upjohn's researchers had discovered a much simpler—and more important, cheaper—method than Pincus had devised. Pincus had promised, lavishly as usual, and Pincus had not delivered.[8]

Searle, a small company that invested selectively in only a few new drugs at a time, had lost this race in an expensive way. On behalf of the Searle Company, Al Raymond was furious. "You haven't done a thing to justify the half-million that we invested in you," Raymond told Pincus. "Your record as a contributor . . . to the Searle Company is a lamentable failure, replete with false leads, poor judgment, and assurances from you that were false." Profoundly shaken at the time, Pincus remained unsettled and worried for a long time, because his survival as a research entrepreneur depended on his relationship with companies such as Searle.[9]

Pincus knew he could not afford to burn his bridges to Searle. Fortunately, Al Raymond soon recovered from his outburst. Searle lost out on cortisone, but it had now become interested in what would become an equally promising avenue of investigation, the testing of synthetic sex hormones. Although a still wary Raymond was not about to invest any big money in Pincus right away, he did contract with him for animal studies on some new compounds.

In the early 1950s, in fact, both Pincus and Rock were testing the same product—benzelstilbestrol, an estrogen that Searle hoped to market under the brand name Monozol. It is not clear for what purpose Pincus was testing the product, but Rock was using it, and several other synthetic estrogens, for female endocrine and fertility disorders. Letters between Rock and researchers at Searle document his and Pincus's familiarity with each other's complementary animal and human testing of similar products.[10] The two men also occasionally communicated directly with each other about the effectiveness of compounds they were both testing, for Searle and other pharmaceutical companies.[11]

Pincus was not conjuring an idea out of thin air when he began to investigate the possibility of hormonal contraception. In 1947, when the National Research Council (NRC) created its Committee on Human Reproduction, it had asked John Rock to set its research agenda, and hormonal contraception was one of the items on his list.[12] And several historical accounts of the development of oral contraceptives have shown how, almost from the moment that estrogen was discovered, scientists began to speculate about hormonal contraception. Actually developing such an agent, however, was a different matter. And since most of the early research into hormonal contraception took place in Central Europe, notably by Austrians Ludwig Haberlandt and Otfried Fellner, working separately, the extent to which Americans were aware of such investigations is unclear.[13]

As long ago as World War I, the idea had begun to take shape. In 1919 Innsbruck, Austria, gynecologist Ludwig Haberlandt transplanted the ovaries of pregnant rabbits into rabbits who were not pregnant. The transplanted ovaries, he claimed, rendered the other rabbits sterile. Haberlandt suggested that such animal transplants into women might also render them "temporarily sterile." Of course, such a technique would hardly have mass appeal. Haberlandt knew it and looked toward other methods. By 1927 he was trying oral preparations of cow corpora lutea on rabbits and full ovarian extracts on mice. He later teamed up with a Hungarian pharmaceutical house to develop an oral preparation, which would be called Infecundin, for possible human use. Throughout this period, European and American laboratories were keeping the abattoirs of Europe busy with requests for the thyroids, pituitaries, ovaries, and testicles of cattle and sheep slaughtered for food, so he would have no problem with supply. Although the evidence is not clear, the product may have been briefly placed on the market just before Haberlandt's death in 1932.[14]

Another Austrian, Otfried Fellner of Vienna, was also experimenting with the ovaries of pregnant cows in the 1920s, and by the end of the decade he had produced injectable extracts and an oral preparation he called Feminin, both of which rendered rabbits and mice sterile.[15] The idea of what Haberlandt initially called "temporary sterilization" did not appear to elicit much immediate interest. Scientists in the United States—Leo Loeb and William B. Kountz at Washington University in St. Louis, who were experimenting on the hormonal sterilization of guinea pigs; William Makepeace and his colleagues at the University of Pennsylvania, who demonstrated the contraceptive properties of progesterone in rabbits; and Pincus, who showed that estrogen injections in rabbits caused the destruction of ova in the fallopian tube—were apparently unaware of their Austrian counterparts' work.[16]

Given the politics of the 1930s, with the rise of Nazism and fascism throughout Europe, producing an injectable hormonal contraceptive could have had chilling consequences. Envisioning the potential appeal to eugenicists does not require much imagination. Medical and legal antipathy toward contraception in the 1930s also played a role, as did concerns even then within the medical profession about the potential health risks attendant on the long-term use of estrogen. And let us not forget the career lesson that scientists could draw from Pincus's experience—tamper with cherished ideas about sexuality and reproduction, even if only with bunnies, and be exiled to Worcester! Whatever the combination of reasons, American scientists did not pursue the idea of hormonal contraception, not even after both estrogen and progesterone had been synthesized, and in spite of clear evidence that American couples were employing whatever methods they could find to control the size of their families in the Depression-era 1930s.[17]

Although American scientists steered clear of hormonal contraception in the years between World Wars I and II, they eagerly embraced general research on hormones in the 1930s and early 1940s. Especially during and immediately after World War II, the major focus of hormonal research was the corticosteroids that control adrenal function. Competition to synthesize such hormones was fierce, as shown by the Searle Company's fury when Gregory Pincus led them down the wrong path.

It is not a coincidence that the same companies competing to develop cortisone products were also involved in creating other hormonal compounds. As the story of the oral contraceptive unfolds, its relationship to the intense competition among the pharmaceutical "houses" (as they were often called because most had roots as family-owned businesses) becomes an important part of the narrative. For that reason, it is important to understand the emerging and increasingly intertwining relationships of scientists, clinicians (especially at research institutions), and pharmaceutical companies in transforming medical research, including that of Pincus and Rock, in the 1940s and 1950s.

. . .

When historians of medicine speak of the mid-twentieth century as the era of "triumphal medicine," they are generally referring to the explosive development of antibiotics. During these years, one magic bullet after another was discovered, synthesized, and put on the market.[18] It began with the discovery of sulfa drugs, the first antibacterials to be marketed as anti-infective agents in the 1930s; they provided a major impetus to the search for similar drugs. World War II dramatically increased the demand for even more effective agents to cure infections and treat disease.

Penicillin, the antibacterial properties of which were discovered by Alexander Fleming in 1928, was isolated and purified in 1940 in Howard Florey's laboratory at Oxford University by Florey, Ernst Chain, and Norman Heatley. The first successful human use was in 1941. By 1944, nineteen American drug companies were producing penicillin, and the major pharmaceutical houses had come to recognize that their prosperity and competitive edge would increasingly depend on the development of an ever-growing pharmacopoeia. But they wanted drugs they could patent, not simply manufacture. As economic historian Peter Temin asserted, during the 1940s and 1950s, the industry changed dramatically, from "a fairly typical manufacturing industry to one based on the continual progress of technical knowledge." New drug development—particularly new products that unlike sulfanilamide and penicillin could be patented and then exclusively marketed by the company that created them—became central to the good health of the companies.[19]

These dramatic changes provided the scientific and economic climate that allowed Hudson Hoagland and Gregory Pincus to build a research enterprise independent of a university structure. Working on contract for several companies, in the 1940s they were involved both in the development of new processes and in the animal testing of new compounds that came directly from the companies. Just as wartime needs helped to spur the development of penicillin, they prompted scientists to study adrenocortical function, attempting to understand its role in physical and mental stress, and to find chemical ways of countering those stresses.[20]

In a war-torn world in which the medical priorities were for agents that could heal the wounded soldier and prevent the able ones from succumbing to physical and mental deterioration, the study and use of the sex hormones, while not exactly ignored, were relegated to the back seat. But the civilian uses of antibiotics and steroids, and the hopes of finding newer and ever more useful ones, outlasted the war. Interest in the sex hormones—especially in their potential to enhance fertility—was reinvigorated during the baby boom. In the postwar years, millions of young American men and women avidly embraced marriage and family life, marrying earlier than their parents and grandparents and choosing larger families over smaller ones. The advent of the baby boom in the United States spurred fertility research and treatment on a large scale, even if no major advances in the pharmacological treatment of infertility would appear until the 1960s.[21]

Most scientists and clinicians who were interested in hormonal research in this period were interested primarily in treating infertility, not developing hormonal contraception. But in some ways, the two went together. That was certainly how Rock had viewed the study of fertility. And so, when Rock came to collaborate with Pincus, he viewed this work as simply another aspect of his life's work on problems of reproduction.

He did not back into contraceptive research inadvertently, even if he had for many years tried to be careful in his public professions of support for birth control.[22] By the time Rock began his collaboration with Pincus, he had already become more overt in expressing his views. He still favored early marriage and early parenthood, assuring "newly married couples" that they "will be happier parents if they have their children young." But he also believed that once a couple decided their family was complete, they should have access to a full range of contraceptive options. After all, he had seen first hand the results of too-frequent childbearing combined with too-few resources. Since he believed that rhythm worked only rarely and that sexual abstinence weakened a couple's love, he became ever more willing to act as a public advocate of contraception. But he never subscribed to the feminist belief that birth control should serve as an instrument of women's autonomy, a tool to enable her to reject or limit childbearing in favor of a career or personal fulfillment. Rather, he was an outspoken family man who maintained that happiness in marriage depended on a couple's ability to support and enjoy as many children as they could emotionally and financially afford.[23]

In Rock's mind, there was no contradiction between his lifelong commitment to alleviating infertility and his growing commitment to the converse.

In the late 1940s, he had become more active in the NCMH. And just after World War II, when the NCMH and Planned Parenthood Federation jointly asked the NRC to oversee a research program in reproductive science and medicine, the NRC created the Committee on Human Reproduction in 1947, with Rock as a founding member.[24]

Widely considered the nation's leading expert in the field of human fertility and endocrine disorders, Rock agreed to set the committee's agenda in that field. His 1948 position paper reiterated his frustration with reliance on animal studies to explain human reproduction. In terse outline form, he derided the scientific understanding of female fertility as "surprisingly obscure . . . Little is known of human reproductive physiology, biochemistry, and hormonology [sic]. Dependence on zoologic analogy is heavy and unsafe." In his judgment there were only about six "fairly good" sterility (his word) clinics in the United States and about the same number of "endocrinologic" clinics. For the most part, he said, the endocrine clinics "occasionally" produced good research and were "steadily improving." He had no kind words for the clinics that focused only on sterility. There, "the research work, with few exceptions, is purely clinical, unscientific, and not worth much."[25]

As befitted a director of a fertility and endocrine clinic, Rock's priorities were the support of research in such institutions and development of a new generation of basic and clinical researchers. His proposed program of contraceptive research included the study of hormonal "*suppression* [of] ovular maturation, ovulation, or conjugation," which were also three areas of high priority in studying the *promotion* of fertility. In other words, understanding more precisely how human ova grew and matured; tracing the process of ovulation, tubal migration, and fertilization itself; and comprehending the hormonal, enzymatic, and other factors promoting or inhibiting the implantation of the fertilized ovum were critical both to promoting and to preventing pregnancy.[26]

Rock provided his colleagues with a full research program, which included hormonal contraception. But it was all for nothing. The committee had been created to develop a research agenda for which the Planned Parenthood Federation of America and the NCMH would serve as the fund-raising arms.[27] The arms were unable to carry the burden, and within four years, the committee had dissolved and researchers sought other funding sources.

And so, after all is said and done, it was not the drug companies, not Pincus (who was already interested but would have needed funding, and Searle wasn't ready *knowingly* to fund the development of an oral contraceptive), not

Rock, but two feminist icons—Margaret Sanger and Katharine Dexter Mc-
Cormick—who were determined to use that hormonal research to devise a
way for women to control their own reproductive lives. One of them was both
willing and able to pay for it.

. . .

Margaret Sanger, still the first lady of birth control in the minds of most
Americans, had loathed the idea of changing the name of what she considered her own American Birth Control League to the Planned Parenthood
Federation. She was right to be offended. The name change did reflect the
stirrings of a growing societal consensus on the use of contraceptive measures, but it was not a feminist consensus.[28] Sanger, whose name had been
synonymous with the birth-control movement for half a century, consistently
maintained that access to birth control on an unfettered, democratic basis
was both a fundamental right of all women and the foundation of social progress. Even as she traveled from youthful radicalism to political conservatism,
she never swerved from those separate but linked convictions. It was her passionate conviction that birth control would free women from having to bear
unwanted children and, almost as important, allow them to enjoy sex without worrying about pregnancy.[29] She insisted, and rightly so, that the name
"Planned Parenthood" did not convey the idea of contraception as a means
of women's empowerment. Without denying that she and McCormick both
believed that impoverished women in the developing world stood in greatest
need for a simple and safe contraceptive, for her to say that the poor should
have fewer children did not conflict with her belief that fewer children would
lead to women's autonomy and general prosperity.[30]

Existing contraceptives prevented pregnancy, but few methods offered
complete security. The two most popular methods—condoms and withdrawal—required the active engagement of the male partner, and men sometimes
viewed them as impediments to their full satisfaction. For some, a condom
formed a barrier to pleasure. Withdrawal required a man to control his responses, not always an easy thing to do.[31] Religious and political opposition
to contraception remained strong in some religions and in some parts of the
country. The Catholic Church vehemently opposed contraception. In several
states, including John Rock's Massachusetts, it was illegal for physicians to
provide birth-control information or devices. Indeed, as late as 1960, thirty
states would still have laws that in some way restricted the advertisement or
the sale of birth-control devices.[32]

Until the prospect of a birth-control pill emerged, Sanger's preferred contraceptive was the individually fitted diaphragm, because it was female controlled. But to obtain a diaphragm, a woman had to visit a physician. (In Europe, nurses fitted diaphragms, but not in the United States; to garner medical support for the diaphragm, Sanger had to agree that physicians would prescribe and fit the devices.) Katharine McCormick, who would fund the development of the pill, left no record of her own sexual attitudes, but when she became involved in birth control, she made it clear that *female-controlled* birth control was her only priority in funding contraceptive research. Although her biographer believes that Katharine's husband was impotent as a young man, others have suggested that his mental illness led her to decide to remain childless. If so, since he would not have been able to take responsibility for contraception, preventing pregnancy would be up to her. In the 1930s, she had even smuggled diaphragms into the United States for Sanger's clinics.[33]

Except within the Catholic Church, cultural opposition to birth control was receding by the late 1940s and early 1950s, in part because such organizations as Planned Parenthood began to persuade the public that birth control was a sensible way to plan a good-sized family and not a feminist plot to overthrow the conventional roles of the sexes. Such attitudes about family planning emerged during World War II and became entrenched in the baby boom era that followed.

In the 1950s, with couples marrying and having their families at young ages, compared with their parents and grandparents, there was bound to be a demand for reliable contraception once they had their three, four, or five children. After all, by then a wife was usually just over the age of thirty, with at least fifteen years of potential fertility still ahead. These couples whose fecundity fueled the baby boom wanted children *and* they wanted to make sure that once they had as many as they wanted, they could stop having them. By 1950 John Rock had spent more than a quarter-century trying to make it possible for the infertile to have the children they often so desperately wanted, but he also witnessed the desperation of women who could never stop having children, even though their economic, emotional, or physical situations worsened with every new birth.

Not only was he used to seeing infertility and overfertility as two sides of a single issue, but by 1950 his ideas about contraception had also become compatible with those of most Americans, if not with his church's hierarchy. In 1949 he had even coauthored a book endorsing birth control.[34] In later years,

Rock would use the specter of world overpopulation to justify his demand that the Catholic Church approve the pill. While "the population bomb" was not an excuse for him—he really did believe that the world was endangered by overpopulation—he nevertheless made it clear to friends, colleagues, the medical students he taught, and the couples he counseled that contraception was likewise for the ordinary couple who wanted to space their children and to stop having them altogether whenever the optimal number of offspring, whatever that was for a particular couple, had been reached.

• • •

Even though the true story of the pill was not filled with the dramatic instances of coincidence and happenstance as most accounts have suggested, its development was, nevertheless, theatrical.[35] Dramatized, it would have as lead characters the two veteran feminists (Sanger and McCormick); the brilliant, original, and brash scientific entrepreneur (Pincus); and the handsome, courtly, and charismatic physician (Rock). The supporting (or sometimes querulous) cast would include two chemists—Carl Djerassi and Frank Colton.

Djerassi, of Syntex, created one of the two chemical formulas that would eventually go into oral contraceptives. In spite of munificent financial rewards from his Syntex stock, Djerassi was convinced that he never received his full share of glory for his accomplishment. Colton, at Searle, was a quintessential company man whose competing formula actually became the first birth-control pill. Rounding out the main characters would be biologist Min-Chueh Chang and the dashing young gynecologist Celso-Ramon Garcia. Chang worked for Pincus, performed all the animal tests, and much like Djerassi considered himself the *real* "father" of the pill, although few outside the Worcester Foundation actually knew who he was. Garcia was Rock's eyes and ears in Puerto Rico, where the first clinical trials would occur, and later became a formidable clinician-researcher in his own right. Ensemble cast members would include several of the too-often unsung heroines of American laboratory and clinical research in the twentieth century—the women who performed the difficult and often tedious technical laboratory analyses, including Anne Merrill at the Worcester Foundation, Rachel Achenbach (Rock's cytologist daughter) at the Free Hospital, and the ever-indispensable Miriam Menkin. It was the interaction of these specific individuals, in the particular context of postwar America, that produced the pill precisely at this time.

Pincus had given serious consideration to the idea of an oral contraceptive before he encountered McCormick. In 1951 he asked Al Raymond of Searle to fund such a project. After the cortisone debacle, Pincus was unlikely to get Searle to agree to provide anywhere near the sums required. He began the research anyway, at a modest pace, relying on the considerable expertise of Min-Chueh Chang. But at the time, Pincus was able only to cobble together some small-scale funding through the Planned Parenthood Federation. By then, the federation was no longer in Sanger's hands but was instead run by professional administrators who did not share her passions. The relatively small amount of funding available to Pincus through Planned Parenthood, amounting to less than $6,500 by 1952, was nowhere near the projected cost of such an ambitious program.[36]

Everything changed when McCormick entered the picture. She was the widow of Stanley McCormick, the youngest son of Cyrus McCormick, inventor of the mechanical reaper and founder of what became the International Harvester Company. Stanley had fallen victim to schizophrenia soon after he and Katharine married in 1904. Katharine McCormick was familiar with the Worcester Foundation, having supported its work on some of the adrenal steroids as possible treatments for the disease from which her husband had suffered.[37] In the early 1950s, after Stanley's death and a family legal battle, she finally gained full control of his estate. Reinvigorating her longtime friendship with Sanger, McCormick confided to her that she was on the verge of making the fateful decision to spend whatever it would take to make oral contraception a reality. Sanger, already familiar with Pincus's ideas, encouraged her enthusiastically.

There is no indication that either of them, longtime champions of the medically controlled diaphragm, had reservations about physicians, not the women taking the pills, controlling access to the new drug. They may not have even realized that the pill would likely be available only by prescription, at least in this country, since both of them had come of age when few drugs fell into that category.

As early as March 1952, Sanger informed McCormick about "what Dr. Pincus is doing on hormones," that is, his contraceptive studies in rabbits and rats, offering to make sure that McCormick was kept informed as the projects progressed, adding, "they have not been finished, of course." McCormick was grateful and sought an introduction to Pincus in spring 1952 by way of her friend Roy Hoskins of Harvard, whose schizophrenia research she had long funded (but dropped abruptly after Stanley died, although she and Hoskins remained good friends).[38] Pincus and McCormick met formally, on a substantive level, at the Worcester Foundation on June 8, 1953, and McCormick offered to fund the development of an oral contraceptive. Within the next several years, she would put more than $2 million (close to $15 million today) into research on the pill.[39]

McCormick's support was critical to this enterprise. Almost no funding agency—not the federal government, not the large research foundations—would have ever agreed to fund avowed contraception research. Both the Committee on Human Reproduction and the NCMH had languished in the early 1950s for that very reason, as John Rock had learned when he unsuccessfully tried to find funding sources for them. Even in this era of dramatically increased support for medical research, when federal and foundation funding was available for general scientific and clinical research on reproduction, the amount allocated did not compare to the funds spent in other, less controversial fields.[40] Because Planned Parenthood had already provided some funding to Pincus, McCormick funneled her initial contributions through that organization. That would make it easy for someone who did not know where the money was really coming from to believe that Planned Parenthood's support was greater than it actually was. However, McCormick soon grew frustrated with channeling funds through Planned Parenthood and began to provide them directly to Pincus. By the time he met McCormick, Pincus was convinced of the contraceptive properties of progesterone, but all he had to go on were animal studies.

This is where Rock came in. In February 1953, some months before Pincus's meeting with McCormick, he informed Paul Henshaw of the Planned Parenthood Federation that Rock and his staff had already "begun some observations with oral progesterone which I supplied to them."[41] Rock would become ever more central to the development of the pill as the focus shifted from the creation and animal testing of various compounds to their use in women.

. . .

Even some historians of the pill have seemed unsure about the exact nature of the drugs being tested as oral contraceptives, and the formulas were changed and adjusted fairly often in the early years. The first thing to remember is that estrogen and progesterone were first isolated in the 1920s and were synthesized—that is, developed in a laboratory—from natural sources in the 1930s. In addition, an inexpensive synthetic estrogen was available as early as 1938. The situation was different for progesterone. Until the early 1940s, it was produced from animal byproducts. The process was expensive, and so was the product. Then, in 1940, American chemist Russell Marker, who had already synthesized estrogen from plant steroids, figured out that progesterone could also be manufactured cheaply, and in large quantities, from similar sources—in this case, the wild Mexican yam, which contained sapogenins. He built a laboratory in Mexico City and founded a company, which he called Syntex, to produce the product.[42]

When Pincus began his search for an oral contraceptive, he had access to effective preparations of estrogen that could be taken in pill form. But progesterone was much more effective when injected. Injections were fine for most therapeutic uses of progesterone, but they would not be acceptable to most women for contraceptive purposes. And even when oral preparations of progesterone did become available in the early 1950s, the effective doses were quite large. When Rock began to use progesterone as an experimental treatment for unexplained infertility, he used injectable forms, but by 1954 he was also experimenting with Syntex's oral progesterone. In December of 1954 he began small studies with the two new compounds developed by Carl Djerassi and Frank Colton: the progestins, which were chemical compounds called 19-nor-steroids. They had a similar biological action to progesterone, but they were effective at much lower doses. It was not until Rock tested these new 19-nor-steroids that he began to believe that the birth-control pill would become a reality. The differences between progesterone and the progestins, as well as the chronology of their use, are important to understanding the story.

In 1952 Rock began exploring more systematically the idea that estrogen and progesterone, used in combination, might be useful in the treatment of so-called unexplained infertility. He had hypothesized that some women did not conceive because they had an underdeveloped female reproductive system. Sometimes, however, a woman managed to become pregnant despite this condition. In such cases, he believed, the pregnancy itself "matured" the reproductive system. This observation led him to wonder if a state of "pseudo-pregnancy" might also develop the reproductive system in such a way as to make pregnancy possible.

To test his theory, he recruited a group of women with long-term, unexplained infertility—"eighty frustrated, but valiantly adventuresome, patients," as he called them—into the study, telling them that he had no idea whether his notion would work or not, but that he thought there was a chance it might. The women took a combination of progesterone and estrogen (diethylstilbestrol) in increasing doses.[43] Sixteen percent became pregnant after the treatment stopped. Rock also experimented with progesterone alone in intravenous and intramuscular preparations.

Initially Rock was optimistic about his findings, but as he later told Paul Rollins, a Seattle doctor of his acquaintance, "the so-called 'rebound' reaction . . . is still uncertain in my mind." On the one hand, "the fact that [the patients] were all of long term infertility, yet became pregnant within a few months after the treatment, made me think that the treatment had something to do with their cure . . . To have sixteen percent, within a limited time and among patients of long exposure, seemed interesting." On the other hand, "The number of cases was small, [and] the number of pregnancies small . . . The percentage itself . . . is not much more than one would expect in a large group of patients if nothing were done." In the end, he said, "I find it hard, myself, to appraise [the treatment]."[44]

Whether progesterone was injected or ingested, it could cause problems. Rock had obtained his injectable progesterone from two pharmaceutical companies, Syntex and Searle, and his oral preparation from Syntex. The large oral doses could be difficult to take or tolerate, and injectable forms had side effects as well. The shots themselves could cause painful reactions; Rock was always looking for the perfect solvent to use for the injections. To get an idea of how the patients would fare, Rock appears to have gotten into the habit of trying new solvents on himself for potential adverse reactions before injecting them into his patients. In a letter to Searle requesting samples of a new solvent, he mentioned his wish for something more innocuous than what they had sent him recently: "I shall shoot some of it into myself first in complete confidence that it won't do to me what the rosin of the intermuscular preparation did."[45]

No matter how the progesterone was administered, the regimen was hard on the women. The high doses of hormones gave them the symptoms of early pregnancy. Desperate as they were to have a child, they sometimes believed they were pregnant, with the inevitable letdown once the hormones were withdrawn. It had never occurred to him to have the women take the hormones cyclically, but when Pincus suggested it for his own purposes, Rock realized that such a change would at least remind the women that they were not pregnant.

After he began collaborating with Pincus, some of Rock's patients received the hormones on a simulated monthly cycle. They would have periods (actually, anovulatory withdrawal bleeding) and would know each month that they weren't pregnant. Meanwhile, the doctors and nurses monitored their reproductive systems while they were on the hormones—through urine tests, evaluation of vaginal smears, and endometrial biopsies. Occasionally, Rock or one of his assistants performed a culdoscopy. (The culdoscope is an instrument inserted through a small incision in the posterior vaginal wall that makes the visualization of the pelvic organs possible without surgery.) In a few instances, a woman had already been scheduled for a diagnostic laparotomy, allowing Rock to look for evidence of ovulation or lack of it.

Pincus had suggested the simulated monthly cycle because he wanted to know for his own purposes that the women were not pregnant.[46] Rock was happy to go along with his colleague both because his own patients often developed the false *hope* that they were pregnant and because Pincus thought that potential pill takers would *fear* the same thing when they did not menstruate monthly. Rock would have been amused to find himself, a half-century later, imagined to have had religious motivations for developing what he and Pincus viewed as a simple solution to two practical problems. Pincus the scientist just wanted to know if the regimen was working, and Rock the kind physician did not want to get his patients' hopes up. But in the early twenty-first century, journalist Malcolm Gladwell characterized their decision as a tortured religious rationalization by Rock and a bad scientific decision. "In John Rock's mind," Gladwell argued in the *New Yorker*, "the dictates of religion and principles of science got mixed up."[47]

Rock had given no thought at all to the Catholic Church when he made this decision, but it comes as no surprise that even today people might still have trouble figuring out his relationship to his religion. McCormick and Sanger, both anticlerical, always found him to be an enigma—a practicing Catholic who not only had no qualms about public advocacy of birth control but also seemed to make up his theology as he went along. Rock once told McCormick that as long as the Church didn't interfere with him, he wouldn't interfere with the Church. She recounted the conversation to Sanger, then added, puzzled, "Whatever that may mean."[48]

Rock did not lose sight of his original aim in the pseudopregnancy studies, to find a way for a subset of the intractably infertile to conceive. But Pincus influenced the treatment protocols for the women. At the same time that Pincus suggested Rock's patients be placed on a twenty-day-on, five-day-off schedule, he also asked Rock to try a progesterone-only regimen to test his (Pincus's) hypothesis that progesterone alone, without added estrogen, would inhibit ovulation. Rock agreed, and in early 1954 began a study using oral progesterone without an estrogen supplement. But after giving the drug to fifteen women for one cycle, eleven had ovulated. Then eight took it for a second cycle, and three of them ovulated. Rock found this discouraging. Although eventually about 75 to 80 percent of the participants appeared to stop ovulating, an ovulation rate of 20 to 25 percent would never lead to a successful contraceptive.[49]

Altogether, through 1954 Rock tried several different progesterone preparations on his patients, including oral and injectable preparations in several different solutions, with and without estrogen. McCormick grew impatient. Rock tried to educate her about the nature of working on a research study with people. Eventually, although she never grew reconciled to what she considered too slow a pace, she was impressed by Rock's clinical exactitude. Both she and Sanger were clinging to a false impression, perhaps fostered by Pincus, that the progesterone studies in women would be relatively straightforward, and that if the drug worked, it would be immediately evident and that would be the end of it.[50] It fell to Rock to explain to McCormick and Sanger that the situation was not so straightforward as they wanted to believe. Regularly, Rock told the ever-restless and always impatient McCormick how important it was to monitor patients closely to ascertain the multiple effects of the hormones on their reproductive systems and overall health.

Given his experience with the progesterone-only regimen, he was right to be so cautious. Not only did ovulation occur in too many cases, but several women also experienced breakthrough bleeding. A contraceptive pill that was not foolproof would be no better than the tried-and-true methods already available. Still, McCormick continued to fret. "It is always so hard to get all the facts one needs about a particular matter," she wrote to Sanger in mid-1954. "I suppose it is because one does not ask the right questions necessary to reach the heart of the matter." Rock spent two hours one day with her, and, she wrote Sanger, "I learned a great deal that I should have known before but . . . had not clearly understood."[51]

Rock would find, however, that the effect of his tutorials were never long lasting. McCormick continued to express her annoyance with what she considered the slow pace of Rock's research, but she was impatient about everything. She often groused to Sanger about how she hated the Christmas holidays because people weren't easy to get hold of when she wanted them, complained about waits for airplanes that most of us would consider trivial, and said she hated to take car trips on Sundays because other cars slowed down her trip. Given her temperament, her impatience with Rock is understandable. She continued to complain regularly that Rock was entirely too much of a perfectionist.

Pincus, who understood less than he thought he did about human reproduction, unconsciously undermined Rock by encouraging McCormick to think the issues were considerably simpler than Rock claimed. Indeed, Rock more than once in the years to come would chastise Pincus for moving too quickly. McCormick saw it this way: "Dr. Pincus is imaginative and inspirational. Dr. Rock is informative and very realistic about medical work."[52]

Rock, by now three decades into a career replete with dramatic intuitive leaps, was not so unimaginative as McCormick seemed to think. But once having made a leap, he wanted to be sure that any answer he had intuited was in fact correct. He continued to fight his losing battle to convince McCormick of the importance of conducting clinical research systematically and methodically. She tried to understand. In one letter, she told Sanger that she had finally understood Rock's reliance on urine analyses and vaginal smears. The determination of the effectiveness of the progesterone, she told Sanger, "is made or broken by them." McCormick also marveled at how time consuming the actual clinical research was, and how important was the cooperation of the patients. "I was surprised to hear that 25 cases took the whole time of one woman doctor" (Angeliki Tsacona, at the Free Hospital), she told Sanger. She also found the study participants frustrating. "The headache of the tests," she complained, "is the co-operation necessary from the women patients.— There is so much of it and it must be accurate. I really do not know how it is obtained at all—for it is onerous . . . Rock says he can get it only from women wishing to become fertile." She thought they should be paid, but neither Rock nor Pincus thought that was a good idea.[53]

In a metaphor quoted almost every time anyone writes about the pill's development, McCormick said that what the research needed was a "cage" of ovulating women. If Rock had ever heard her say that, he would have been appalled. It was true, he once told a group of his friends, that the infertile were good research subjects because they were desperate for a chance to conceive. But their plight, he believed, made it all the more important that no one ever abuse their trust. Whenever he asked "people who want babies and can't have them" to participate in a research study, he said, it was critical for them to "know that they're not being exploited—that everything that is being done is done in their interests and not just for an abstract research thing." Rock simply would not compromise on this point. The single-minded McCormick realized that she would have to accept it, but she neither liked nor understood what she considered his overscrupulous attitude.[54]

McCormick remained bemused by Rock's insistence that the study participants be treated as human beings with real problems. She was also frustrated by his demand for meticulous detail in the study of the various combinations of hormones. She just wanted results. Her letters to Sanger about Rock are by turns baffled and admiring. At one point she praised him for "being exacting about it [his research]—if it is not done right the results are not only useless but misleading." In theory she realized the importance of clinical accuracy, but she didn't always like it. "Dr. Rock is a martinet in his clinical work,—very demanding and not easily satisfied."[55]

Yet, Rock seemed to have a double standard by not insisting the entire study follow the rules he demanded in his own studies. While Rock was testing the progesterone formulations on his infertile patients in Brookline, Pincus inaugurated another study at Worcester State Hospital. Unlike Rock's subjects, all of whom were volunteers in the fullest sense, these subjects were mentally ill women (and even some men). This study was morally suspect and ethically questionable. Although Rock did not participate in it, he agreed to train the physician who conducted it. And although the families of the patients consented to the experiment, the patients were not consulted and were probably not competent to consent on their own behalf. Pincus seems not to have cared; in this era, the mentally ill were all too frequently made unwilling participants in medical research. Or he may have believed that the consent of the patients' families was enough. As for Rock, perhaps he did not want to intervene because they weren't his patients.[56]

Katharine McCormick did not care one way or another who the study participants were or what they thought. She just wanted the pill. She was truly single minded, and in her mind the pill was the most important thing in the world, which meant, of course, that she believed it should be the most important thing in the world to Pincus and Rock. Because of McCormick's enormous financial support for the WFEB, Pincus tended to cater to her and tell her what she wanted to hear. She had more trouble with Rock, but since he was the clinician making the medical decisions, she felt the need to exercise her influence with him, too, whenever possible, taking advantage of every minute of his that she could command. She once apologized to Sanger for refusing to take her long-distance call (in an era when long-distance phone calls were not an everyday matter), telling her later, Rock "had just come in when you telephoned, and I did not want to leave him for fear he would escape!"[57]

...

Rock didn't really understand what drove McCormick, and even if he had, he was unlikely to dance to her tune—at least not yet, and maybe never. He took his work on the pill seriously, but in the mid-1950s, it was still a relatively minor project for him. He remained far more focused on the problem of infertility. Frequently profiled during these years in popular magazines such as Look, Coronet, and Reader's Digest, he enjoyed an enviable reputation with the public and his colleagues.

Rock seemed to be everywhere in these years. Despite having lived with heart disease for a decade, he had the vigor, energy, and appearance of a man at least ten years younger than his sixty-plus years. Ever since his first heart attack, he had watched his health carefully—no salt, little fat, no tobacco. He had to give up smoking (addicted to a pipe, he now packed it with corn silk), but, he was grateful to learn, he did not have to give up his cocktails. Although these measures would not prevent additional coronary episodes, the regimen worked for him in the long run. His beloved twin, Nell, died shortly before the two of them would turn sixty-five, but he would live another thirty years.

And now, with the baby boom turning infertility into a national preoccupation, he was in the vanguard of a new specialty. His name was so firmly linked to the study of infertility that even though he had been working with Pincus for two years by 1954, Margaret Sanger was outraged to learn that Planned Parenthood had named him chair of its research committee. As she wrote to her old friend Abraham Stone, "Abram, Abram [sic] what has happened to you to allow the enemy to walk in the front door. You know as well as everyone knows that John Rock's interest is increasing the power of the fertility of the woman, and by no means giving his interest to the control of that function."[58] She knew Rock was working on the pill. She still didn't trust him.

The field in which Rock pioneered is now called reproductive medicine, but it was so new when its practitioners were creating its first professional organization that they weren't sure what to call their society. They settled on the rather prosaic American Society for the Study of Sterility. Founded in 1944, the group sought to claim the mantle of professional authority in all matters of fertility and reproduction. Today called the American Society for Reproductive Medicine, it was the first medical and scientific organization for specialists in fertility and infertility. Rock was one of thirty founding members.

The organization brought together some of the older pioneers in the field —including I. C. Rubin, who developed tubal insufflation, and early birth-control advocate Robert Latou Dickinson—with men of Rock's slightly younger generation and a sprinkling of more recently minted physicians. By the time of the society's second meeting, in 1946, the first woman had been admitted, and by 1950, there were eight women in a society that numbered just over a hundred. Among them were infertility specialist Sophia Kleegman of New York and Georgeanna Segar Jones of Johns Hopkins University. (In 1981 Georgeanna Jones and her husband, Howard Jones, would be responsible for the United States's first in vitro birth.)

When the society was founded, all its members were physicians and nearly all came from gynecology. Two years later, a few basic scientists—PhDs rather than MDs—were welcomed into the group, including Carl Hartman, late of the Carnegie Institution, who had recently joined the Ortho Research Foundation, and John MacLeod, an expert on semen analysis and "male factor" infertility. Still, membership remained heavily tilted toward gynecologists. In the early 1950s, only 7 percent of the physicians limited themselves to the treatment of male "sterility," and only 11 percent were from the basic sciences, as opposed to clinical research and practice.[59]

Over its first decade of existence, the society would define the new field. As the first national organization to focus specifically on reproductive questions across a range of disciplines, by the 1950s it increasingly brought together clinicians, medical researchers, and basic scientists. Its journal, *Fertility and Sterility*, was launched in 1950, with Rock as one of the authors of the first issue's lead article, "Dating the Endometrial Biopsy," an extension of the pioneering work Rock had originally performed with Marshall Bartlett in the 1930s. Coauthors this time were Rock, Robert Noyes, and Arthur Hertig. Their analysis included more than eight thousand biopsies conducted for more than a decade and confirmed Rock and Bartlett's earlier findings. The authors concluded that "examination of [the] endometrium during the secretory phase [the period after ovulation could be presumed to occur] gives more information about the time of ovulation, degree of progestational change, normality and abnormality of [the] endometrium than any other single test done in sterility studies." As late as 1994, this article was the most cited article from that journal.[60]

By 1955, the membership of the society had grown five-fold to more than five hundred (by 1960 it would have nearly a thousand members). In that same year, the society created the title of honorary vice president to recognize the accomplishments each year of one outstanding figure. John Rock was the first to be so honored.[61]

By this time Rock had been investigating and treating infertility for thirty years. During the Great Depression, his sterility and endocrine clinic had seen only about two hundred patients a year—the desperately infertile who tried various treatments year after year, waiting for a miracle, and women suffering from numerous disorders of the menstrual cycle. In those years Rock generally had one resident and a medical student under his direct supervision, and he would have loved to have devoted himself to problems of reproduction. But he couldn't—he could never have made a living. Medical practice, even for most specialists, was very different from what it is today. As late as 1944, Rock was still delivering babies. Not until his first heart attack that year did he stop doing obstetrics, and he never would completely give up general gynecology. Still, after World War II he was able to devote the majority of his time to what interested him most. In the baby boom that followed the war, his interest in fertility was matched by two things—a national preoccupation with having babies and an almost religious faith in the progress of medicine.

By the end of the 1940s, the Fertility and Endocrine Clinic, one of about half a dozen medical-school-affiliated infertility clinics in the United States, was generally regarded as the most important fertility research and treatment center in the nation.[62] After the war, its patient base had exploded to about two thousand a year, with most coming for infertility workups, and by 1954, it was adding patients at the rate of about two hundred a year. In the early years, most of the funding for the clinic had come from the hospital and some donations; after the war, grant funds for research in reproduction, although not for contraceptive research per se, came from the Committee for Research in Problems of Sex, the Committee on Human Reproduction, and the Carnegie Corporation. The pharmaceutical houses provided various hormonal preparations, experimental drugs, and the antibiotics used in several of the studies.[63]

In the words of sociologist Paul Starr, academic medicine "radically changed" in the postwar years. The federal government became a major funder of medical research, overshadowing although not completely eclipsing support from foundations and pharmaceutical companies. Although funding for research on reproductive questions lagged considerably behind other fields, there were new opportunities for both specialized practitioners and the young physicians who competed for residencies and staff positions with eminent authorities.[64] Rock was now one of the preeminent figures in the field at one of the preeminent universities in the nation.

At last, he could spend most of his time in reproductive medicine. His correspondence files beginning in the early 1950s bulge with letters from physicians across the country seeking advice and information on his surgical procedures.[65] By 1954 and 1955, doctors at infertility clinics, now sprouting up all over the nation, sought Rock's counsel; other medical schools sought to emulate Rock's Free Hospital clinic. Rock played host to scores of doctors who wanted to observe his clinic's methods and modes of operation.[66] With patient demand for infertility services booming, gynecologists in the United States and around the world were eager to have some knowledge of the new specialty. From Switzerland, Greece, and Latin America, young and established physicians sought to spend six months or a year at the Free Hospital to enhance their expertise in this area. Aloys Naville, a young Swiss physician, later wrote Rock that "the tremendous influence you had on me . . . changed my whole outlook on life."[67] And Rock served as a mentor to several young American doctors who would make up the next generation of specialists in reproductive medicine, including Celso-Ramon Garcia and Luigi Mastroianni, who in later years were partners in developing the program in reproductive medicine at the University of Pennsylvania.[68]

Hart Achenbach, Rock's son-in-law, worked with him in the early 1950s and remembers the clinic as an efficient operation. The nurse escorted each patient into the examination room and conducted the initial interview, took a blood pressure reading, and obtained a urine specimen. Next, one of Rock's fellows took the medical history, after which Rock entered the examining room. As he conducted the examination, he dictated his findings to the nurse.[69]

It bears repeating that during these years his work on the pill was only a small part of his vastly expanded research and clinical operation.[70] In 1954, even as McCormick lay in wait to capture a few moments of his time for what was most important to her—limiting births—his daily life was still taken up mostly with infertility problems. For nearly a decade he had enjoyed the assistance of a team of research fellows, in addition to the medical students who worked on research projects and the residents and young attendings who saw a significant proportion of the clinic patients and collaborated with him in research studies. Until 1952 there had only been one or two fellows a year, but there were three in 1953 and four in 1954. The fellows did everything. They assisted at surgery, took sperm counts, and did postcoital tests, often called PK tests, which involved examining sperm from a woman's vagina following intercourse. Overworked and no doubt often underappreciated, a number of the fellows from this era would go on to enjoy distinguished careers in the field of reproductive medicine, including Somers Sturgis and Herbert Horne as well as Garcia and Mastroianni.[71]

During the 1950s Rock wrestled most often with three problems: two in women, ovulatory disorders and tubal occlusions, and one in men, infertility caused by inadequate sperm production. For ovulatory disorders, he experimented with a host of hormonal preparations, for the most part without success. His own ongoing studies of the endometrium, particularly the use of endometrial biopsy, had helped to make ovulatory abnormalities easier to diagnose. Still, the therapeutic value of such knowledge in the short run was limited, since such dysfunctions remained difficult to treat. Some women did not ovulate at all, or only irregularly. In the 1930s and 1940s, Rock, like many of his colleagues, had made liberal use of animal gonadotropins, but he had become much more skeptical of their efficacy by the 1950s. And of course, his experiments with estrogen and progesterone, alone or in combination for both ovulatory disorders and unexplained infertility, had led him to Gregory Pincus.

He also treated some ovarian disorders surgically, such as those resulting from Stein-Leventhal syndrome (polycystic ovarian syndrome) or cyst formation caused by endometriosis. However, the patients rarely conceived. In one series of fifty-six ovarian resections between 1946 and 1958, only four of the women became pregnant. Many of his colleagues were even more cautious about surgery, which had taken a back seat to medical therapies since the 1920s, when endocrinology burst on the infertility scene. More surgery was done on women than on men, but even on women, among the most advanced infertility specialists, surgery was rarely the first resort.[72]

But surgery was hard to avoid in the face of damaged fallopian tubes. If the ovum and sperm could not meet in the tube, fertilization was impossible. By now Rock had abandoned the idea that he could make progress in in vitro fertilization and decided against any revival or modification of the Estes operation. So what could he do instead? Would a new surgical technique for reconstructing the tubes be feasible, he wondered?[73] In the past, even when a skilled surgeon could reconstruct and open a damaged tube, it would often close soon after the operation, before a pregnancy could be established. Overall, patients could expect about a 5 percent chance of conceiving after surgery.[74]

Rock was more optimistic about the efficacy of surgery than some of his colleagues, even if he often cautioned that only after a careful study "of all factors of fertility . . . and assiduous attention toward perfecting them—short of surgery—will a conscientious gynecologist" begin to consider resorting to the operating room.[75] Still, unlike many of his colleagues who had come into infertility treatment from endocrinology, he had trained as a surgeon. Even when surgical treatment of infertility went out of fashion in the 1930s and 1940s, he never gave up on it. He continued to perform diagnostic laparotomies, in spite of new diagnostic advances, such as the invention of the culdoscope, that would appear to have made them less necessary. Rock performed culdoscopy, but when it failed, he did not hesitate to employ the more complicated procedure.

For damaged fallopian tubes, surgery was a tempting proposition for both patient and practitioner. Many women specifically requested surgery because, as one gynecologist remarked, "there is always the patient in a 'hopeless case' who has children." The decision on whether to operate, insisted Harvard gynecologist Fred A. Simmons, should be left to the woman. Many physicians concurred. But some women, unfortunately, were unable to give up the idea of motherhood until they had been operated on repeatedly. Their doctors would often keep on agreeing to do so because they believed they could beat the odds. Rock hoped to find a method that would work at first try. Along with his junior colleague William Mulligan, whom he was grooming as his successor as director of the Fertility and Endocrine Clinic when Rock retired, he attempted to develop more effective tubal surgery. Mulligan, Rock, and another physician, Charles Easterday, developed a technique employing tiny tubing and "hoods" made out of a new plastic—polyethylene—that would be used to keep the fallopian tubes open after surgery.[76]

Rock was initially optimistic about this new technique, leading him to offer—even in advance of the study's publication—to send details of the procedure to colleagues in other parts of the country who inquired about the technique. When Texas gynecologist H. O. Padgett asked his advice about a specific case, Rock replied in some detail. "I still believe this to be a highly technical procedure," he said, "not yet standardized to the point where it can be confidently used by those who have not had a great deal of experience in tuboplasty." Nevertheless, he promised to send more detail, after which Padgett could decide whether he had the experience to try it. If Padgett did not want to do it himself and his patient could "bear the expense of a trip to Boston," Rock wrote, "I will be glad to operate on her in the Free Hospital, where she can pay if she is able, but will be charged nothing if she is not."[77]

Rock's high hopes notwithstanding, tubal surgery was rarely successful, with or without the plastic. Take the case of eighteen-year-old Mrs. S, who came to his clinic in 1953. Both fallopian tubes were blocked. Her first surgery was unsuccessful, and she returned again in 1955. Her youth made the doctors wish to try again. Once again they failed. Another woman who refused to give up for eight years also underwent two unsuccessful surgeries. Of the forty-eight women in one series of cases, only four got pregnant.[78]

. . .

Rock hated to see women undergo needless procedures and had often complained about men's unwillingness to come in for testing. The men's clinic Rock had organized in 1949 at the Free Hospital met on Saturdays, a day off for many men. This clinic was an acknowledgment of a renewed attention to male fertility problems, influenced in large measure by the baby boom ideology and optimism about medical progress. The imperative to treat male infertility was driven by another factor as well, a pervasive though unverifiable sense that the condition of combat during World War II had negatively affected male fertility. Soldiers had faced exposure to radiation and hazardous chemicals, as well as high scrotal temperatures, which researchers believed could have affected their production of sperm. Rock's records indicate that in the postwar period, the number of men receiving infertility treatments was increasing.[79]

Rock drew on his training in urology when he worked on the problem of infertility in men. Experimenting with almost every new treatment that came along, he also developed some of his own. He was one of the first practitioners to attempt sperm freezing. He also continued to work on his technique for concentrating semen for use in artificial insemination. During the 1950s, reproductive specialists attempted without success to come to some agreement on what exactly constituted male infertility. Everyone agreed that a man with a seminal emission of more than 2.5 cubic centimeters, a sperm count of at least 100 million sperm per cubic centimeter, and a high proportion of the sperm active and normally shaped, was fertile. And they agreed that a man with no sperm at all was sterile. But in between, disputes continued. When the American Society for the Study of Sterility had attempted to standardize diagnoses by providing guidelines in the late 1940s that set the fertility standard at 60 million sperm with 60 percent active and 75 percent normally shaped, its definition met resistance. Some clinicians believed infertility started at 80 million sperm, others argued for 40, and a few insisted that a man with only 20 million sperm per cubic centimeter, as long as most of them were normal and active, was fertile.[80]

If a woman married to a man suffering from untreatable sterility wanted to bear children, donor insemination was the only option. Donor insemination had been around since the late nineteenth century but remained controversial, although physicians in major urban centers tended to have more favorable attitudes than those in small towns and rural areas.[81]

Fertile women in infertile marriages drove the requests for donor insemination. Some religions approved its use, and others did not. Mainstream Protestant denominations, including the Episcopal Church, tended to be the most accepting, while Orthodox Judaism, Catholicism, and the Anglican Church remained opposed to its use. But even though his church condemned donor insemination, Rock had been using the procedure at least as early as the 1930s both in his private practice and in the clinic.

In the 1950s, there were no laws covering the issue. Not a single state prohibited, permitted, or regulated donor insemination. There were only a few legal cases, all arising from divorce. None made it to a level where a precedent could be set, and the courts took different positions. In one case, although the husband admitted to having consented to the procedure, his wife was declared an adulteress. In another, the child was declared illegitimate; nevertheless, the husband was required to pay support because his agreement implied a promise of support. These two cases spurred the American Society for the Study of Sterility to take its first controversial stand. Despite members' misgivings about its reception by Catholic doctors in the United States, at the society's 1955 business meeting, a resolution passed 79–8 declaring donor insemination an "ethical, moral, and desirable form of medical therapy," as long as a couple sought such a procedure, the physician found "a biologically and genetically satisfactory donor," and "careful study" by their doctor concluded that the "couple will make desirable parents." Moral and legal ambiguities notwithstanding, many couples viewed donor insemination as a medical solution to male sterility. An article in the *Medico-Legal Digest* in 1960 estimated the total number of children born through donor insemination at 50,000.[82]

After the war, although many men still resisted the idea that they might be the cause of their wives' inability to conceive, Rock's correspondence indicates that others were more than willing to undergo treatment if there was any hope of a cure. As an analogue to the idea that progesterone therapy for women with either immature reproductive organs or unexplained infertility might produce a rebound effect—the so-called Rock rebound—and promote conception after the treatment had been discontinued, men were given testosterone on the same principle. The testosterone, either in the form of testicular implants or injections of megadoses over several months, completely suppressed sperm production temporarily. The hope was that once the treatment was stopped, sperm production would rebound well beyond the pretreatment levels. The regimen had been successful in animal studies. The chief proponent of testosterone therapy was urologist Morris Heckel, who reported remarkable results in a series of cases. In the early 1950s, testosterone therapy was all the rage.[83] Rock was among the practitioners who conducted studies of testosterone therapy, but neither he nor other clinicians could replicate Heckel's results. Rock was more optimistic about new techniques of artificial insemination that would try to improve the fertilizing power of men with low sperm counts. He and his colleagues tried several methods. They centrifuged the semen, sometimes suspended it in solution, and tried various methods of placement (in the vagina, cervix, or different parts of the uterus).

Another technique that Rock favored in the early 1950s was one developed in the 1940s by James Whitelaw, which used a cap placed on the external cervical os (opening of the cervix). But by the middle of the 1950s, reporting on a comparative study of all the methods he had tried so far using both untreated semen and the washed and concentrated preparation, he and his collaborators reported that in the end, "simple vaginal placement of untreated semen was the most successful."[84]

Rock was also a pioneer in sperm freezing in the 1950s. Although it would not be fully perfected until the 1970s, cryopreservation would enable clinicians to take the process of separating the more active and vigorous sperm from the malformed or sluggish ones in cases of oligospermia one step further by making it possible to cull the most promising sperm from several ejaculates and use this augmented sample for insemination.[85] In these years Rock was claiming a success rate of 8 percent overall in cases of artificial insemination using the husbands' semen. (But not all artificial insemination was a response to male infertility, since the technique was also used to bypass a problem cervix.)[86]

For those men whose sperm seemed perfectly adequate, but where postcoital testing of their wives revealed that most or all of the sperm were not moving, he did not think that male infertility was the problem. Instead, he attempted antibiotic therapy on the women to treat a possible cervical infection.

These experiments proved about as inconclusive as the trials with polyethylene had on tubal blockages. With his research fellow Herbert Horne (known as "Trader" and later a prominent gynecologist in his own right), Rock gave women, whose cervical mucous seemed to be killing their partners' sperm, large doses of terramycin, one of the newly developed antibiotics. Of the thirty-five women treated with six grams of terramycin for three days preceding their expected day of ovulation, who had no other diagnosis for their infertility than what Rock called "poor or absent spermigration in women whose husbands' semen is normal," ten became pregnant, encouraging Rock to suggest that others might like to try the same method.[87]

Rock kept hammering at the problem, but the intractable nature of male infertility continued to vex him. In a rueful moment in the mid-1950s, Rock told an informal gathering of fellow physicians that he believed little progress had been made in the treatment of male infertility. With characteristic humor, he told his colleagues how he advised men to eat large amounts of lettuce (because of its high concentration of vitamin E), and after all, look how prolific rabbits are! He said he put men on diets, having read a study that lean dogs were more fertile than fat ones. He had given them vitamins. He had prescribed testosterone in doses large and small. He had injected gonadotropins (hormones capable of promoting gonadal growth and function) from various sources. He had given thyroid extracts. He had also tried the new steroids, he said, but was "shocked" to find they caused azoospermia and led to a disinterest and eventually the inability to engage in sexual activity, although "fortunately," he concluded, "the results were reversible." But no matter what he tried, he concluded regretfully, he had found few ways to help infertile men. After generations of research on the semen of bulls and boars, stallions and rams, he said, clinicians still knew "pitifully little that was of practical value" when treating men.[88]

· · ·

Although these questions occupied much more of Rock's time and energy than did the birth-control pill in the mid-1950s, he had not lost interest in the oral contraceptive. He remained involved but refused to be rushed unduly. McCormick could badger him all she wanted, but as far as he was concerned, she was just going to have to wait until he was satisfied that the time, the drug, and the proper testing location were right.

That said, right from the start he and Pincus were on the watch for appropriate sites for more extensive testing once they had found a suitable compound to test. In 1953, when Rock was conducting his first small-scale clinical trial of oral progesterone, Planned Parenthood's Paul Henshaw suggested setting up a trial in Jamaica.[89] Pincus demurred. Sanger wanted to let her friends in Japan and Hawaii do the trials, but Pincus and Rock were both reluctant. Pincus was holding out for Puerto Rico, and he finally persuaded Rock. Eventually McCormick came around as well, and by the summer of 1954, she was telling Sanger, "I had not thought of Puerto Rico at all seriously as you know but I may have to."[90]

All this was before they had a drug reliable enough to test on a sizeable population! Up through the end of 1954, Rock's clinical studies at the Free Hospital and Pincus's own (directed by Dr. Alexander Freeman) at the Worcester State Hospital were using progesterone, and some of the women still appeared to be ovulating even on the highest doses. But then, in late 1954, everything changed. Pincus and Chang became quite enthusiastic about the new compounds known collectively as the 19-nor-steroids.

These new drugs, which would be called progestins, were synthetic analogues to progesterone. In the body, it was hoped, they would have the same biological action. There were several, of which two seemed most promising in animal studies. The first was called norethisterone (now norethindrone). This one had been developed by Carl Djerassi and patented by Syntex. The other was norethynodrel. This one was Searle's formula, developed by Frank Colton.[91] Pincus and Chang thought the Syntex compound was slightly androgenic (causing the physical development of masculinizing characteristics) in rats. The Searle compound, they said, did not have that effect. What Pincus and Chang did not know at the time was that the Searle compound had inadvertently been adulterated with a small amount of estrogen, which likely caused the different activity.

Rock began to study both the Syntex and the Searle compounds in December 1954. In September 1955, he wrote to Searle's clinical research director Irwin C. Winter that he intended to report soon on his results with their product (which was then called SC-4642).[92] He wrote again a month later, telling Winter, "It [SC-4642] looks pretty good." Rock decided, therefore, to enlarge the numbers of women in his Brookline study in hopes of "more definitive results."[93] Winter was still not sure how he wanted to proceed. Before Searle expanded even its experimental use by providing the drug to other researchers, Winter said, he needed to understand more about the drug's safety and mode of action so that he could explain them to his colleagues at the company. His fellow scientists, Winter told Rock, remained puzzled about how the drug actually worked, and he did not understand it well enough to explain it to them.

Indeed, just how little was known of the action of the new 19-nor-steroids can be seen from some of the comments and questions Winter fielded. One researcher, for example, told Winter that he believed that Rock's early findings regarding endometrial changes using SC-4642 on four patients "might be interpreted as due entirely to an estrogenic effect." What did Rock think? "I very much doubt it," Rock replied, because "the change is in the progestational direction and not in the proliferative." In other words, he explained to Winter, the endometrial changes are "not characteristic of an estrogenic effect." When a woman was taking this drug, he explained, her uterus looked just like a uterus under the influence of natural progesterone. The fact that Rock was widely recognized as the preeminent expert on the endometrium, at a time when endometrial changes were the only sure way for clinicians to measure women's cyclic hormonal changes, gave his views great credibility.[94]

It was now the fall of 1955, and Rock had tested what would become the first birth-control pill on only *four* women. Not surprisingly, he did not want to commit himself publicly to any claims about its effectiveness.[95] Pincus, however, was not so reluctant. Based on these four cases, he was convinced that the oral contraceptive had been found. He even went so far as to announce its development to the world—or at least to the international birth-control movement—at the International Planned Parenthood Federation meeting in Japan in October 1955. Rock did not attend because McCormick had refused to finance his trip. Although she was willing to let Pincus go, she wanted Rock in Brookline overseeing the women taking the progestins.

When Rock learned what Pincus had done, he was furious. The publicity, he fumed, was vastly premature. He feared that Pincus's grandstanding would cause more harm than good.[96] Pincus was just being Pincus. His willingness to trumpet results before Rock thought it was prudent to do so would continue to vex the more circumspect clinician and remain a major cause of discord between them. Although Rock was willing to go along with Pincus and announce preliminary results of their research in *Science* in 1956, Rock wanted more data before declaring publicly that they had developed an effective oral contraceptive.

Pincus's willingness to stick his neck out, on the one hand, and Rock's caution on the other, would continue to cause friction in their working relationship, but that friction, resulting from their differing temperaments and working styles, probably also contributed to making theirs such a productive collaboration. McCormick, although she could be surprisingly blinkered in her understanding of both men, shrewdly assessed their importance to "her" project. Pincus was essential, she told Sanger, because "without [him], we should be stopped in our tracks." At the same time, she was absolutely convinced that "if anything should happen to Rock we should be in a predicament" because unlike any other clinician "he knows all the terrible practical difficulties that occur in the female reproductive system."[97] On the whole, she preferred Pincus's style, because his impatience more nearly matched hers, but she respected Rock's breadth of experience and knowledge, even though she found his caution annoying.

Rock's participation would become ever more critical as word of the pill trickled out to the medical profession. Rock held the title of clinical full professor at Harvard. He was an eminent medical researcher and practitioner. Gregory Pincus, brilliant as he was, had never entirely shaken his maverick reputation. His institutional home, the Worcester Foundation, was still viewed in some circles as an upstart institution. In spite of some exceptional research accomplishments, the foundation had not yet attained the distinction it would enjoy in the 1960s and beyond. And of course, Rock's reputation rested on his success in promoting human fertility, not repressing it. They also had very different personal qualities. Whether he was this way in fact or not, Pincus *seemed* impulsive and perhaps even rash. Rock, in contrast, whether he was this way in fact or not, appeared deliberative, cautious, and calm. His association with the pill research promoted its respectability.[98]

Rock's Catholicism cannot be ignored, either. When McCormick found out that Rock had not left the Church, she exclaimed, "How they [the Catholic Church] manage to put up with him I do not know!" But he was then and would remain a practicing Catholic who counted several priests among his friends.[99] His open avowal of his faith also confounded some opponents of contraception who were not sure what to make of his involvement. Criticizing someone like Rock, by now known to his patients, the public, and the medical establishment alike as a dedicated and caring physician who specialized in helping the childless to conceive, would be more difficult than criticizing Pincus, known to the public as the scientist most famous for creating "fatherless rabbits." Even Margaret Sanger came to view Rock as an asset to the program, in spite of her virulent anti-Catholicism.[100]

In general, Rock and Pincus worked well together in spite of their disagreements. Still, although Rock respected Pincus's scientific acumen, he said later that he found him "a little scary . . . He was not a physician and knew very little about the endometrium though he knew a great deal about ovulation."[101] This was a more damning observation at the time than it would be now. In the 1950s, being able to explain endometrial changes was perhaps one of the two most critical elements in understanding the process of reproduction.[102] In addition, perhaps because Pincus was not medically trained, he never completely acknowledged the complexities of dealing with research on human beings. What Pincus viewed as Rock's excessively scrupulous attitude about conducting drug tests on human subjects would be seen by others as one of Rock's positive attributes.

Rock's involvement reassured those who mistrusted Pincus's tendency to rush to judgment, a group that seems to have included some of the people at Searle, a few of whom remembered the cortisone fiasco. Rock knew that he would be forever linked to these new compounds, and he wanted to be absolutely assured both that they worked, which he had already come to believe, and that they would be safe, about which he was initially somewhat less sure.

Overall, however, Pincus and Rock were a good team. They met frequently to talk about the progress of the research. Soon, once Rock was satisfied that the new 19-nor-steroids prevented ovulation and did not appear to have deleterious effects on the female reproductive system, they would choose a place for larger trials. Pincus had rejected Jamaica. He and Rock, pressed by Sanger to let her Japanese friends conduct trials there, agreed privately that Japan, where they would be unable to monitor the work personally, would not be a good venue for their major trials. Pincus did agree to train a Japanese physician in their methods but had no intention of relying solely on his results. They were also willing to let Planned Parenthood physicians engage in a trial in Hawaii, but this never happened because the physicians refused to spend the time at the WFEB to learn the techniques that Pincus and Rock believed essential. In their own ways, Pincus and Rock were both perfectionists who knew that they would not have as much confidence in results reported by others as they would in their own. They were also facing reality, knowing as they did that once they proclaimed success, their every claim would be scrutinized and criticized. If they were to have confidence in the results, they would have to control the clinical trials.

Except among the desperately infertile, most women had little patience for participating in research where they had to take their temperatures, save their urine, come in for regular vaginal smears, and submit to the occasional endometrial biopsy. Taking the pills would be the easy part—it was the medical tests and evaluations that were onerous. Pincus had considered trials in Puerto Rico as early as 1953. It was close, with frequent and direct flights between New York and San Juan. He had good connections at the medical school of the University of Puerto Rico, in particular his friend David Tyler (brother of Los Angeles fertility specialist Edward Tyler). The faculty at the medical school was, as he called it, "American" trained—that is, had been educated on the mainland—so they and the Pincus-Rock group shared the same general scientific and medical assumptions. Puerto Rico also had another advantage. It was an American territory where birth control had been legal since 1937. In that year, an earlier law making it a felony to disseminate contraceptive information or devices had been repealed. There was a court challenge to the repeal, but the court decided to uphold the legality of contraception, with only one exception: contraception would remain illegal if prescribed for "social and economic reasons" rather than medical ones. However, "medical indication" for birth control was interpreted thereafter very broadly, since poverty and ill health often went hand in hand.[103]

Rock was a bit more cautious about Puerto Rico than Pincus was, since he continued to maintain that all the clinical trials should follow his full protocols and wasn't sure that could be guaranteed at such a distance. Rock not only wanted, as McCormick told Sanger, "ovulating *intelligent* subjects, . . . [who] can be relied upon to carry out the procedures," he also wanted to be there to know firsthand if they were doing what they were supposed to be doing. But he would never have given up his own work to supervise a field trial. So although he expressed his doubts to McCormick about getting the participants to do everything he wanted, he also told her that "he has great confidence in the men there and in the terrific need they face and are anxious to meet, so he thinks it is worth the try."[104]

After consulting with faculty and administrators at the University of Puerto Rico, Pincus and Rock designed a clinical study that would enlist women medical students and student nurses at the university as research subjects. But soon after they visited Puerto Rico to set up the study, things began to go wrong. Students failed out, dropped out, and were too busy to save their urine, come in for smears, or take their temperatures. Many of them found the whole regimen simply too inconvenient. The researchers at the university next approached a women's prison. Initially, some of the prisoners agreed to participate, although whatever may constitute "agreement" by inmates can hardly be the same as agreement by nonincarcerated people. But then they changed their minds, and the project could not proceed.[105]

Very soon, however, another opportunity presented itself. Pincus was ready, and in early 1956 Rock also agreed that the new progestin compounds were ready for larger field trials. McCormick breathed a sigh of relief, telling Sanger how "encouraging" it was "to have John Rock so enthusiastic."[106] One of the most controversial field trials in twentieth-century pharmaceutical history was about to begin.

Edward Doisy. In 1923 Doisy, working with Edgar Allen, produced estrogen, which was called at first the ovarian hormone. Six years later, Doisy isolated estrogen in a pure crystalline form. Courtesy of the National Library of Medicine.

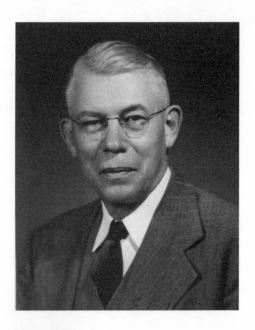

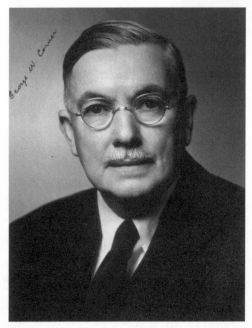

George Corner. In 1929 Corner, then of the University of Rochester, led the team that produced the first "corpus luteum extract," which would later be called progesterone. In 1940 Corner succeeded George Streeter as the director of the Department of Embryology at the Carnegie Institution of Washington. Courtesy of the National Library of Medicine.

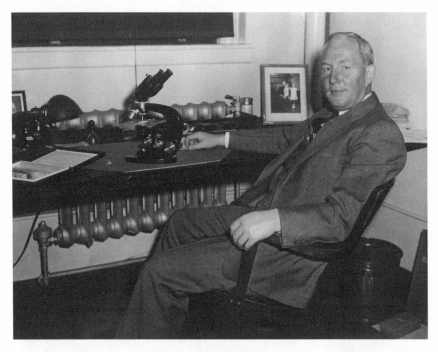

Arthur Hertig, who collaborated with Rock on the embryo studies, in an undated photograph (probably late 1950s or early 1960s). Courtesy of Rachel Achenbach.

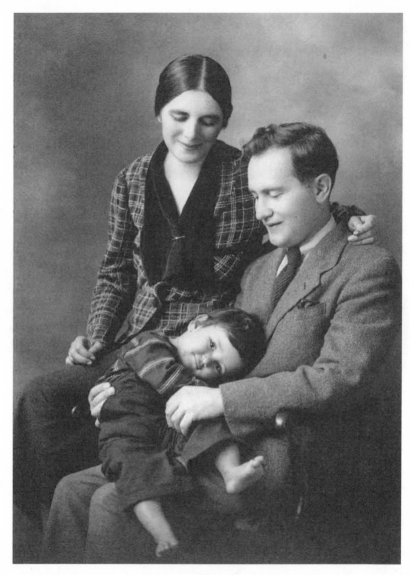

Miriam Menkin, Rock's laboratory technician and collaborator on the in vitro fertilization studies, shown here in the 1930s with her husband, Valy, and son, Gabriel.
Courtesy of Gabriel Menkin.

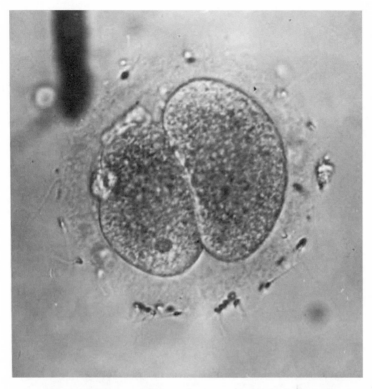

Original photograph from the first successful in vitro fertilization of human eggs, 1944. This one is in the two-cell stage and was one of four eggs success-fully fertilized in vitro by Rock and Menkin. The notation on the back is in Menkin's handwriting. Courtesy of Rachel Achenbach.

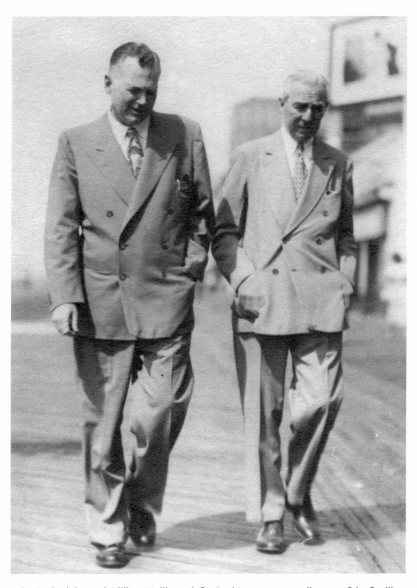

John Rock (right) and William Mulligan (left), Rock's successor as director of the fertility and endocrine clinic at the Free Hospital for Women, sometime in the late 1950s. Courtesy of Rachel Achenbach.

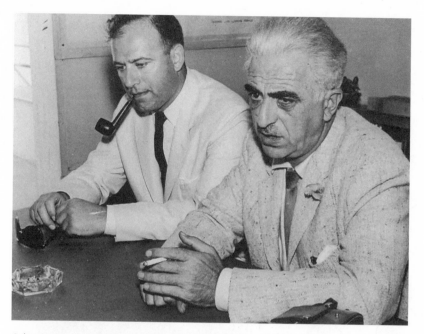

Celso-Ramon Garcia (left) and Gregory Pincus in the early 1960s. Courtesy of the Department of Obstetrics and Gynecology of the University of Pennsylvania School of Medicine.

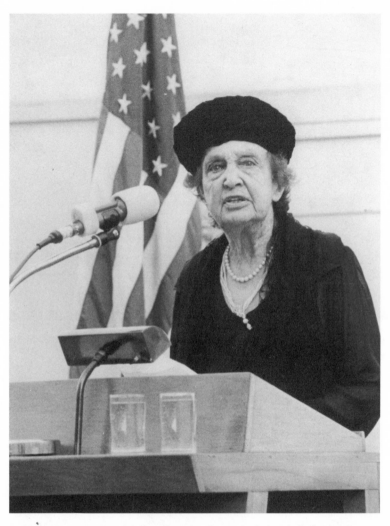

Katharine Dexter McCormick (in 1963), who almost single-handedly funded the development of the oral contraceptive. Courtesy of the MIT Museum.

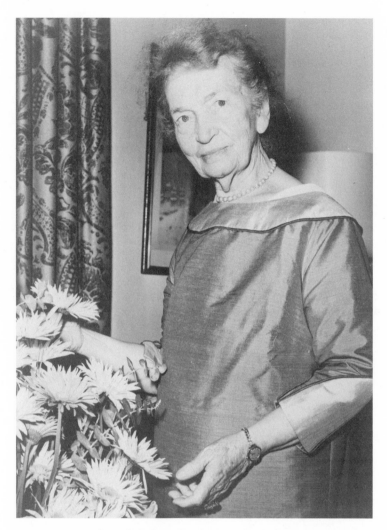

Margaret Sanger, the nation's foremost advocate of birth control, in 1961.
Sanger and McCormick have been called "the mothers of the pill." Courtesy of
the Library of Congress.

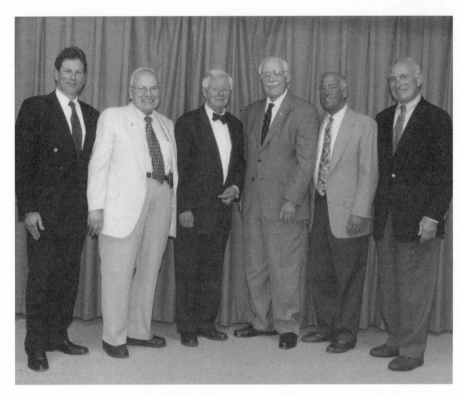

From left to right, Jack Ludmir, Celso-Ramon Garcia, Luigi Mastroianni, John Mikuta, Robert Israel, Edward Wallach, June 2002, on the occasion of the annual S. Leon Israel Lecture, delivered by Mastroianni, entitled "Ethical Issues in Assisted Reproduction." Robert Israel is S. Leon Israel's son; Edward Wallach had once been a fellow under Gregory Pincus; John Mikuta is a gynecological oncologist; Garcia and Mastroianni are two of Rock's most distinguished protégés, and Jack Ludmir, who trained under Garcia and Mastroianni, is Wanda Ronner's department chair at Pennsylvania Hospital. Courtesy of Jack Ludmir.

Chapter 7

THE ERA OF THE PILL BEGINS

Brookline, Massachusetts, 1955. Forced at age sixty-five into mandatory retirement from Harvard and the Free Hospital for Women, John Rock decides to found his own reproductive study center.

Rio Piedras, Puerto Rico, 1956. Field trials of the oral contraceptive, directed by Edris Rice-Wray, MD, begin on April 1.

Washington, D.C., 1960. The Food and Drug Administration approves Enovid as the first oral contraceptive, available only by prescription at a cost of ten dollars per month.

The inauguration of the oral contraceptive field trials in early 1956 opened a new chapter in John Rock's life. But before that could happen, he had to deal with an unwelcome, though inevitable, transition in his professional life. Harvard University had a mandatory retirement policy—no exceptions—and John Rock reached the milestone of age sixty-five in 1955. Thirty years before, he had become director of the sterility clinic at the Free Hospital for Women and over the course of three decades had turned it into the nation's leading fertility clinic. He had known retirement loomed, of course, and the Free Hospital had even allowed him to designate a successor—his protégé Bill Mulligan, who had already taken over nearly all his surgery cases. But still, it was a difficult transition. Here he was, at the peak of his influence in the field of fertility research and practice, forced into what Katharine McCormick referred to as a "hovel" in order to continue his work.[1] Over the next few years, it would become increasingly evident that the Free Hospital did not relish having to compete with Rock's new enterprise. Rock was not, however, going to be herded into the pasture without a fight. And for the moment at least, he had McCormick and her millions in his corner.

Leaving his lifetime professional home was not the only difficult transition Rock was facing as 1955 came to an end. He was grieving over the loss of his beloved twin sister, Nell, who had died on March 10, two weeks before their sixty-fifth birthday. Born within minutes of each other, John and Nell had spent much of their childhood in each other's company. They remained close. She had been dogged by ill health since the 1930s, and—as he had done for Charlie—Rock watched over her medical care. At least Nell, unlike Charlie, had survived her first major stroke. But while her end did not come totally unexpectedly, Rock felt as if he had lost a part of himself. He grieved in private, as he had for his son. He did have one confidant in this sadness, however, one of his cousins. Once Lizzie Rock, now Elizabeth Quirk, she had grown up with them in Marlborough. Writing Rock a few months after Nell's passing, she said that his description of his sister's last days "helped me to be more reconciled to [her] death."[2]

John kept up a steady correspondence with Elizabeth, who remained a beloved link to his past. He still felt close to her, even though she lived in Florida and he rarely saw her. Elizabeth made up a bit for the loss of Nell, perhaps for family more generally. He remained estranged from his older sister, Maisie. He did keep in touch with the ever-good-natured Harry, but Harry was no substitute for Charlie, dead now these fifteen years. The two surviving brothers did not have a great deal in common. Harry was the only one among the siblings not to cut ties with Maisie and Delia, so John could always be sure of hearing about them whether he wanted to or not. John continued to miss Charlie, who had been more of a father to John than Frank ever was.

If Charlie had been John's mainstay in the family, John had been Nell's. Since childhood, John had assigned himself to be her confidant and protector. And now Charlie and Nell were both dead, and Maisie might as well have been, as far as he was concerned. John wished that the hated Delia would get out of his life too, but she was still a presence. His sense of obligation to his father led him over the years to respond to her requests for physician referrals, and even for financial assistance, but beyond that, he had as little to do with her as possible. He would rejoice openly when she died.[3]

Once Nell was gone, Rock's emotional ties became even more centered on Nan, their children, and the grandchildren. All their daughters were grown now, and all except Ellie were married, with children of their own. Their empty nest freed Nan to travel with Rock even more often to conferences and on lecture tours, particularly when they took him away for more than a few days. The summers brought them at least a month's vacation, often with daughters, sons-in-law, and grandchildren coming and going.

Rachel, the eldest of the children, shared her father's enormous energy and his dry sense of humor. She had a no-nonsense approach to life, an attitude he valued and strove to project himself.[4] Her husband, Hart Achenbach, whom she had married in 1948, had been one of Rock's fellows, and he would go on to have a long and productive career as a general surgeon. Rachel, a skilled cytologist and the mother of a growing family, was working with her father and his associates on several projects, including the progesterone studies.

A. J. and her husband Hank Levinson had moved to New York. Very close to her mother, A. J. had chosen Nan's alma mater, Bryn Mawr, for college. Martha had attended Wheelock College, but then she had married a man, Rock told a colleague, who had developed a mental illness and become a danger to the children. Martha, in effect, was a single parent.[5] His youngest, Ellie, had attended the University of Chicago but never graduated. (She spent too much time on good works, Rock later complained, and not enough time on her studies.) She also worked for Rock on and off in the mid to late 1950s and had a strong spiritual bent; she became active in Opus Dei, the ultraconservative and now controversial Catholic society. Her father seemed bemused by what he called her "sacerdotal obligations, which start with Mass every morning and, I daresay, end with prayers for her sinful relations at whatever . . . hour she finally turns in." She also apparently had quite a temper, which Rock found difficult to handle. Having hired her to manage his office for a time in the late 1950s, he was troubled by her moodiness.[6]

Rock had not encouraged any of his daughters to take up medicine, telling them he did not really approve of women physicians. Still, he did not always behave as he claimed to believe, praising those women physicians whom he thought especially gifted, such as New York infertility specialist Anna Southam. Rock publicly lauded Southam's accomplishments, referred numerous patients to her, and sponsored her for membership as a fellow in an exclusive and heavily male medical society. Rock also accepted women fellows in his clinics at a time when it was difficult for them to acquire experience in areas of specialization, such as Rock's, that were dominated by men.[7] His first "official" woman fellow, Lillian G. Wheeler, came in 1946, and there were several more in the 1950s. He continued, however, to insist that as a general rule, women did not have the temperament to be doctors.[8]

Rock never shed his conventional attitudes toward women, even though his own experiences should have suggested to him that his views were too simple. After all, Nan had an unconventional streak, with her intellectual interests in physics and mathematics and her adventurous youth. Even as a wife and mother, she occasionally worked outside the home to round out the family income, particularly during those early years when Rock was building his practice and his reputation. But she never had a career and considered her role to be supportive of his. The Rocks raised their daughters to follow their mother's path rather than his.

. . .

The field trials of the pill began on April 1, 1956. Pincus was the organizational genius behind the trials. Rock served as medical director, charged with designing the research protocols, overseeing the data sent back to the Free Hospital, and supervising the study of tissue samples and biopsies. Rock traveled to Puerto Rico relatively frequently, but he did not directly oversee the medical examinations conducted on the island. That task fell to a young physician who had come to Brookline in 1955.

Celso-Ramon Garcia would become a leading expert in reproductive medicine. He grew up in New York and majored in chemistry at Queen's College, after which he entered medical school, completing his MD in 1945. He started out in pathology but quickly moved to obstetrics and gynecology. In 1955 he was thirty-three years old and for two years had been an assistant professor of obstetrics and gynecology at the University of Puerto Rico. Gregory Pincus recruited him to work on the first of the pill trials, the ones that never got off the ground. Garcia was then selected for the highly sought-after Sydney Graves Fellowship at the Free Hospital.[9] Garcia supervised the trials from Brookline. In Puerto Rico, day-to-day operations were the responsibility of Edris Rice-Wray, an American-trained physician with a graduate degree in public health, who at the time was medical director of the Family Planning Association of Puerto Rico, and Iris Rodriguez Pla, a social worker.[10]

By this time Rock was working out of a building provided by Harvard and located on the grounds of the Free Hospital. He called his new operation the Rock Reproductive Study Center and hoped that in creating a research and clinical facility adjacent to the hospital, and continuing to work closely with the medical staff there, he would not have to disrupt either his research or his patient care. This was the facility McCormick routinely described as "the hovel," or "that miserable little building." She regularly expressed anger that Harvard and the Free Hospital would put such a distinguished researcher in so dismal an environment. But she kept her eyes firmly on her own holy grail, the oral contraceptive, and put nearly $100,000 (more than $750,000 today) into renovations to the building. Rock did not complain about his situation and chose to make the best of it.[11]

It was frustrating for Rock to reorganize his professional life just at a time when, for the first time in his entire career, significant funding was available for the kind of research he conducted. Although Harvard did not pay him a regular salary, and his income from the Free Hospital remained negligible, he could now count on funding from both the drug companies and the federal government for some of his projects. The funds helped to support technicians and fellows and paid some of his salary, although most of his income came from his private practice. Luckily for him, during the baby boom his private practice had grown seemingly exponentially, so that even he, a physician who never seemed to care whether his patients actually paid their bills or not, could command a good living.

Rock was not at all concerned that leaving the directorship of the clinic would affect his private practice, but he was worried that he could lose momentum in his research. The "artificial" hormones, he believed, would open up new contraceptive options and treatments for infertility. How to induce ovulation was still as critical an issue for Rock as how to suppress it, and he became especially interested in the prospect of an oral contraceptive for men, which he believed would be just as important as the one they were developing for women. How vexing for him that just now, when a host of new compounds were pouring from the pharmaceutical labs, that he had to find a new institutional home.[12]

When these first field trials began, Rock had no idea how much the pill would eventually dominate his life. From their inception, the trials sparked controversy. Even a half-century later, disagreement continues to swirl around the entire process of the pill's clinical testing and approval for sale, in part because of its enormous ongoing cultural impact. The Puerto Rican field trials have often been used as a paradigmatic account of how villainous researchers took advantage of illiterate, impoverished women, duping them into taking drugs that no one knew were safe. The women, so the story goes, were powerless human guinea pigs, taken advantage of by arrogant doctors and soulless businessmen, shabbily treated and ignorant of the risks they were taking, who suffered so that affluent American women could have the benefit of freedom from pregnancy.[13]

True, false, or a bit of both? That is a complicated question. It *was* true that the women in the trials were poor, and some were illiterate. And it was true that the researchers did not know for sure how safe it was to take such drugs for a long period, since no one had done so. And it was also true that many of these women, mothers of more children than they wished for, were desperate for a workable form of birth control that their husbands or partners either would agree to let them use or that they could use clandestinely.

The first women to take the pill came from families who had recently moved into new publicly funded housing in Rio Piedras. Because this housing was highly desirable, and families lucky enough to be living here intended to stay for a while, the study would have a stable population who could be closely monitored as the study progressed. Women accepted for the study had to be under age forty, with one or more children, and obviously neither pregnant nor surgically sterile. The plan was to have 100 participants and another 100 controls, although Rice-Wray actually put 125 women in the initial control group with the idea that at least a hundred of them would "match" the study group in terms of age, years married, and number of pregnancies and live births.[14]

Keeping track of this group of matched women proved difficult. Women who were not taking the drug had few incentives to stay involved in the project. After a few months, Rice-Wray decided she could more confidently count on women who had once been participants to continue to provide the needed information, so she told Pincus that she would use their data as the control data. Her decision was later characterized as an attempt to mislead the Food and Drug Administration (FDA), but Rice-Wray's decision was neither sinister nor illogical, and surely not, as investigative journalist Barbara Seaman later charged, the height of irresponsible medicine.

The controls in this case were matched with study participants so that the researchers could assess the reproductive patterns of women of similar age and parity as the study participants. These women were not clinical controls in the way that we think of controls used for contemporary double-blind trials. Seaman seems genuinely to have misunderstood the difference between matched and clinical controls, and she further misunderstood the timing of their selection, reporting (incorrectly) that the selection of these matched controls came late in the study, after the Searle Company had submitted its application to the FDA. According to Seaman, it was the FDA that insisted on a "control group . . . and when the recruiter at the Family Planning Association in Rio Piedras could get no volunteers, Pincus instructed her to re-label the drop-out folders as 'controls.'" Seaman believed this was a deliberate attempt to mislead the agency, but she misread Rice-Wray's actions.[15]

Pincus, Sanger, and McCormick all believed that conducting large-scale trials among women here would predict the worldwide acceptability of the pill. Pincus viewed the overcrowding and poverty of the island as one of its advantages as a testing site. If Puerto Rican women could successfully use the pill, he reasoned, impoverished women throughout the world could be expected to follow suit. (Critics of the Puerto Rican trials make the same point but use it as evidence of the reprehensible behavior of the scientists and physicians who tried this drug out on indigent and "ignorant" people.)

Pincus was correct in surmising that women in Puerto Rico would welcome the pill, but he was wrong about the reasons. The pill trials, as Rock would later remark to several friends, worked not because Puerto Rico *was* a typical underdeveloped society, but because it *wasn't*. As long ago as 1940, as Annette Ramirez de Arellano and Conrad Seipp have noted, the health and economic prospects of the island's residents were improving. This in turn led the island's inhabitants to become not just "aware of new possibilities but . . . sensitized to the kind of rational calculation necessary to take advantage of them." With more and more children living to adulthood, Puerto Ricans had become "receptive to the idea of family planning." By the mid-1950s, these authors concluded, "a comprehensive strategy for remaking Puerto Rico into a modern society [had] evolved."[16]

The controversy over the field trials began almost the minute the first woman swallowed a pill. Because Puerto Rico was claiming its own identity, having had home rule for almost a decade, its leaders and journalists, as well as its people, were sensitive to incursions from the mainland. Within weeks of the trial's start, El Imparcial, a popular newspaper, accused the project's sponsors of conducting a "neomalthusian campaign," and local doctors told their patients that the pill was dangerous.

Once Rice-Wray learned of the story, she quickly informed Pincus that a newspaper reporter had discovered the project and published a damning article. The reporter claimed that under his pointed questioning, Rice-Wray had "confessed" to Dr. Juan A. Pons, the secretary of health, that she was involved in the program. Pons, the reporter continued, condemned the Family Planning Association for employing "public officials of the State" in a "neomalthusian campaign," and for using the "State Government . . . as bait for contraceptive campaigns of private agencies."

Referring to the journalist's attack as the "excitement," Rice-Wray admitted that she was somewhat worried about Pons's reaction, since "after all, he is my boss," and it was an election year. She was relieved that Pons did not call her on the carpet, and she was pleased to receive the support of another cabinet official (Rivera Santos, the secretary of agriculture), who told her, "If they start putting any pressure on you let me know. You are not alone. We will back you up." But her problems did not dissolve. At least one doctor in the municipal dispensary was telling the patients that the pill was "no good."[17] The negative publicity caused some women to drop out of the study, but Rice-Wray had a long waiting list, and new participants were quickly enrolled.

Rice-Wray's relief was premature. Eight months into the trial, she was forced out of her position and had to leave the island to find another job. Her successor, Dr. Manuel Paniagua, would also face accusations that he and the other researchers were using Puerto Rican women as if they were experimental animals. Eventually, in an effort to counter the accusations, Paniagua appeared on television in a program sponsored by the Family Planning Association of Puerto Rico. Deliberately playing the devil's advocate, the interviewer told Paniagua, "Around here they say that these pills have been used only in animals in the United States and only here have they been given to women. Is this so?" "Completely false," declared the doctor, and to another ostensibly pointed question, "Would you give this pill to your daughter?" Paniagua was able to respond not only that he would do so, but also that many American doctors were giving it to their own family members as well.[18] (Indeed, as early as 1957, Pincus was personally sending pills to his young married relatives.)[19]

These criticisms reflected the island's complex reality. The Catholic Church, of course, opposed the pill trials, but so did some in the newly emergent, democratically elected government. This antagonism toward the pill trials may have had as much to do with the growing sense of autonomy of the island as with the belief that poor women were offered what some officials considered an inadequately tested drug to control their fertility. Without denying that the conduct of the pill trials would not be compatible with our present-day conduct of clinical trials, we do not believe they were either immoral or unethical according to accepted standards of the era. Rock and Garcia designed the same protocols for the women of Puerto Rico as Rock had used for his own patients in Brookline. In spite of slip-ups in the field, the researchers strove to adhere to Rock's instructions.[20]

Nominally Catholic, Puerto Rican women did not always share their church's views on contraception, but there was still some wariness about open defiance of the Church. Before the pill, sterilization—la operacion—was probably the most common form of birth control in Puerto Rico. It was a sin, but it was only one sin, to be confessed and have forgiven. Once forgiven, a woman was freed from both further sin and further childbearing. With almost every reversible form of birth control, in contrast, a woman committed sin repeatedly. But a pill seemed different. After all, when a woman inserts a diaphragm or a man puts on a condom, it is pretty clear what is about to happen, and what consequences are being prevented. But if a woman took a pill every morning, that did not necessarily mean she planned to have sex in the evening. Sophistry? Perhaps, but it salved the conscience.[21]

It is patronizing to characterize the women who chose to take the pills, or to participate in other birth-control studies, as unwitting dupes. Just because women are poor, or illiterate, does not mean they are unintelligent or unable to make rational choices. As historian Lara Marks recounted, at least in the experience of Adeline Satterthwaite, the field physician in the second of the two Puerto Rican trials, the women she attempted to enroll in her studies "argued with the doctor or quit if they did not get their way."[22] And just because Pincus, Sanger, and McCormick believed these women to be ignorant as well as impoverished doesn't mean that the scientist and the two feminists did not also firmly believe in the pill's safety and efficacy. (Pincus otherwise would not have liberally handed out the pills to his own family members.)

To assert that the women in the field trials were not victims of medical perfidy, however, is not to say that the experiments were free of risk. In fact, even as the researchers geared up to begin work in Puerto Rico in early 1956, Rock and Garcia were still in the midst of completing a study of fifty women at the Free Hospital. Rock, although he now was convinced that both SC-4642 (the Searle compound) and SN-759 (the Syntex preparation) were effective and *believed* they were harmless, still had some concerns about the effect of long-term use.[23]

. . .

The women in the pill trials were not very different in their economic and marital difficulties from many of the women Rock had treated over the years at the Free Hospital, those thousands of poor and overly fertile women whose reproductive systems had been damaged from repeated childbearing. Río Piedras resident Señora J. G. was only thirty years old when she began taking the oral contraceptive in 1956, but she already had ten children, the oldest sixteen and the youngest just ten months. Her husband drank heavily and insisted on daily intercourse but claimed to be too ill to work. She supported the family by doing "odd jobs" and was delighted to have access to the pill, which she took faithfully, asserting that she "had no reactions" and was "very happy with the results." Señora H. A. was just two years older and had only half as many children, but her husband was frequently hospitalized for mental illness. Reading between the lines of officialese, we gather that he posed an actual danger to the children. Señora A. was unwilling to leave her husband, and since he refused to allow her to be sterilized, she asked for the pill as well. Women in these situations could not count on their husbands to take responsibility—not for contraception, not for much of anything. Both Sanger and Rock, from their different vantage points, would certainly have drawn satisfaction from the success of the pill in enabling women like these to stop having children.[24]

From the start, the Puerto Rican trials confirmed Rock's conviction that the 19-nor-steroids prevented ovulation, but he continued to be concerned about their potential long-term effect on the ovary. So Rock insisted, against Pincus's wishes, that a comparative study of the ovaries of treated and untreated women be undertaken. Worried that the drug might reduce the production of ova in the future, he wanted to be sure there were no follicular changes in the ovary itself. And so that same year, just as the Rio Piedras trials were under way, Rock conducted a study among a small group of patients at the Free Hospital, using the Syntex compound SN-759. He was satisfied with the results, but the numbers were small—only nine women.[25]

At least one respected researcher in the field of clinical hormone research, Robert Greenblatt, attempted to reassure Rock that the ovary would not be damaged by the pill. Greenblatt knew the ovary about as well as Rock knew the endometrium. (In 1961, Greenblatt would make reproductive history with his discovery that clomiphene citrate could induce ovulation, and he also conducted pioneering work in the United States on the use of human menopausal gonadotropin for the same purpose.) Greenblatt was convinced that the small-scale results Rock reported from Brookline would hold up under further scrutiny. "As to [your] fears that continuous administration of progesterone-like substances might cause damage to the ovaries, we may be able to put [your] conscience to rest," he said publicly. His own experience led him to "believe that the small doses of progesterone-like substances employed by Dr. Rock will not cause ovarian damage." Greenblatt's assurances carried significant weight with Rock.[26]

Still, Rock believed that he ought to make sure for himself. He would begin a second study the following year, comparing ovarian tissue from untreated women in their twenties and thirties with that of women who had taken the pill. For the first group, he intended to use two sources. One would include women at the Free Hospital undergoing laparotomy for various conditions; they could relatively easily have a biopsy of one of their ovaries taken. If a patient was having a hysterectomy, common practice was to remove one of the ovaries, so in such cases the entire ovary could be studied. A second group, he hoped, would come from one of the clinics in Puerto Rico performing tubal ligations. The surgeon in charge had agreed to perform ovarian biopsies on women requesting sterilization who had not taken the pill. They would constitute the controls.

Performing ovarian biopsies on women taking the pill was a bit more complex, but not impossible. Several Rio Piedras women were participating in the trials of the pill while they waited to be admitted to the hospital for a tubal ligation. Demand for la operacion remained strong in the mid-1950s, which meant that women sometimes waited months for their surgeries. Rice-Wray told Pincus in late 1956 that "we are watching for any of our cases who request sterilization so we can send them to Dr. Carasquillo." The samples would be sent back to Rock for comparison with the untreated ones.[27]

Rice-Wray submitted her first (and, as it would turn out, last) full-scale report in January 1957. While this report was not able to address Rock's concern about the pill's possible impact on the ovaries, it did confirm that the pill was a highly effective contraceptive. At the end of 1956, the project had data on 221 women who had taken the pill, without a single pregnancy that could be caused by, as Rice-Wray put it, "method failure." In terms of providing other data, however, these women were not always "compliant," to use the word doctors favor when talking about patients' decisions about following (or not) medical instructions. Sometimes they failed to save their urine for testing. An even larger number resisted coming in for endometrial biopsies. (Of twenty-two biopsies scheduled, doctors succeeded in getting fourteen.) The procedure was unpleasant, but in addition to women being "afraid of the examination," Rice-Wray told Pincus, they often had "no one with whom to leave the children."[28]

Rice-Wray's most serious negative finding, and one which in different circumstances might easily have jeopardized the whole project, was that almost 23 percent of the original group, and 17 percent of the entire number, had significant unpleasant side effects. Dizziness and nausea were the most common, but headaches and vomiting ran a close second. Half the women who experienced these reactions did so in the first three months, but in the remainder, the problems came anywhere from the fourth to the eighth month. Twenty-five of the women withdrew from the study because of the reactions, leading Rice-Wray to conclude that although the compound "gives 100% protection against pregnancy" when taken according to directions, "it causes too many side reactions to be acceptable generally."[29]

Pincus was not to be cowed. He simply disregarded Rice-Wray's conclusion that the side effects were too great a drawback. The expert on rats and rabbits diagnosed the human reactions as psychosomatic. He ignored the bad news and reacted with unalloyed elation—the pill worked, and that was all he cared about. But Pincus was not a physician. Rats and rabbits, after all, can't complain if they have headaches or nausea. Rock took the complaints more seriously. Some of the symptoms were known reactions to estrogen. And nausea, which pregnant women often experience, could also have been a reaction to the progestin. Perhaps, he said, getting rid of what was then called the estrogen "contaminant" would eliminate some of the more severe reactions. Without the estrogen, some side effects did diminish, but participants experienced more breakthrough bleeding. Bleeding as a side effect would surely deter widespread acceptance of the pill for contraceptive use. It was decided to put the estrogen back in and standardize the amount, and to provide participants with an antacid for the nausea. The nausea did decrease, but neither it nor the other side effects were eliminated in the original 10 milligram pill. They remained a serious problem.

Dramatically reduced dosages would eventually minimize many, but not all, of these kinds of reactions. For the short term, however, women who had side effects either learned to live with them or stopped taking the pill. Because the desire for contraception was so great among the women of Rio Piedras, replacing those who went off the pill because of the side effects posed few difficulties.

Rice-Wray left Puerto Rico soon after she filed this report. Although not fired outright, she was "forced to resign," as she put it. "It's obvious that I caused Dr. Pons too much discomfort," she told Pincus. "I was told by someone on the inside, 'They respect you but they are afraid of you.'" Rice-Wray next accepted a position with the World Health Organization and moved to Mexico, and Manuel Paniagua took over.[30] But she had not soured on the birth-control pill and would later assist Pincus and Rock in developing a field trial in Haiti. Even after what had happened to her in Puerto Rico, she was still willing to take a risk. "I can't be involved in Birth Control activities until the member nations give us the green light . . . Also I am there [in Haiti] to work on my job and not do something else." Despite danger to her livelihood once again, however, she believed so strongly that poor women should have access to the pill that she continued clandestinely to support the pill trials.[31]

Pincus's cavalier dismissal of the significance of the pill's side effects was just one example of his rather casual attitude overall about human experimentation. This was not the only time he played down problems that his clinical colleagues took more seriously. A few years later, Rock would complain to a Searle scientist about being kept in the dark by Pincus about some Searle compounds sent to Brookline from Worcester for testing on humans without, in Rock's view, a full disclosure of their properties and possible effects. Having tested one of Pincus's compounds, taking at face value that the safety studies were in order, Rock told I. C. Winter that "we had two very unpleasant reactions" and he was unwilling to do this again. Winter responded, "I share your scruple in this regard, and we here have long been disturbed by the apparent casualness with which materials go from Dr. Pincus's animals to your patients."[32]

In this instance, Pincus had asked Rock to test a compound without providing complete data on the formula or its possible toxicity. Winter confirmed Rock's fears about these particular compounds. They had indeed not gone through Searle's "quite elaborate procedure involving both Biological and Clinical Divisions [of Searle] prior to their release for administration to humans." Winter, in fact, "did not know" whether the drugs were safe.[33]

Rock's public caution about the pill masked to some degree his growing confidence that it worked and was harmless; nevertheless, he wanted to be sure and continued to insist that the researchers explore diligently every possible potential flaw in the new compounds before reporting success. In expressing these views, he was mindful of both his own legacy in reproductive medicine and his hopes for the future development of new and even better contraceptives. Proven efficacy and long-term safety of the pill, he believed, would guard against complaints by fellow researchers and physicians that Pincus and Rock had been overly quick to report success.

And critics there surely were, right from the start. One of the earliest and most vocal was Carl Hartman, by the mid-1950s the research director at Ortho Research Foundation. Rock and Hartman had known each other since the early days of the Rock-Hertig study, when Hartman was a scientist for the Carnegie Institution. One of the leading experts in reproduction in nonhuman primates, Hartman was a laboratory scientist, like Pincus, not a clinical researcher. This was not the first time he had been critical of Rock's work; he now argued forcefully that the pill was not safe. "I am sure that you cannot safely raise or lower the secretions of one endocrine gland without affecting all of them," he told Rock, Pincus, and Garcia, adding darkly, "I would call your attention to the pathology involved." Although Hartman had no clinical research experience, he refused to let such a lack prevent him from strongly expressing his opinion, which, as events would prove, was wrong. When in the 1960s a really alarming complication arose, it would turn out to be something neither the proponents nor the critics anticipated.[34]

It is easy to make judgments in retrospect, but how could either Rock or Pincus be sure of the pill's safety in those early stages? Rock himself had already been annoyed by Pincus's propensity to make public pronouncements prematurely. He had been angry with Pincus for declaring in Japan in 1955 that an oral contraceptive had been developed. Rock was a bit mollified when it turned out that no one at the Japanese meeting had actually understood what Pincus was driving at, so his announcement had fallen on deaf—or at least uncomprehending—ears. Still, when Pincus made this announcement, Rock had tried the Searle compound on only four women, so Rock's belief that Pincus was out front on the pill far too early is certainly understandable.[35]

Rock did not present any official data on his work with the new compounds until 1956 at the Laurentian Hormone Conference in Canada. The paper, based on Rock's Free Hospital studies and coauthored with Pincus and Garcia, bore the coy title of "Synthetic Progestins in the Normal Human Menstrual Cycle." After assessing progestin's effects on the human female reproductive system in detail, Rock said only that "we are led to suspect that ovulation has been inhibited in at least a very high proportion of cases." Even with such a deliberately low-key statement, his fellow workers in reproductive science knew exactly what he meant. And then, in late 1956, still relying on the Brookline data, Rock and Pincus published preliminary reports on those initial Free Hospital results in *Science*. This was the first official peer-reviewed scientific publication proclaiming the effectiveness of these compounds in preventing ovulation. Now the scientific community was alerted to the fact that the 19-nor-steroids were "effective ovulation-inhibitors in women."[36]

Rock kept trying to make Pincus care as much about the conventional protocols involving the publication of research findings as Rock himself did. But Pincus was irrepressible. Rock wanted first to inform other scientists and medical researchers, in careful scientific language, of the possibilities that lay ahead for oral contraception. Pincus, in contrast, wanted to shout the results from every possible rooftop. When Pincus went to Sweden in June 1957, he declared in a widely reported speech that he "had developed an almost 100 percent effective pill for preventing pregnancy." Rock felt the reverberations all the way in Boston, when, as Pincus's known collaborator, he was bombarded by the media. He cabled Pincus, "Mild Storm Brewing Your Speech. Suggest Buttoning Up." Then he reluctantly dealt with the American press, which publicized the story throughout the country. He also had to placate Planned Parenthood's Medical Committee, which deplored what it considered premature publicity. Rock did get a small laugh at the misspelling of Pincus's name. Throughout the U.S. press, he turned up as "Dr. Pincer."[37]

Rock followed his cable to Pincus with a letter to him conveying his irritation with what he saw as irresponsible behavior. In addition to numerous press inquiries, he told Pincus, he had received a reproving letter from Allan Guttmacher, writing in his capacity as chairman of the Planned Parenthood Federation of America Medical Committee. Guttmacher told Rock in no uncertain terms of "the concern which we feel here in New York in regard to the uncritical releases Pincus has made to the lay press regarding the pill." He urged Rock to remind Pincus of the committee's "fear that if additional trials unearth a flaw, such as adverse side effects or undesirable ineffectiveness in certain refractory women, such premature and uncritical statements may backfire on you, Pincus, and the whole movement." This was just what Rock wanted to avoid, and he told Pincus that it would do neither of them any good to have people "think that we are either going off half-cocked, or trying to grab publicity."[38]

Pincus shrugged off Rock's concerns. Rather than agreeing to "button up," he went on to assert the same claims about the pill two months later in a *Ladies' Home Journal* article by a friend, medical journalist Albert Q. Maisel. Once again, Rock sent a curt note to Pincus, to which he attached a letter he wrote to I. C. Winter at Searle, placing responsibility for this article squarely on Pincus. His letter to Winter expressed his exasperation over Pincus's public statements. If anyone besides him had a right to be annoyed, Rock told Winter, they should be irritated only "out of commiseration for me." Still, he expressed his regret if the article "caused you any discomfort."[39]

Undeterred, Pincus took off for a tour of South America, ready to proclaim his successes to as much of the world as might not know an oral contraceptive had been developed. By now Rock seemed almost—not quite, but almost—resigned, writing to J. William Crosson at Searle that "as you know, Pincus is touring South America, practically with station stops. I shudder to think of what he is saying about the contraceptive value and clinical safety and dependability of the new steroids." But he consoled Crosson, and himself, with the hope that "eventually, all will go well." After all, there was nothing else for him to do.[40]

Once the article in *Science* appeared, which was widely considered the appropriate first step in announcing a new discovery, Rock became a bit more reconciled to Pincus's statements to the press. The first official report to breathe the words "oral contraception" came in the 1957 published version of Rock's 1956 presentation to the Laurentian Hormone Conference. And it was not Rock but Georgia fertility specialist Robert Greenblatt who was bold enough to say it out loud. "Dr. Rock," he proclaimed, "has unwittingly given us an excellent oral contraceptive." Not so unwittingly, we know, but at this point Rock had still been retaining his pose of public reticence.[41]

Publicly reticent, perhaps, but Rock was privately expressing his full confidence in the pill. His friend Mary Faulkner told him in October 1957 that when she "went down to the Planned Parenthood annual meeting last week" she "detected a slight disapproval of the pill." Rock already knew that. Some of his colleagues, he told her, still were unable "to conceive that this thing would work." But the pills did indeed work, he insisted, and they were safe as well. "I think that the only legitimate questions are those which I raised a year and a half ago," he continued. "I wanted to be very sure that [the pill] didn't affect other ova than the one that was going to be ripened and discharged in the particular month during which the pills were taken." Although "I was quite ready to find that there would be disadvantages," he concluded, "we're unable to find any."[42] He was not entirely right, as later events would prove, but the side effects that would so concern the nation in the 1960s had not yet become evident.

. . .

The public reports of the pill's effectiveness, needless to say, made Katharine McCormick ecstatic. Although she continued her persistent complaints that the research proceeded much too slowly, she was now convinced that the pill was birth control's magic bullet, which would enable poor women around the world to control their fertility and thus bring about social and economic progress.

Although Pincus, Sanger, and McCormick were all persuaded that the pill would prove a panacea for world overpopulation, Rock did not agree. He doubted that the pill would be a solution for poor women around the world, particularly not in those rural areas where women and girls had no access to education, no rights, and no privacy. Having been to Puerto Rico, and having treated poor women all his life, Rock knew the difference between being poor and being poor and subjugated better than his collaborators did. The Rio Piedras trial was a success, he told a group of his friends, because the women who took the pill possessed "a moderately high degree of culture" and were able to articulate goals for themselves that would be attainable with a smaller family. Perhaps not every one of them was literate, but they were all certainly numerate and could understand both how to take the pills and why taking them might be a good idea.[43]

For poor women in places such as rural India, for example, he was far more skeptical than the others. "I don't believe [the pill] is the answer to India at all," he said in 1957, although "probably in the urban areas" of India and other developing nations it was likely to be more successful than in the countryside. Rock did not believe that the pill was the ultimate contraceptive solution. He was, however, confident that the success of the 19-nor-steroids would open up an entire new world of contraceptive potential—for longer-acting compounds, for a pill or injection for men, for things not yet thought of. For him, the pill just opened a door. "That's why," he told the trustees of the center he had established after retiring from Harvard, "I'm so insistent on learning more about how everything works."[44]

He hoped that McCormick would be interested in supporting some of these new ideas, but as far as she was concerned, the female oral contraceptive was the end of the road. Once she was sure of its success, she would lose interest in the entire subject. She did continue to support the WFEB, although on a less grand scale, out of gratitude and because as a savvy fundraiser Pincus, unlike Rock, always made sure to stay on her good side, but she had moved on. She next became as obsessively involved with building a dormitory for women students at the Massachusetts Institute of Technology as she had been with the development of the pill. If Rock had been a little less focused on his own goals and a little more willing—or able—to curry favor with McCormick, he might have been more successful with her. Or maybe there was nothing he could do once she had the pill. But in 1957, they were all still immersed in its development.

Rock had moved from Harvard to his new clinic. He had no lack of patients and was as busy as ever: In that year he and his small clinic staff were seeing 500 new patients a year, about 3,500 visits total. About half the clinic's patients were infertile couples, the other half equally divided between obstetrics and gynecology. (Although he no longer practiced obstetrics, the younger doctors did.) The medical staff performed about 100 major surgeries and 120 minor ones. In addition, Rock supervised residents and fellows at the Free Hospital, where they had an additional 190 patients with 700 visits. Medical students and residents had the opportunity to participate in the research, see patients, and attend clinical meetings. Rock continued to be swamped by requests from fellow physicians, both the less experienced younger doctors seeking training and the senior gynecologists who wanted to observe the clinic and learn from him.[45]

Rock's infertility practice was absolutely booming in the new center, and he wanted to continue to work on the kinds of challenging problems he had met at the Free Hospital.[46] First, however, he had to figure out a way to support his work. So he gathered a group of his wealthy and connected friends and sought their help and advice. "Since I moved from the Free Hospital and brought with me the appeal which I had for people who couldn't afford to pay," he told them, "the load of non-productive patients has increased considerably. And they have to be paid for somehow. And, if we're going to fulfill the purposes which I have in mind, which is to take everybody for whatever they can afford to pay, then we will need some money eventually."[47]

Rock's lower-income patients had simply followed him from the Free Hospital—hardly a surprise, given his reputation for treating everyone with compassion and dignity and for never fussing about being paid. Since he had no intention of turning these patients away, he wanted to find a way to subsidize their care. His intent was to create a nonprofit corporation so that he could both apply for research grants from federal agencies and foundations, and receive donations for patient care "from the Community Fund or from one of the large charitable trusts."[48]

Realizing that his own history of managing money did not augur well for his ability to raise funds on his own, in 1957 Rock asked a group of his friends and supporters to serve as incorporators of his center. His board members included men and women from leading Boston families—Saltonstall, Deane, Storey, and Faulkner—New England blue bloods who belonged to the same clubs as Nan and John, all of them longtime supporters, and some of them his patients.[49]

The lawyers on his board prepared and filed incorporation papers and waded into the swamp of state bureaucracy to try to move his application through the system. Others provided moral and financial support. Mary Faulkner, the most generous among them, gave an anonymous gift of $50,000 to the center in 1959, the same amount as McCormick provided. Still, Rock had no genius for management and little patience with administrative minutiae. Incorporating his enterprise was a nightmare for him, and it took several years for the center to emerge in its final entity as the Rock Reproductive Clinic (RRC), a nonprofit medical institution. Until he was able to get to that point, however, Rock could not apply for federal grants. Thus, at the very time that federal funding had become critical to financing medical research, Rock lacked even the ability to apply to these agencies when his other sources of funding were grinding to a halt.

The process of incorporation was well along when the state's Bureau of Hospitals threw up a roadblock, two of them in fact. As it happened, in the late 1950s, physicians in private practice all over the state had begun to incorporate to mitigate their personal liability risks, and the director of the bureau failed to see the difference between Rock's enterprise and a private practice. A second problem was a licensing one. Rock's was not the only clinic attempting to both create a separate entity and preserve its links to a medical school or hospital. As the bureau's director put it, he had "quite a number of requests for the organization of sub-clinics of hospitals as corporations and it gave rise, he said, to a proliferation of licenses," a practice which the bureau wanted to stop.[50]

Publicly, Rock expressed considerable optimism about the potential for raising research funds for his new center; he allowed himself to hope that being released from the structure of the Free Hospital could be an advantage. As an institution, he said, the Free Hospital was "only mildly interested in problems of reproductive physiology. They are interested in morbid processes—in diseases—referable to the generative tract of the female, but they're not particularly concerned with the things that I think are by far the most important things that confront humanity today." Although the hospital had "always been very hospitable to me and cooperative," most of its staff did not share his interests. "I have, since 1925, had to do all the work myself." One of the reasons he wanted to create an institutional base for clinical reproductive research, he said, was to see his work carried on. It would be "a pity" if it were "allowed to drop down if I drop out."[51]

McCormick's entire philanthropic history suggested that once she either lost interest or believed a project was complete, she simply moved on. Worse, from Rock's perspective, was the behavior of the Free Hospital and Harvard, neither of which showed any inclination to smooth Rock's path. Rock and the Free Hospital's trustees squabbled so much over financial arrangements for his new center that Nan had to step in, hiring a management consultant to deal with the hospital on Rock's account. Through it all, however, Rock retained his relationship with Bill Mulligan, his successor as director of the Fertility and Endocrine Clinic, and always insisted, at least publicly, that the hospital's intentions were never malign. Still, relations with the leadership were difficult. The Free Hospital and Harvard viewed Rock's new clinic as a competitor. It would have been clearly in the institutions' interest for Rock to have retired from practice rather than move next door.[52]

It took considerably more legal maneuvering than Rock expected, but his board did manage to get the facility incorporated. He remained, however, overly reliant on McCormick to support his operation and on the Searle Company to fund studies of its products. McCormick never ceased being amazed, not to mention irritated, at how labor-intensive human research was. Since neither Pincus nor the Searle scientists conducted research on humans, they didn't really understand either. Rock tried to explain his practices to Searle executive I. C. Winter, noting that for him "to keep a patient load large enough to include a sufficient number of the particular kind of patient as is needed for observation of particular effects; that is, regular ovulation, anovulation, amenorrhea, hypermenorrhea, etc.," he'd had to expand his "practice far beyond the limits of what is called 'private practice.'" And even though the participants in these studies tended not to be typical clinic patients by the 1950s, Rock did not believe it was fair, when conducting clinical research, to make the women "pay the cost of very frequent office visits, and all that this entails, in secretary, nurse and doctor service, which must be supplied" to them.[53] Rock's representations moved Searle to double its grant funding, from $5,000 to $10,000.

It wasn't until the early 1960s that Rock would be able to distribute his brochure for the RRC. Welcoming "the responsibility of helping the over-fertile and the infertile couple" alike, Rock's clinic was prepared to subvert, although not to take on directly, the laws of his native state, which still prohibited any form of contraception except rhythm. While acknowledging that fact, Rock informed potential patients that even in Massachusetts, doctors could prescribe the pill for numerous gynecological conditions, including what might be called menstrual cycle regulation. Patients also would have the opportunity to participate in research studies. "Therapeutic trials and physiological investigations," he assured them, would be "made only with the consent of the informed patient and when there is possible benefit to them in the specific procedures."[54]

Drawn by Rock's reputation, patients had been pouring in to the clinic from around the world even before the various legal matters had been settled. But money always fell short. Rock and his various administrative secretaries issued streams of instructions to the staff regarding their work hours, the clinic's appearance, office routines, patient records, and the importance of treating patients with dignity and respect. Rock valiantly tried to keep the

budget under control, and his secretary tried equally valiantly to collect patient fees. Both were losing battles. He enjoyed money and liked to spend it,
but he could never get beyond his own ingrained conviction that a doctor's job
was to heal, and he refused to think about healing in connection with money.
Rock billed his patients, but whether they paid him or not still seemed almost
immaterial. Even when his clinic became hopelessly strapped, he would tell
his patients not to fret if they had outstanding bills. Don't worry about threatening letters from my secretary, he told them. Come see me anyway and we'll
work it out somehow. Even before McCormick's grants stopped at the end of
1960, the clinic could not pay its way. Of the $50,000 given by Mary Faulkner
in April 1959, only $15,000 remained at the end of the calendar year.[55]

Things would only get worse financially.[56] Rock's fame was at its height,
but his years as a researcher were drawing to a close. Even if his clinic had
been eligible for federal funds earlier, he might not have gotten them. The National Institutes of Health, awash in money, was willing to provide grants for
basic research into fertility but not for contraceptive research. It would surely
not have funded, for example, the development of an oral contraceptive for
men, a form of birth control that only now, in the early twenty-first century,
may be on the horizon.[57] Could he or another researcher have done it then?
Perhaps. Searle and other pharmaceutical houses were turning out a huge variety of synthetic hormonal compounds. If Rock could have teamed up with
another Pincus, and if resources had been available to them, maybe he could
have done more than putter about. But he could not do anything by himself.
His vigor notwithstanding, not only was he about to turn seventy, but he also
now had more limited access to the research services of the medical students,
residents, and fellows at the Free Hospital.

Throughout the last years of the decade, Rock's refusal to give in to his clinic's precarious financial situation helped to keep him in good enough spirits
to keep on working. Although often "fearful of falling through the thin financial ice on which I'm skating," he called himself "an optimist at heart"
who refused even "to let legitimate worries confound me."[58] His ambitious
research program included—in addition to the ongoing testing of the contraceptive 19-nor-steroids—efforts to develop a male hormonal contraceptive,
clinical testing of some of the new ovulation-inducing compounds, developing an increasingly successful technique for the freezing of human sperm,
and continuing his clinical research and treatment of the intractably infertile
couples who always seemed to find their way to his office. Although increasingly concerned with contraception, he never turned away from the problem

of infertility and always considered his contraceptive and fertility research to be two aspects of one intellectual problem.[59]

McCormick provided funding for most of Rock's operating expenses during the early years of his new enterprise. She also subsidized his salary and would continue to fund the clinic until 1959. As a result, much of his time was taken up with the extension of the oral contraceptive trials, as well as preparing and reviewing papers for publication. He also continued to treat importunate infertile couples, welcome the increasing numbers of physicians who wanted to observe the infertility clinic, and find room for the several research fellows who arrived from the United States and around the world to work with the increasingly famous Dr. Rock.

In 1957, the FDA approved the drug Enovid in the 10 milligram dose for use in gynecological disorders including endometriosis, dysmennorhea, and "regulation of the menstrual cycle." In so doing, the FDA relied on the research of a growing number of experts in reproductive medicine, including Rock and the increasingly prominent Edward Tyler of Los Angeles. The nation's practitioners were not, however, precluded from prescribing it as a contraceptive. Once the FDA approves a drug, physicians can prescribe it for other purposes than the ones for which the drug has received formal approval. But it was difficult for doctors to know what they should be doing about the pill, and they besieged both Rock and Pincus for information. As a doctor wrote Rock after attending one of his lectures, "Several of my patients have asked me about the long awaited pill to prevent pregnancy." Could Rock advise him? Responding to this as well as hundreds of other inquiries from practitioners, Rock replied that he would forward his letter to the Searle Company, noting that Searle was not the only manufacturer producing the pills. However, Rock informed his colleague, the other firm, "Park, Davis, & Company has some reluctance in promoting Norlutin as a contraceptive so I am not appealing to them." In forwarding the request to Searle, Rock also suggested that Searle might want to have its "detail man" (who would now be called a pharmaceutical rep) "call on Dr. Heiges" as well.[60]

Rock attempted to respond to all letters from fellow physicians. He was also deluged by mail from men and women who had read his name in one or another of the newspapers or magazines that described the pill. As he told Winter, by late 1958 he was "getting mail from all over the world asking about the 'pill.'" He and the Searle Company agreed that he would respond to each that the writer contact Searle directly for information, but that the pills could "be used only under the supervision of the patient's own doctor." Hereafter,

Rock would refer all inquiries to Searle's Lee van Antwerp, a physician who had become, Winter told Rock, "our official buffer between the Company and the laity."[61]

Once the pill was approved, even though not yet for contraception, women were asking their doctors, as well as John Rock and Gregory Pincus, where and how they could have access to it for birth control. But the initial FDA approval was not intended to serve as backdoor approval for the oral contraceptive; this case had to be presented to the FDA on its own merits. Despite the fact that McCormick began to celebrate when the first *Science* article appeared, the journey was far from at its end. The contraceptive pill, as numerous historians have reminded us, was unprecedented—the first drug that did not attempt to cure anything but was deliberately designed to be taken by healthy women for an indefinite time for what today we call lifestyle reasons. Even though the FDA had a more casual approach to drug approval in that era than it would after the thalidomide tragedies in the early 1960s, everyone knew how important it was to have the best evidence possible. And that meant adding more studies, particularly since they hoped to have the pill approved at dosages not only of 10 milligrams but also 5 and 2.5 milligrams as well.

Rock had hoped to initiate trials in Mexico. He and Nan visited at least one village outside Mexico City in early 1956, even before the field trials began in Puerto Rico. Fearing disapproval by the Church, he was surprised to find the project thwarted instead by the Communist village government, which refused to permit Rock to proceed. "Isn't it a scream," Katharine McCormick wrote Sanger, "that we should have bumped into Communism instead of Catholicism in Mexico! Such a pity, too, when the lay-out was so propitious for carefully matched tests." Rock was prepared to try again in Mexico two years later, but that project, too, seems not to have come to anything.[62]

Clarence Gamble funded an additional study in Puerto Rico, with which Rock was not involved; Rock did oversee two others, however. In 1957, Pincus, Rock, and Garcia initiated a project in Haiti, modeled on the trials in Rio Piedras, with Rock personally traveling to Haiti to set it up. Haiti, however, was not Puerto Rico. Although the appearance of democracy prevailed, and Francois "Papa Doc" Duvalier won the presidency in the fall of 1957 with an enormous majority, election fraud was rampant and Duvalier was beholden to the military for his victory. The fact that he had been popularly elected, as well as his background as a physician trained in public health, however, led Rock and Pincus to believe not only that the impoverished nation would be politically stable but also that Duvalier would be receptive to birth control. Apparently Duvalier did sanction the study at first, but as a leader, he proved to be a power-mad, brutal, and capricious dictator, his domination undergirded by the Tontons Macoutes, who acted as Duvalier's "secret police and instruments of terror."[63]

The Haitian doctors did what they could, but the study was difficult to manage. Physicians left or were replaced, sometimes suddenly, and the project lurched forward in fits and starts. The women who enrolled were different from the Puerto Rican volunteers in their habits and aspirations. The Puerto Rican participants, particularly in Rio Piedras, lived in a society that was interested in modernizing and transforming its rural subsistence existence. In Haiti, the lives of everyone, but especially the lives of women, were much more precarious. Treated like chattel, and with little incentive to curb births since children could be put to work by the age of five or so, a number of the women, while interested in contraception, were unable to translate that interest into the reality of systematic participation. When one's very existence hangs by a thread, calculations of future benefit can be difficult to achieve. In the end, the researchers managed to gather usable data for just 121 women.[64]

Rock was more successful in rural Kentucky, as a result of the support of Mary Breckinridge (a member of the prominent Kentucky family that had produced distinguished legislators and journalists as well as the celebrated settlement worker Sophinisba Breckinridge). Mary Breckinridge had founded and in the late 1950s still headed the Frontier Nursing Service (FNS). She and Nan Rock were old friends, having come to know each other in France, when in the aftermath of World War I both worked for the American Committee for Devastated France. Nan was a young driver. Breckinridge was a senior administrator, serving as director of the committee's nursing department. But Breckinridge was the kind of leader who made everyone feel important and valued. Their age difference (Nan was fifteen years younger than Breckinridge, who was born in 1881) was no bar to friendship. Nan served on the FNS board. Breckinridge frequently stayed with the Rocks when she came to Boston.[65]

Breckinridge, as a young widow of twenty-four, decided to become a nurse and completed her training at St. Luke's Hospital in New York in 1910. In 1912 she married for the second time, to a college professor. She and her second husband had two children. When both children died, first her newborn baby girl and then her adored four-year-old son, her marriage unraveled. She divorced her second husband and resumed her maiden name. She began to search for meaningful work to fill her life and volunteered in postwar France, where her experience encouraged her to devote her life to serving the health needs of children and their mothers.[66] Training formally as a nurse-midwife in England in the early 1920s, she then traveled to Scotland to observe the operation of a health service in a remote area staffed by nurse-midwives. After her return to the United States, she settled in the mountains of Kentucky, in part because of her deep family ties to the state, but also because she saw enormous need for health-care services in this remote, impoverished region. She founded the FNS in 1925.[67]

At first, she staffed the FNS with nurse-midwives trained in Great Britain, but when war broke out in Europe in 1939, she lost eleven of her nurses. Undeterred, Breckinridge began her own school, with a class of two to start, that same year. By the 1950s, the FNS provided health-care services to men and women, adults and children. It was a stable institution, having served the region for three decades, and it was staffed by highly trained nurses who knew well the people who came to them for medical services. When Breckinridge invited Rock, who was a member of her National Medical Board, to visit the FNS in 1958 to talk about clinical trials with Enovid, Nan joined him, and they traveled to Kentucky in late May.[68]

Breckinridge thought highly of Rock, and he in turn—in one more example of his ability to transcend his own conventional attitudes about women—thought highly of her. He learned to accept that here in the FNS, female nurses performed the work that male doctors usually did everywhere else, and she learned to tolerate in him some behavior that she normally disapproved. She didn't drink, and she didn't approve of those who did. Still, she sat with John and Nan every evening of their visit while they enjoyed their predinner cocktails. And despite her longstanding opposition to providing contraceptive services, she made an exception in this case.[69] Although her colleagues remembered her as being rather unbending and slow to accommodate new ideas, particularly in her later years, Rock always received a warm reception. She may have come to realize that times were changing even in rural America. Perhaps she believed that the pill would be more acceptable to her community than more traditional contraceptives.[70]

The families served by the FNS tended to be quite large. Eight or ten children were common, and a few families had more than a dozen. Some couples shunned contraception for religious reasons. As Rachel Bowling, interviewed for the service's oral history project, said, "We had ten children. We never did do nothing to keep from having children 'cause thought it was wrong. I believe it is yet. [That's what] the good Lord put us here for . . . that's our punishment he put on Eve."[71] Others simply valued their large families. Descriptions of their lives bring to mind images from seventeenth- and eighteenth-century North America. As one of the nurses remembered, in the 1950s "there were people who lived in hollows who hardly ever came out of them. Certainly the women didn't . . . People grew their own gardens. They canned their own foods. They killed their own hogs and had their own chickens. Had their own milk cow."[72]

And it was the women who did most of the work. Helen Browne, who succeeded Mary Breckinridge as director of the FNS, recalled that the "men turned over the sod in the garden. Maybe helped [their wives] plant the seed, but from then on she was completely responsible for tending it. For gathering the crop when it was ready."[73] The older children would have been a big help to their mothers. The school year generally ended in February in the mountains, in part because the high waters made getting to school difficult, and in part because the children were needed for planting. By the time children were ten, girls could cook beans, make cornbread, and milk the cow, and the boys would bring in the water (houses did not have plumbing), the wood, and the coal. Boys and girls both helped in the corn patch. "They were all needed," Browne remembered, to raise, process, and cook the food, gather the eggs, butcher the pig.[74]

If the older children were valued for their ability to help, the babies brought joy. The youngest was always spoiled until the next one came along. Birth control in such a climate was a hard sell. It would become easier when the economy began to change in the 1960s, with more job opportunities particularly for young women, but Rock's appearance antedated the changes. At first, Rock planned a study of only twenty women. Rogers Beasley, the medical director of FNS, was the physician in charge; Breckinridge assigned the day-to-day supervision of the project to the highly regarded, no-nonsense Anna Mae January. "Miss January," as everyone called her, had a near legendary reputation as a trusted diagnostician and was much loved by the people she treated. They said she was "just as good" as a doctor, or even better, since many of the patients said "they'd just as soon have her as a doctor." January took personal care of each patient. If any of the women in the trial would come in to the clinic when she was off duty, January would insist on coming in anyway. Eventually she allowed some of her more trusted staff to dispense the pills, but she handled everything else herself.[75]

The FNS, in spite of its clientele's preference for large families, seemed to encounter no difficulty in recruiting participants for the Enovid study. Some of the women had ten or twelve children already. Others had serious physical ailments that made it dangerous for them to bear more children. The pills also could be taken in private, and at least some of the women, it seems, took the pills without telling their husbands. The nurses were surprised at the willingness and ability of the participants to adhere to the study protocols. "I think a lot of us had questions about how regular[ly] people would take them," nurse Mary Penton said, but "we found they did very well. Even some of the ones we thought might not remember as well as others." These rural white American women added another layer of positive results, but the data wouldn't be used immediately. This study was not complete at the time of Searle's first request for FDA approval of Enovid as a contraceptive. Also, many of these women were taking the 5 milligram dose, and the FDA was willing at the outset to consider only the original 10 milligram formulation.[76]

...

As Rock's early confidence in the pill evolved into firm conviction, he became significantly more committed to assisting the Searle Company to bring Enovid to market as a contraceptive. In return, Searle's scientists became ever more reliant on his advice. Although Rock was not the only clinical investigator to test the pill, the record indicates that Searle researchers often sought him out whenever a situation turned awkward or troublesome. For example, when Edward Tyler, prominent infertility practitioner and powerful West Coast voice in the national Planned Parenthood Federation, continued to express reservations about the pill's efficacy and safety, Searle asked Rock both to explain to *them* the exact nature of Tyler's objections and to talk personally to Tyler.

Tyler simply was not persuaded that the pill was as effective or as safe as Rock and Pincus had claimed. His own early studies had a 9 percent pregnancy rate (he started the pill several days later in the cycle than Rock thought prudent, however) and a high dropout rate because of the same side effects that Rice-Wray had found. He had also used the Syntex formula to prevent miscarriage and found that a few of the female children born had androgenic abnormalities (Rock told his colleagues that unlike Enovid, the Syntex formula was slightly androgenic). Tyler reported to Planned Parenthood that in his view "oral contraceptives have a reasonably good degree of effectivity, but he personally does not agree that the safety of the method has been established, particularly with regard to long-term effects on pituitary, liver, and adrenals."[77]

Tyler was not the only early skeptic. Across the Atlantic, prominent British gynecologist Gerald Swyer disputed the progestational action of Enovid on the endometrium. Geoffrey Venning, who ran Searle's British division, had known Swyer since their student days at Oxford. Swyer was, Venning said, "the leading authority in the country on the action of oestrogen and progesterone on the endometrium." Swyer forcefully insisted that Enovid did "not, repeat, not [have] a progestational effect" on the endometrium, and Venning's data did not change his mind. Venning wrote Winter with some urgency, and Winter in turn asked Rock, arguably the United States's leading authority on the endometrium, for help. Rock quickly responded with two pages of detailed technical information, as well as several illustrative slides, for Swyer to review, although Swyer proved unpersuadable. In 1958 Rock had become a committed believer in the drug's efficacy and safety and spared no effort to convince doubting fellow physicians.[78]

Tyler's specific worries about the pill were never borne out, nor were the ones he would express in 1960 about the possibility of an increased incidence of endometrial cancer as a result of pill use. The most serious complication that did emerge in the 1960s—thromboembolic disease from which some women died—was never predicted by even the pill's severest naysayers in the 1950s. And Rock was correct about the progestational effect of the pill. It continues to be the dominant hormonal influence in oral contraceptives even today.

Searle's executives believed in Rock's superior understanding of the way hormones functioned, and they trusted him. Rock, in turn, although he does not seem to have realized it, had gradually become much less of an independent voice on the pill and more of an advocate for it and the company that made it. While we wouldn't go so far to call him an apologist for the pill at this stage, he was well on the way to becoming so. Still, unlike Pincus, he was not in the company's employ. In the mid-1950s, while publicly maintaining the image of an independent scientist, Pincus was actually a full-fledged salaried Searle employee. Rock didn't know this, and neither did McCormick, but Pincus had all the perks of employment, including stock options and a Searle retirement plan.[79]

Rock, in contrast, had no financial stake in the fate of the pill. Searle did not fund Rock's research; McCormick did. Rock believed that a clinical investigator should not be tempted by the profit motive when testing a particular drug. He knew and liked the Searle researchers and investigators with whom he worked, and Searle, like all the drug houses, provided its compounds without charge and provided grants to conduct studies. Companies also sometimes paid part of the salaries of a technician or secretary involved in assessing or tabulating data.

The relationship between Searle and Rock was mutually beneficial, however; Rock's grants from Searle amounted to $10,000 to $11,000 per year (around $75,000 today) in the late 1950s. (To compare, McCormick's funding for Rock, at $50,000 per year, would be the equivalent today of around $350,000.) Because of his reputation for integrity, his belief in the pill became a valuable commodity in itself for Searle. Now that the pill had moved from the laboratory to the practitioner's drug closet, Searle had more need of Rock than of Pincus. Rock, however, on nearly every public occasion credited Pincus for the "inspiration" that led to the pill and for "extraordinary administrative and executive talents," without which the pill would never have come to fruition.[80]

Nevertheless, Rock was already far along in his transition from pill researcher to pill advocate. One of the early signs of his new role was his willingness to help when Searle turned to him for advice on how to make the pill socially acceptable to the American medical community and to the public. Searle's Lee van Antwerp asked Rock for his advice on how best to "introduce Enovid for ovulation control—if, as and when that time arrives. What should we say to the doctor? Should we have printed instructions for the doctor to hand his patient if he wishes? If so, what do we say (thus indirectly) to the patient?"

Nowadays, from the mandated patient inserts to the printed information from the pharmacy every time we pick up a prescription, we have access to a great deal of information on every medication we take. But not then. (In fact, women health activists opposed to the pill would make the first inserts a reality.) But in 1958 the whole idea of directly informing patients about a drug was inconceivable. And explaining a pill designed to prevent pregnancy even to doctors seemed a monumental enterprise. This was all new—for the drug companies, for the doctors, and for the public. It was not modesty but anxiety that led van Antwerp to confide to Rock that "Enovid for such a purpose falls far outside our not-too-narrow experience." Any ideas from Rock were therefore "most welcome."[81]

The Searle Company remained uncertain about the reception of a drug boldly promoted for birth control, and John Searle himself had bandied around with Rock several euphemisms, which Antwerp also asked Rock to recall for him. Rock was more than responsive. He was eager to try his hand at describing this new concept of oral birth control, but he warned van Antwerp, "I am not experienced in this kind of promotional work," and so "I don't expect you will approve" of the results.[82] Nevertheless, Rock threw himself into both efforts. To avoid the term contraception, he suggested, substitute "child spacing," or "postponement of pregnancy," or even "suppression of ovulation,"[83] although surely not every woman knew she ovulated, or if she did, that ovulation was necessary for pregnancy to occur. Searle would soon settle on the most clearly understood euphemism for birth control, "family planning."

Rock's rough draft of possible wording for an informational brochure for physicians offers an insight into what a specialist in reproductive medicine expected a general practitioner to know. Assuming that many of his colleagues might not understand the role of the corpus luteum and progesterone in ovulation, he took a page and a half describing the menstrual cycle, comparing the "reign of the corpus luteum" after ovulation to the dominant member of a "politburo," who "achieves dominance" by "suppress[ing] his potential rivals and liquidates other actual contenders. Similarly in the ovary, during the fortnightly reign of a corpus luteum, its potent progesterone causes regression of the unsuccessful competing follicles which leads to their eventual disappearance, and holds in abeyance the progress of those less well developed," he noted. The practical information on Enovid is compressed into less than a third of his draft. Enovid, he says, "completely mimics" the action of progesterone. It prevents ovulation and "non-pathologic uterine flow" during the three weeks it is taken, after which "flow, in all but a rare case, will appear after about 3 days."[84]

In fact, Rock seemed to believe that women knew almost as much about their bodies as their general practitioners did. His draft wording for patients begins, "Enovid is an artificially made hormone that is chemically quite similar to the two hormones, *estrogen* and *progesterone*, naturally produced in the human ovary." Although "ten times stronger" than progesterone, "its [Enovid's] action on various organs is quite like that of the natural hormone," he said, prefiguring the argument about the pill's naturalness that he would later make to the Catholic Church. Without ever using the terms contraception or birth control (nor did he in the draft for the doctors), he wanted to make clear that "as long as the medication is taken daily, no female germ cell—no ovum—is set free. This means, of course, that the woman, even though married, cannot expect to become pregnant."[85] By 1958, the Searle research staff was coming to Rock routinely for help in understanding the various uses—noncontraceptive as well as contraceptive—for Enovid and the company's newer pills. "I know we are asking you to write more and more," I. C. Winter apologized in one letter, and a few weeks later said again, "I seem to be always increasing your already heavy load."[86]

Rock, having invested his considerable credibility in the pill's efficacy and safety by the end of the 1950s, all the more eagerly assisted Searle because he had become emotionally invested in proving that the medical opponents of the pill were just plain wrong. He found Edward Tyler's views especially rankling. Now in his forties, Tyler was ambitious, talented, and a rising star in the field of reproductive medicine. In the early 1950s he had juggled his medical career with one as a television comedy writer for Groucho Marx, Milton Berle, and Jack Paar. Like Rock, Tyler enjoyed the limelight and had a flair for the dramatic. (And unlike Rock, he didn't try to pretend otherwise.) He was a driving force in the Planned Parenthood Federation and had conducted clinical trials in Los Angeles on the oral contraceptive. He was also, although neither Rock nor Searle knew it at the time, the FDA's principal independent expert on the pill.[87]

Tyler was also a member of the board of the American Society for the Study of Sterility. When he invited Rock to speak at the society's annual meeting in 1960, it would be the first time, as Searle's William Crosson said, that "this Society will recognize the existence of an oral contraceptive." Rock declared that he did not want to go, but Crosson flattered him into it. If you don't speak, Crosson told him, then Tyler would give the presentation himself. "If this occurs, I can envisage the development of a situation that could obstruct general acceptance of the oral method for several years or more by this rather powerful group of clinicians."[88]

The appeal to his professional pride—and his rivalry with Tyler—worked. Rock grumbled, but he agreed to go and promised to "write Tyler and accept his gracious willingness to use me for his not too obscure purpose. I hope, at least, I shall be able to keep my temper on leash."[89] Pincus and Tyler had clashed publicly over the pill, and Rock knew of Tyler's report to the Medical Committee of Planned Parenthood. Whether he also knew that the FDA considered Tyler a "more neutral" and therefore more trusted voice than Rock on the safety of the pill, a fact not revealed until the early twenty-first century by historians Suzanne White Junod and Lara Marks, is doubtful.[90]

• • •

There have been conflicting accounts of the process of FDA approval of the pill. Journalists, including Morton Mintz and Barbara Seaman, accused the researchers and Searle of foisting false and misleading data on the FDA, lying both about the numbers of women involved in the study and the way the study was conducted, and concealing evidence of side effects and even serious complications. There is no evidence, however, of lies or medical misconduct, although it is true that Pincus, in the excess of his delight at finally having developed an effective oral contraceptive, greatly minimized the unpleasant side effects.

As fall edged into winter in 1959, everyone at Searle, as well as Pincus, Rock, and Garcia, whose research formed the core data for the application, remained on tenterhooks. On July 29, 1959, Searle had submitted its application for FDA approval of Enovid as an oral contraceptive, to be prescribed for up to twenty-four months. Now, they awaited the outcome.[91] Searle's application contained twenty volumes of detailed clinical data, the largest New Drug Application (NDA) ever submitted to the FDA up to that time. The FDA, overwhelmed by an enormous number of NDAs in the 1950s (it was, after all, the era of the antibiotic and steroid revolution), did its best to cope with just three full-time physicians and four part-timers who were still in their residency training. Enovid was assigned to Pasquale DeFelice, one of those young physicians, who was just completing his residency.[92]

The FDA, critics have maintained, would go on to approve a drug that it knew had not been tested extensively. Mintz, for example, insisted that the pill was approved after testing on only 132 women, and that figure was quoted repeatedly. He, other journalists, and some scholars have also complained that the researchers misled practitioners and the public about how many women actually took the pill by stating their findings in "woman years"; however, "woman years" was generally accepted nomenclature in the statistical assessment of any contraceptive's effectiveness and not an attempt to distort the numbers.[93]

How true are the critics' claims? Although only 132 women had taken the pill continuously for at least one full year to three full years, Searle actually submitted 897 cases of women who had taken Enovid at its 10 milligram dose at the time it sought approval for the drug as a contraceptive in July 1959. Additional data from the next six months raised the total to 1,200; another 995 women had taken the 5 milligram dose. In addition, between 1957 and 1959 an estimated 500,000 women had used Enovid to treat gynecological disorders. By early 1960, the number of women from the three Puerto Rican studies who had taken "one dosage form or another" of Enovid for twenty-four consecutive cycles or longer stood at 66—38 of whom had gone at least thirty-six consecutive cycles, some of them as many as fifty-two cycles.[94]

Such numbers would not be acceptable today, but as Suzanne White Junod and Lara Marks have pointed out in their authoritative study, by the standards of the day, the pill was thoroughly tested. As a comparison, in the same year that Enovid was approved by the FDA, so was Librium, a powerful tranquilizer and antianxiety drug. That drug was approved for use for various psychiatric symptoms after being tried on 570 patients, with no indication of the duration of treatment, and it was approved for use in epilepsy after being tried on only three patients.[95]

DeFelice may have been young and inexperienced, but he clearly recognized the importance of this application. Not wanting to make a mistake as he traversed uncharted territory, he did what any good official would in his place—he asked questions and requested more information. After all, Searle was asking the FDA to approve a drug, he said, "to treat a normal condition, ovulation," and not a disease. Is it safe for use "even for 24 months"? he wondered. "Premature menopause," he told Crosson, "is a real possibility." And what about "carcinogenesis, . . . inter-glandular activity [sic], and the potential for future pregnancies"? Finally he wrote, "We seriously question the validity of the use of a progestational agent . . . for the inhibition of ovulation, a normal body function, when there are so many unanswered questions concerning the potential for harm. This is especially true in view of the lack of advantage over other presently available contraceptive agents." The upshot was that DeFelice rejected the submission as "incomplete and inadequate."[96] At the heart of this refusal to rubber stamp the application without additional data was the young physician's reluctance to treat a normal biological process as if it were a disease or even a medical condition.

Bill Crosson was furious when DeFelice declared Searle's application "inadequate," and he fired off a pointed response. DeFelice might have had a more conciliatory answer from Searle researchers if he had not made the mistake of declaring that "inhibition of ovulation" was a new claim. Whether DeFelice had misunderstood the original application, or simply expressed himself clumsily, Crosson, assistant director of clinical research for Searle, pounced on that statement in his four-page single-spaced reply: "Inhibition of ovulation after the cyclic administration of Enovid is not a new claim, . . . but an inherent action of the drug . . . clearly outlined in our original N.D.A. . . . We have had numerous cases of nausea, some of breakthrough bleeding, of mastalgia and even of weight gain (all . . . carefully delineated in our Reference Manual)," he told DeFelice, "but we have had no single case reported to us where Enovid was implicated in premature menopause, in carcinogenesis, in adverse modification of 'inter-glandular activity' or of interference with future pregnancies or even of persistent disturbances of post-treatment menstrual cycles."[97] Crosson agreed with DeFelice that "unanswered questions" remained, but he pointed out that while "we by no means compare the importance of Enovid to digitalis and morphine, it is fair to point out that these two drugs which have been known, which have been studied and which have been in therapeutic use for many years still have many 'unanswered questions' concerning their activity."[98]

True, but morphine and digitalis were not intended to be taken by healthy individuals, and that seemed to be the great difficulty for DeFelice. He did not want to recommend approval of a drug—to be taken by people who were not ill—that might have unfortunate aftereffects, unless he was as sure as he could be that he was doing the right thing. Comparing the birth-control pill, which would be taken by healthy women, to morphine and digitalis, which were taken for relief of extreme pain and heart disease, respectively, may seem a bit extreme now, but in the 1950s the developers envisioned the pill as a drug for married women to space their children for economic or emotional reasons, and to curb overpopulation, which was increasingly being viewed as an environmental and public health crisis. No one foresaw the pill's actual social and cultural effects.

Having written his letter, Crosson turned next to Rock for help, asking him to accompany him and I. C. Winter to Washington to meet with the medical officer. Rock agreed, and a meeting among the four took place. What actually happened when the four men finally gathered is a matter of dispute.

Interviewed some twenty years later, Winter recalled the meeting as being held on a bitterly cold day in December, with Crosson, Rock, and Winter standing "in a barren little entryway for more than an hour and a half until DeFelice showed up. I felt at the time that we were left waiting to discourage us." After this literally cold beginning, according to Winter, the meeting proceeded, with Rock countering some of DeFelice's reservations by questioning his experience. Winter recalled Rock repeatedly referring to DeFelice as "young man." For example, when DeFelice raised a question about cancer, Rock told him, according to Winter, "I don't know how much training you've had in *female cancer, young man*, but I've had considerable!" Rock remembers being extraordinarily put out, recalling two decades later that DeFelice "was a nondescript, thirty-year-old from Washington. Can you imagine, the FDA gave him the job of deciding. I was furious." Rock also recalled that at the end of the meeting, when DeFelice said that he would review everything they discussed, Rock "grabbed him [DeFelice] by his jacket lapel and . . . said, 'No, you won't take it all home with you. You'll decide right now.'" According to Rock, DeFelice responded, "'Oh, all right,'" and, Rock reminisced, "I don't think he knew the significance of what he was doing."[99]

Rock told the same version when he was interviewed for the FNS Oral History Project in 1979.[100] DeFelice, however, recalled the meeting—and the entire approval process—somewhat differently. He was indeed young, only thirty-five at the time, and remembered being very conscious that the pill was an entirely new kind of drug. As he told journalist Loretta McLaughlin, "Everything up to that time was a drug to treat a diseased condition. Here, suddenly, was a pill to be used to treat a healthy person and for long term use. We really went overboard. Even though the pill had been through more elaborate testing than any drug in the FDA's history, there was a lot of opposition . . . Penicillin went through the FDA process very easily even though five hundred people a year still die from penicillin reactions. With the pill, however, the FDA had to come out of the licensing process absolutely clean!" In his recollection of the meeting, "Rock was a gentlemen about the whole thing . . . I've only met about three doctors in my entire life who I would trust with anything. Rock was one of them." But, he said, he still did not give approval on the spot.[101]

Letters during this period between the key players in this drama suggest that everyone involved had some accurate recollections and some misremembering. The only meeting that we can document was held on October 23, 1959, shortly after Crosson responded to the FDA's requirement for additional information. There is no contemporary record of any meeting in December, which is not to say one didn't occur; however, given the volume of correspondence among Crosson and Winter and Rock, it is hard to imagine that not one of them would have remarked about their seeing each other, even if they did not mention the purpose of the meeting. But there are no such remarks.

Rock's participation in this October meeting was critical to their ultimate success, according to both Crosson and Winter. They "got very much further with Dr. DeFelice than we could possibly have without you," Crosson told Rock. Rock responded that he hoped he had helped. "I guess I did enough blowing off." However persuasive, and whatever his memory, Rock was unable to coerce DeFelice into an immediate approval. Instead, the Searle Company modified the application to remove the 5 and 2.5 milligram doses, and DeFelice sent the amended application to an "outside referee." Searle did not know who that would be, but it was probably Edward Tyler.[102]

After the meeting, and the submission of the amended application, the impatient wait resumed. According to FDA rules, DeFelice would have had 180 days from October 29, the date of the amended application, to inform Searle of his recommendation. In February Edward Tyler told Crosson that "medical representatives" of the FDA would be making "personal contact with those who have had clinical experience in the use of Enovid as a contraceptive agent." Crosson doubted that Rock would be one of them, "since you have already expressed your opinion rather firmly."[103] In what Junod and Marks call "an unusual but not wholly unprecedented move," DeFelice wrote to seventy-five obstetrician-gynecologists "at leading medical schools"—all of whom had used Enovid clinically—asking them to evaluate the drug.[104]

DeFelice asked whether such side effects as nausea and breakthrough bleeding would make the product undesirable or whether the medication would affect future fertility, perhaps increase the danger of a future miscarriage, or produce congenital abnormalities in subsequent children. Might it cause premature menopause? Should there be "any concern about the possible carcinogenicity after long-term use?" And finally, he asked, "Do you feel that Enovid or Enovid like products should be available on prescription for contraceptive purposes?"[105] DeFelice was being prudent, and rightly so.

The Searle executives and Rock were letting their anxiety that DeFelice was somehow out to crush the pill's approval affect their judgment. Crosson underestimated DeFelice, who as a matter of course included both Rock and Pincus (who was not even a physician) among the experts solicited. After responding clearly and directly to each of the questions, Rock asserted his position that only "failure to learn the proved physiological effects of this product" would result in denial of the NDA. Alluding directly to their shared Roman Catholicism, and indirectly to his fear that DeFelice would disapprove the pill on religious grounds, he concluded, "Since my pleasant interview with you in Washington I happily disbelieve that extraofficial prejudice against contraceptive measures [i.e., the Catholic hierarchy] can have any influence."[106]

After reviewing all these responses as well as information provided by Edward Tyler and others, DeFelice moved closer to a decision. Finally, Dr. Gordon Granger, chief of the Drugs and Devices Branch of FDA, met with Tyler, who now gave the pill his endorsement. In early April, Crosson wrote Rock that Searle had not heard anything, and Rock responded that "I . . . am prepared to war with them [the FDA] if [the decision] isn't favorable." No war was necessary. By the end of April, Searle received word that DeFelice would recommend approval; the FDA announced its decision on May 9, and approval became final on June 23, 1960.[107]

The Searle Company was happy, although feverishly working now to get the new lower doses approved. Rock was gratified. McCormick, having griped for years about how long the whole process was taking, began to lose interest. The media gave the approval's formal announcement prominent but relatively brief notices, although more stories about the pill were in the works. *Newsweek* headlined its four-paragraph story "Is This the Pill?" and called it "the long-awaited, much-debated oral contraceptive," noting its cost (a relatively pricey ten dollars a month). And the *New York Times* emphasized that the FDA made its decision on the basis of safety, not on its "own ideas of morality."[108]

And maybe that was right. By now the pill seemed nearly ho-hum news. The media had been covering the pill at least since its 1957 approval for gynecological disorders. It would be in the next decade that the real battles—cultural, medical, and religious—would be fought, and Rock's professional life would once again change dramatically, as he transformed himself into an international advocate for the pill. So, too, would his personal life change dramatically. His wife, Nan, was diagnosed with cancer.

Chapter 8

THE FACE AND VOICE OF THE PILL

Brookline, Massachusetts, 1961. Nan Rock dies of colon cancer in August.

New York, 1963. Knopf publishes John Rock's *The Time Has Come: A Catholic Doctor's Proposal to End the Battle over Birth Control.*

Belgium, 1964. A Catholic journal carries an essay by Father Louis Janssens, professor of moral theology at the University of Louvain, which credits Rock's book with having provided a way for the Catholic Church to change its birth-control policy.

When Nan Rock was diagnosed with colon cancer in the summer of 1959, she and John were determined not to give in to despair. She underwent surgery and for the next year and a half seemed free from recurrence. In public, Rock handled himself as he always did in times of personal crisis—he kept his feelings to himself, and the world saw only what he wanted it to see, a man calm and confident that the surgery had removed all the cancer. Nan also refused to be defeated and was making it a point to live her life to the fullest. By remaining brave and strong herself, she helped John to act that way. Few people outside the couple's circle of close friends knew about her illness. As far as many of Rock's professional associates were concerned, during these years his only concerns had to do with the pill.

...

Once the FDA had approved Enovid, Katharine McCormick congratulated herself on achieving her goal and moved on. Gregory Pincus, whose scientific acumen and organizational skill had brought the pill from animal testing to doctors' offices in less than a decade, was enjoying the boost in his reputation provided by such a spectacular success. For both of them, the pill represented a job well done. For John Rock, it was different. Although the pill had not been central to his work in the 1950s, by the early 1960s it would come to dominate his professional life in a way it had not done during the years of its development and testing. Within a few years, Rock would appear on television screens and magazine covers around the world, becoming the voice and face of the pill.

In the 1950s, Pincus had been the pill's outspoken champion, Rock the behind-the-scenes voice of caution. But by 1960, things were different. Rock was becoming an increasingly valuable asset for the Searle Company. Its executives and scientists had already come to appreciate his medical judgment; they now came to value the obvious publicity value of having a strongly observant Catholic expert in reproduction as one of the pill's leading advocates. Margaret Sanger's oft-quoted comment about Rock—that he was "a good R. C. and as handsome as a god," and as a result could "just get away with anything"—may not have said it all, but it said enough. R. C. was a pejorative term for a Catholic, and Sanger never hid her anti-Catholic bigotry. But it was getting harder to display such open prejudice. Rock was handsome and persuasive, the very image of the trustworthy doctor. As Catholics had become more numerous in the United States, they had also become more powerful politically; and Sanger captured in this one pithy phrase a key aspect of Rock's value to promoting the acceptability of the pill.[1]

During the next few years, Rock would become more receptive to taking on a larger role in the promotion of the pill, for three reasons. In the first place, he was at a crossroads in his professional life. Since everyone who worked for Harvard was forced to retire at sixty-five, he couldn't take personal offense at his own forced retirement. But he really had not wanted to leave. Instead of going away quietly—to write his memoirs, enjoy a more leisurely pace in his private practice, and maybe take up a consulting position—Rock had simply packed up and moved next door. With McCormick's money, he had founded his own clinic, where he planned to continue playing a critical role in the ongoing development of the field of reproductive medicine. McCormick knew that Rock's pill studies were at a crucial stage, so he could still count on her for funding. So far, so good. She remained Rock's shield against the Free Hospital's designs on his research fellows, his practice, and his patients. But this was about to change, once the pill was approved.

In the second place, Rock was truly persuaded that the oral contraceptive could solve the birth-control problem for Catholics. His coreligionists in working-class Boston were among the heaviest sufferers from the ill effects of too many children and too little money. Most of the patients at the Free Hospital's rhythm clinic were Catholics, trying to avoid conception through the only means allowed by the Church. But successful use of the rhythm method requires not just close attention. A woman must also have regular ovulatory cycles. A number of things can throw off ovulation—an illness, stress, a change in weight—so even among the regular ovulators, rhythm was never foolproof, and for those with irregular cycles, it was impossible. Rock, however, had kept the clinic going for so many years because, marginally effective though it was, it was the only form of birth control allowable to Catholics, at least until now.[2] The oral contraceptive, he believed, provided an induced "safe period" that was the equivalent of the natural safe period that women experienced every month.

And finally, Rock's personal life would be torn to shreds in 1961, when Nan's cancer returned. The return of her illness, and her death that same year, would unmoor him completely. He needed to keep busy, the busier the better.

It was the confluence of these several factors—the Searle company's recognition that Rock's Catholicism, combined with his medical reputation, would be a major asset as the company marketed their new drug; Rock's forced retirement from the Free Hospital and subsequent difficulties in reestablishing an institutional base; the devastating loss of his wife; and his conviction that the oral contraceptive could be used by observant Catholics—that transformed Rock from pill researcher to the leading advocate of the drug he had helped to create. In these early years of the decade, from 1960 to 1964, Rock truly had some grounds to believe, as he often said, that American Catholics could "end the battle over birth control."

For many years, Rock had enjoyed a cordial relationship with Searle executives and scientists, especially with I. C. Winter and Bill Crosson. The company's president, John Searle, also admired him, although they knew each other less well. Winter and Crosson routinely came to Rock for explanations of the workings of the female reproductive cycle. Even in the late 1950s, some of the Searle scientists had only sketchy knowledge of how their new contraceptive pill actually worked. When stumped by either a question about or an outright contradiction to their understanding, they increasingly turned to Rock.

When Crosson cajoled Rock to take Tyler up on his invitation to speak about the pill at the 1960 annual meeting of the American Society for the Study of Sterility, Rock made headlines. Addressing more than four hundred of his colleagues as well as most of the national media's medical correspondents, Rock endorsed the pill as safe and effective. And there was more. Rock described the pill as "a means of modifying a woman's monthly cycle," then went even further, as *Time* magazine's correspondent noted in surprise. Here was Rock, in *Time's* description "an active Roman Catholic," promoting the pill as "a morally permissive variant of the rhythm method."[3] The Searle executives could not have been happier.

Once they had gotten over the hurdle of FDA approval, Searle's executives believed that the principal problem would be the moral acceptability of the pill. Within two years, the company would also have to deal with safety concerns, and Rock would once again come to the pill's defense. Searle had earned his gratitude. The company had come to his rescue when others were letting him down. And perhaps no one was letting him down so much as the leadership of the Free Hospital.

After he moved to the "hovel" on the grounds of the Free Hospital, and once McCormick saw to it that the building was properly renovated, she continued to provide him with $50,000 annually in operating expenses, including $10,000 toward his salary. She also paid Celso-Ramon Garcia's salary, but she always begrudged having to do so. In her own mind, she made a distinction between supporting the research (which was acceptable to her) and paying the researchers (which was not). She could not understand why she should fund any part of Rock's salary; she believed his income should come from his private practice. In vain did Rock try to get Pincus to explain to her that if she wanted him to spend more time on the pill, he would necessarily have much less time for his medical practice. She was convinced, all of Rock's explanations to the contrary, that the women he studied should be no more trouble than Pincus's rats and rabbits. And of course, she must have reasoned to herself, she wasn't paying Pincus's salary. If she had known that Pincus was on Searle's payroll by the mid-1950s, her attitude might have been different.

· · ·

At the end of 1960, Rock was in a tough situation. McCormick had no further use for him. The Free Hospital coveted his patients. Harvard wanted to consolidate its reproductive services and thought of him as an impediment to that process. He was having difficulty creating his new organization. Nan's good sense had preserved him from total disaster in his negotiations with the hospital, but Nan would soon be gone.

Her cancer was casting its malevolent shadow over everything. In 1959, after her surgery, Rock told his cousin Elizabeth Quirk that he and Nan were determined to live their life to the fullest, to try to forget as best they could that her cancer had invaded it. They went together to Bombay (now Mumbai) in the fall of 1959 for a meeting of the International Planned Parenthood Federation, where Rock and Pincus presented data on the oral contraceptives.[4] From Bombay they traveled through Europe. But in the midst of his extraordinarily hectic professional life—the pressures of seeking approval for the birth-control pill, the preparation of reports on the pill trials for publication, and the administrative headaches involved in running his new clinic—the threat of Nan's cancer returning accompanied him everywhere.

In August 1960—just over a year after she was diagnosed—the Rocks took a vacation to Guatemala, revisiting the location of his formative early experiences. This was where young John had first glimpsed a future he could embrace, where he had begun to find himself. It was a nostalgic journey, with Rock sentimentally evoking the memory of his "very dear old friend, Dr. MacPhail." The United Fruit Company provided the Rocks with a car and driver so that they and MacPhail's sister Jessie—who had moved to Guatemala to be near her brother and remained after his death—could visit Quirigua, the location of MacPhail's former hospital. John and Nan also visited Mayan ruins and spent some time in Guatemala City. Rock and MacPhail had kept their friendship alive for as long as MacPhail lived. MacPhail had delighted in Rock's growing reputation and took some credit for starting him on his way.[5]

Six months after they returned, the health of both Rocks took a turn for the worse. In January 1961, Rock had another heart attack. And Nan's cancer soon returned. During his own recovery, the two spent most of their time together. By late spring, he was trying to run the clinic from home, rarely leaving Nan's side. It was clear she was failing. Her pain was great, as Rock's log of her condition during her last weeks dramatically illustrates. She died on August 8, 1961. One of the family's first calls was to Rock's friend Monsignor Francis Lally, who came almost immediately to give the desolate Rock what spiritual comfort he could.[6]

Nan had anchored John's life. He loved his daughters and delighted in his ever-growing flock of grandchildren, but they had their own lives, and besides, no one takes the place of a beloved spouse. After her death he sought solace in work, always Rock's anodyne when tragedy struck. Searle scientists and executives continued to call on him to help them answer questions about the oral contraceptive. Already a well-known public figure, Rock was again becoming a media darling, turning up everywhere, including in *Newsweek*, *Time*, and *Good Housekeeping*, and appearing on CBS and NBC. While Pincus had not been eclipsed completely, the press most often turned to Rock. After all, he was a medical doctor who actually treated patients. He was both photogenic and telegenic, putting to good effect his long years of acting in Tavern Club productions. Rock had a stage presence that came off as natural and effortless. And his Catholicism always could be counted on to provide a journalist with something controversial for readers or viewers.

. . .

The social and cultural history of the oral contraceptive is heavily interwoven with the history of the sixties—sex, drugs, and rock and roll, as the cliché goes. Historians have spilled gallons of ink disentangling cultural from technological influences, charting changes in the behavior of the married versus the unmarried, and chronicling the revolt against authority that could be applied to the papacy just as easily as to national policy, to medical authority figures just as easily as to parents. To many who lived through the experience, 1960 and 1968 seemed hardly to belong in the same century, let alone the same decade.[7] Indeed, the first half of the 1960s belonged more to the 1950s, culturally speaking, than to "the sixties." And during this time, the pill belonged to the married. Perhaps more significantly for John Rock, it represented an important element in Catholic assimilation into the mainstream of the American middle class.

In 1960 Catholics represented a quarter of the American population, and one of their own was running for president. But in some ways, they remained culturally distinct. Heeding the words of their priests and bishops, most Catholics still believed that the purpose of marriage was to raise children, and the purpose of sex was to procreate. Companionship, happiness, and joy in family life were all well and good, if they happened, but they were certainly not essential, perhaps not even particularly important. If a couple couldn't afford to rear more children, well, then, they could try rhythm, and if that didn't work, they would just have to stop having sex. Indeed, it had been only a decade before, in 1951, that Pope Pius XII had given formal sanction to the rhythm method.

Fast forward to 1968: American and Western European priests would be defying the hierarchy and giving their married parishioners permission to use birth control, and almost no one but the disgruntled (and celibate) hierarchy would still be insisting that the only purpose for sex was procreation. The oral contraceptive had a major influence on the attitudes and behavior of married Catholics. And John Rock was both a driver and a symbol of this particular transformation.

Until the 1960s, Catholics had been pretty much left out of the twentieth century's reproductive transformation, continuing to have families that were consistently larger than the families of white Protestant and Jewish couples.[8] During the baby boom, Catholics had simply kept on having larger families. They just stood out a bit less when everyone else was producing more children. But in the 1950s, Catholics were becoming more assimilated into American culture in other ways, too. They suburbanized, took up the anticommunist cause, and their religion seemed less of a barrier to their acceptance. A Catholic would even be elected president in 1960.

While Catholics were moving toward the mainstream, so too was the birth-control movement, once the province of self-proclaimed radicals.[9] As one journalist described the latter change, in 1916 Margaret Sanger was considered a criminal for distributing birth control, and by 1949 she was being awarded honorary degrees by elite colleges for it. Her brilliant cooptation of the medical profession was of course one factor; another was the middle-class and urban desire for smaller families as the economic need for large broods of children became relegated to rural areas. But perhaps a bit less recognized, until the fissures within Christianity broke open so publicly in the late 1950s and early 1960s, were the ways in which most Protestant denominations had been moving toward approval of the use of contraceptives by married couples. (Within Judaism, only the Orthodox disapproved of the use of contraceptive devices.)

The Unitarians and Universalists, predictably, had been among the first to approve of contraception, the latter in 1929 and the former a year later. The Anglican Church was a bit more tentative but was also moving in the same direction. Although contending that abstinence was the "primary and obvious method" for a couple to use if they did not desire a pregnancy, the 1930 Lambeth Conference also proclaimed that "other methods may be used, provided that this is done in the light of . . . Christian principles." Congregationalists followed with a more ringing affirmation of contraception the following year. By the 1950s nearly all mainstream Protestant churches could agree, as the magazine *Christian Century* stated, that "Christians should feel no qualms about using such devices to prevent conception as have been made available by science."[10]

"Birth control" had become "family planning," and almost everyone took for granted that companionship and sexual pleasure were nearly as important to a couple's happiness as their joy in their children. An opinion survey among white married women, conducted by *Scientific American* in the mid-1950s, had discovered that an overwhelming majority of Jewish wives (nearly 90 percent) and a somewhat smaller majority of Protestant women (73 percent) approved of the use of any contraceptive method for married couples.[11]

The fact that white Protestant and Jewish couples, as well as middle-class African Americans, took advantage of the contraceptive methods available reflected the shift in beliefs about the meaning of marriage and parenthood. In the 1950s, few married women remained deliberately childless. Women, indeed, turned motherhood into a career of sorts, at least while their children were young. Birth-control methods allowed them to plan and space subsequent births. Protestants and Jews, and their spiritual leaders, believed that contraception, used in this manner, fostered a couple's love and commitment. Romantic love and sexual intimacy fueled happy marriages and were expected to bring feminine fulfillment. These attitudes were at the core of the baby boom. The fact that everything changed within a decade or so may certainly belie the reality behind those beliefs, but it does not make them less heartfelt at the time.[12]

Most Catholics, especially but not only the clergy, viewed the purpose of family life quite differently. In the *Scientific American* poll, two-thirds of Catholic wives approved only of rhythm, and even that not completely.[13] In fact, no matter how similar in education or income, Catholics were "less likely to practice family limitation" of any sort, including rhythm, and if they did, they used it much less consistently. Only one factor brought Catholic wives closer to the rest of the nation and that was working outside the home. "The differences based on religion," the researchers noted, were "smallest among wives who have worked at least five years since marriage." But only a minority of women in the 1950s worked outside the home when their children were very young.[14]

If even rhythm made the Catholic hierarchy uncomfortable, diaphragms and condoms were beyond the pale. Most Catholics believed that Protestants and Jews were in error when they justified the use of contraceptive devices under any circumstances. Protestants could argue all they wanted that acceptance of or objection to contraception was a matter "of religious persuasion." Not so, said the Jesuit magazine *America*. "The Catholic Church teaches that contraception is against the natural law, and [obedience to the natural law] is . . . a matter of universal obligation." Contraception, therefore, was inherently evil. That "evil is not limited to the adherents of any particular religious creed but is independent of religious persuasion." Protestants and Jews were, quite understandably, bewildered by the Catholic Church's insistence that the "natural law" as the Church defined it "transcends civil legislation." As far as the Catholic Church was concerned, it was not a question of simply allowing Protestants, Jews, and others to go their own way. If the Catholic teaching was the only correct one, then the Church had to stand firm.[15] Catholics could be tolerant of those in error, the Church taught, but they need not agree to let them pass legislation that would embody their error.

It is particularly interesting that just as Catholics were moving into the mainstream of American life, the Church would throw the gauntlet down before the issue of family planning. But so it was. Lurking beneath this attempt to hold back a tide of belief and practice contrary to their own was the fear that contraception was born of, and led to, an ethic of marital pleasure and mutual fulfillment that was inimical to the restraint and self-denial so exalted in principle by the Catholic Church. The raison d'être for marriage, the Church stated flatly, was the "procreation and education of children," and a couple should have no reason to have sex if procreation were not a possible result. After all, "to participate in sexual intercourse, but at the same time to take steps which would interrupt the normal consequence of that act, is to obstruct the natural processes for which marriage was primarily intended."[16] Seminarians who believed their textbooks learned, even as late as the 1950s, that "the sexual act [was] a thing filthy in itself," and that all marriage did was to give couples "the right to perform indecent acts."[17]

The Catholic Church made no apologies for organizing campaigns to keep draconian anti-birth-control legislation in place in Connecticut and Massachusetts, or for intimidating public hospitals in largely Catholic cities into prohibiting doctors from offering contraceptive advice or devices. No stranger to this controversy, Rock had criticized the hierarchy's position for more than a decade, telling *Time* magazine as long ago as 1948 that physicians should be free to provide contraceptive information. "I don't think that Roman Catholicism forces a man to interfere with other people's freedom of conscience and action within their own moral principles. In a democracy such as ours, a man's religion does not oblige him to force legal restrictions on another man's freedom of action."[18]

By 1960 or so, much of the Catholic lay press had caught up to Rock's 1948 position. *Commonweal*, the leading nonclerical Catholic magazine, began taking a much more conciliatory stance in encouraging its readers to be more tolerant of Protestant and Jewish views. This softening of Catholic lay press views had much to do with the presidential aspirations of John F. Kennedy.

It was important for Kennedy to distinguish his faith as a Catholic from his possible actions as a president. With the nation's official Catholic spokesmen (and men they universally were) insisting that the Catholic position on contraception, while a minority view, was the only correct one, and with Catholic majorities continuing to support rigid anticontraception laws in Connecticut and Massachusetts, Kennedy found that his fellow Catholics were fueling opposition from those who believed that a Catholic president would be in bondage to Church positions.

Commonweal, however, was on Kennedy's side and began running articles in 1960 insisting that Catholics were not "bound to support existing anti-birth control laws" and certainly had "no obligation to put them on the books where they do not already exist."[19] The magazine also published letters from Catholics who disagreed with the Church's stance, and by 1962 its editor called the Connecticut law against birth control "particularly odious, since it makes a crime of not only the dissemination but the use of contraceptive material. To put it bluntly," the editor continued, "I want to keep the state out of the bedroom. The marriage relationship is a personal and a sacred one, and this legislation gives powers to the state in an area where I am quite unwilling" to have it do so. Having the state involved in sexual matters in any way, he concluded, is "an obvious and serious danger, and I am unable to understand Catholics who do not see it."[20]

Such dissenting voices, within both the laity and the priesthood (including some theological experts), did not, in the early 1960s, sway the views of the Catholic hierarchy, which doggedly refused to move an inch on the issue of birth control. Conceding that overpopulation in the developing world was a problem, the hierarchy called for scientists to develop new food sources and for the developed world to be wary of imposing its views on nations inhabited largely by poor people of color. As for married couples in the United States, they were simply told to trust in God and curb their lustful natures. At this point, Catholics in great numbers had not yet begun to defy their church. Certainly they did not in Massachusetts, where year after year the Catholic vote prevented repeal of the half-century-old ban on the sale of contraceptive devices.

Rock was preparing for his public campaign to "end the battle over birth control," as he would say time and again during the next several years. He believed that the pill, a different kind of contraception from mechanical or chemical barrier methods, should pass muster with the Church. Within the

next few years, Rock would become one of the prime movers in making it possible for Catholic couples to justify the use of birth control to each other and
their consciences.

He began to promote this idea in the early days of the pill, in the guise
of considering menstrual irregularity as a treatable gynecological condition.
Some Catholics agreed with him, at least in part. In 1958, only a year after
the pill was approved for use in gynecological disorders, the *New York Herald
Tribune's* science editor, Earl Ubell, claimed of the pill that "the compounds
may solve the problem of birth control in this country." Ubell even quoted
an unnamed priest in the Catholic archdiocese's chancery who said "that the
church would not consider it a sin if a Catholic woman regulated her menstrual period with such pills and thereby increased the rhythm method's effectiveness." In this very Catholic city, however, he cautioned his readers that
"according to the Chancery Office priest, the rhythm method may only be
practiced by Catholics with permission of confessors where there is economic
or health justification, consent of husband and wife, and when it does not lead
to other sins."[21]

Although Rock had no moral qualms about birth control, as late as 1959 he
still had not decided how much of a public stir he was willing to create and
seems to have sought spiritual advice. To one correspondent he wrote that
although he was persuaded that the Church would have to change its mind
on the birth-control issue, he also wanted to "fight this battle in my own way
and without . . . avoidable embarrassment."[22] By 1960, having expressed his
anxiety to the Searle executives over whether Pasquale DeFelice's Catholicism
would make the FDA physician unwilling to approve the pill, Rock moved on
to initiating private conversations with several priests who were more expert
in Catholic law and doctrine than he was. He did not want them to advise him
about what position he should take, however. What he really wanted to know
was how to justify theologically the one he had already adopted.

Soon after Rock told the 1960 meeting of the American Society for the
Study of Sterility that he believed the pill would be acceptable to Catholics,
his remarks evoked a public attack from Jesuit priest John Lynch. Father Lynch
insisted that if the pill were used with "contraceptive intent," then its use was
a sin. The pill, he said, was "direct sterilization," and he was sure that any
"competent theologian" in the Catholic Church would "reach the same conclusion." Rock seemed taken aback and wrote to Dom Gregory Stevens, a distinguished theologian at Catholic University. Was it possible that Lynch was
correct? Rock asked. Dom Gregory equivocated, his own thoughts still being

formed. On the one hand, Father Stevens saw no difference in "contraceptive intent" between couples using rhythm and women taking the pill. On the other hand, the pill did appear to him to be a form of "chemical [albeit temporary] sterilization." In short, he needed to give the question more thought. Rock, however, after a dialogue with the priest lasting nearly half a year, was increasingly sure of his position. In October, after visiting Dom Gregory in Washington, Rock wrote, "I want, desperately, to be, and to set things, right." What he really wanted, as he made clear, was to persuade Dom Gregory to agree with him. "I hope you'll think I am right already," Rock wrote, "and should, therefore, push ahead on my present course."[23]

Rock did just that, addressing Planned Parenthood associations in 1960, promoting the pill both in the *Journal of the American Medical Association* and in *Good Housekeeping* in 1961, and fielding hundreds of letters from physicians, pharmacists, and ordinary Catholics, women and men. In *Good Housekeeping*, Rock praised those Catholics, both clerical and lay, who believed that Catholics should not stand in the way of people from other religions having access to birth control. In other words, "All restrictions, written or unwritten, should be lifted" in the public arena, including in hospitals and outpatient clinics. "No one should be compelled to accept birth control, or to participate in a birth-control program, against his will. All methods—including the rhythm method—should be offered so that the communicant of any faith will be able to choose a method in accord with the dictates of his own conscience." Citing statements from a group of Nobel laureates and "scientific and public leaders," he predicted that unless birth control became part of an international solution to the problem of global overpopulation, the people of the world would experience the emergence of "a Dark Age of human misery, famine, undereducation and unrest, which could generate growing panic, exploding into wars fought to appropriate the dwindling means of survival."[24]

By now, Rock was regularly expressing his "confident hope" that the oral contraceptive "will prove acceptable to my church." The pill, he said, "simply duplicates the action of" progesterone, "this natural hormone" that is supplied by a woman's body "when nature seeks to protect a fertilized ovum or growing foetus from competition" by preventing the release of another ovum.[25] He said it publicly. He said it privately. Whenever he wrote to Catholic couples, he said it forthrightly. To one he wrote, "You ask about my church. There are many members of the clergy who are quite willing to express their approval of these pills to me in private," although not yet publicly.[26]

One of his correspondents was a woman who became pregnant twice in as

many years while practicing rhythm, and whose priests had denied her newest baby baptism because she told them she was using contraception. Rock
responded with sympathy and reassurance. It was true that the "official position of the Catholic Church" was that any form of birth control, except for
rhythm, was wrong. But that did not mean she had to agree, since "this point
of view is not covered, as far as I know, in canon law, nor has the Pope issued a statement covered by his infallibility." Rather, the pope had simply "expressed the opinion on which the official position of the church is based." In
case she missed his point that the Church was in error, he said further that "in
my conscience" the use of the pill was perfectly acceptable, encouraging her
to "do only what your conscience clearly tells you after you have considered
your priest's advice." He said the same thing whenever a Catholic physician
questioned his stand on contraception.[27]

The fact that Rock was speaking in theological terms about fallibility and
infallibility showed the influence of his friends and associates among the
priesthood. Many of them, like Rock, had come to believe that the Church's
position on contraception should change. Unlike Rock, however, they still
would not speak out in public. They hoped that the Church would change its
mind and they would never have to do so. But Rock's clerical friends were in
the minority among American priests in 1960 and 1961. The idea that the pope
could be fallible on birth control was not something the American hierarchy
was willing to entertain.

In 1962, Rock became the literal face of Catholic support for contraception
when he was featured on national television in a special CBS Reports program
on "Birth Control and the Law." He no longer pulled his punches. He later
remembered that a rapt national television audience heard him proclaim that
"I approved of [the pill] and that the Church ought to approve of it and that I
was very sure they eventually would." His appearance prompted an avalanche
of mail, including letters from Catholic women who wanted to use the pill
but wondered about its morality. He responded personally to as many as he
could, telling them to remember that the pope had not spoken infallibly on
the issue. Papal pronouncements, therefore, "need only to be considered carefully by Catholics in the formation of their consciences. It is their consciences
which must finally tell them what is right and what is wrong in matters of
faith and morals on which the Pope has not already spoken under the mantle
of infallibility."[28]

. . .

What had begun as Rock's opinion had now become his crusade.[29] After Nan's death, he traveled the United States and South America, and crossed the Atlantic Ocean during the next several years, to promote his views. He argued that the oral contraceptive really was a form of contraception that could be made acceptable to the Catholic hierarchy. He promoted the intrinsic importance of sex to a couple's happiness. And he had become increasingly involved in the issue of what was perceived as a global population crisis.

It is difficult to say precisely how important what was sometimes called the "population bomb" was to Rock. His familiarity with the idea of a potential for a world crisis due to excessive population growth was of long standing. As far back as the late 1940s, environmentalist William Vogt, who served as the executive director of Planned Parenthood, had raised the specter of overpopulation as part of his organization's message. Over the course of the twentieth century, advances in public health had helped most of the world lower the death rate, but the birth rate kept on climbing.

As cold war anxieties replaced the threat of fascism in the minds of many Americans, some of those concerned with increasing population described the developing world as the next battleground between communism and capitalism. Atomic metaphors abounded: Hugh Moore, Dixie Cup magnate and cold warrior, fanned the fears of communism with his 1954 pamphlet, "The Population Explosion." The more moderate John D. Rockefeller III led the Population Council, which he had founded in 1952. While the Population Council developed demographic data to chart the growth of the world's population, Moore gained attention by his claims that Communist control of the underdeveloped world was a foregone conclusion unless the population of these nations was brought under control.

Rock would also have discussed the population issue with Katharine Mc-Cormick and Margaret Sanger. The two venerable feminists and members of the International Planned Parenthood Federation believed that contraception would lead to women's emancipation in the developing world, while the mainstream philanthropists argued that fertility control translated into stable societies. The anticommunists, of course, feared the takeover of an ever-larger "third world" by the followers of Marx and Lenin. All in all, advocates of providing contraception to the poorer nations of the world proliferated in the 1950s.[30]

The issue also aroused considerable interest among Rock's fellow experts in human reproduction. In 1956 Rock wrote to Karl Sax, a colleague at Harvard, to congratulate him on his new book, *Standing Room Only*. Referring to the "terrifying urgency" of the global population problem, Rock noted the importance of "speeding up intensive research for the ideal contraceptive," on which, of course, Rock was working.[31] Very soon, Rock would see how socioeconomic development and fertility control were interconnected in Puerto Rico.

A conventional Republican voter for most of his life (he would start voting for Democrats in his very late years), Rock's correspondence in general showed little passion for any political issue except those connected with his own work. The population issue did touch on his area of expertise, but he was interested in it for other reasons as well. A more or less reflexive anticommunist, he adopted cold war rhetoric to justify what seemed natural to him, that extreme poverty led to disease, unhappiness, and, yes, social unrest. As he worked on the pill, he became sensitive to the issue of overpopulation, although he never saw the pill as a panacea for the rural, illiterate, and innumerate poor nations in Asia and Africa. Once he began to care about this issue, he made it his business to try to make sure he truly understood the matter. When he was planning his trip to Bombay for the 1959 meeting of the International Planned Parenthood Federation, for example, he asked his friend and college classmate Christian Herter, at the time Dwight Eisenhower's undersecretary of state, to have someone at the State Department brief him on the problems in India. Both his personal and professional correspondence clearly demonstrate that the population "explosion" was an issue for him.[32] Still, it was not the only, or even the most important, reason for his decision to become the Catholic face of the contraceptive revolution.

For nearly his entire professional life, Rock had borne personal witness to the evils that could result from too many children combined with too little money. He had treated the indigent and the struggling for more than thirty years. Some patients came to him after having been driven to abortion. Others barely coped, sometimes having their children sent off to foster care when their burdens became too heavy. Still others endured alcoholic husbands, or supported incapacitated ones. Some of the men, reportedly too ill to work, were nevertheless capable of repeatedly siring offspring. What he had first witnessed in Boston he saw repeated in Rio Piedras and rural Kentucky. Even among the many fortunate couples who loved each other, repeated pregnancies and the nagging fear of pregnancy caused tensions and worries.

Rock wanted every couple who wanted a child to be able to have a child, and he wanted every couple who had children to be able to enjoy sexual intimacy without the constant fear of pregnancy if they were not ready to have another child. Since the Catholic Church allowed married couples to have intercourse during a woman's "safe" period, and since, in his view, the pill simply guaranteed an extended "safe" period, then the Church should allow couples to use the pill. Rock had long approved of diaphragms and other contraceptive methods, but he saw the pill as particularly good for Catholics because it created no mechanical or chemical barrier between sperm and egg. Having this belief confirmed privately by priests and theologians he trusted, he grew ever more confident. A number of priests, he told Searle's Bill Crosson, "down deep . . . agreed with me; but of course they cannot allow themselves to do it in public . . . If I can stay on the job I shall do my best to wear them down and break their fetters for them."[33]

. . .

John Rock was already a household name in the United States in 1963, thanks to nearly nonstop media coverage of his views, but he was about to become an international celebrity. In that year, Knopf published Rock's second book on birth control, *The Time Has Come: A Catholic Doctor's Proposals to End the Battle over Birth Control*. Much of the book covered the history of contraception and the problem of global overpopulation. It was the final section, endorsing the pill as a legitimate form of contraception for Catholics, that had a major impact nationally and internationally.

Late in his life, Rock recalled that the book had been the brainchild of the Planned Parenthood Federation of America, not his own, although he soon threw himself into the project. In his old age he recalled it as the book "that was published many years ago with my name as author." Two professionals, both of them working for Planned Parenthood, did most of the writing. One was Frederick Jaffe, then the organization's public information specialist, and the other was Winfield Best, who in 1963 was its executive director. Experienced writers and public relations experts, they shrewdly recognized that the book would carry much more weight if it appeared to come solely from Rock's own mind and heart.[34]

Rock's voice emerges quite clearly in this book. Even if he did not actually do the bulk of the writing, he put a great deal of time and effort into the project. Several drafts of the manuscript survive, including sections in Rock's handwriting. Among them are pages of additions, corrections, and comments from him, as well as correspondence from Jaffe. Rock did not hesitate to overrule their suggestions when he disagreed. "I did spend quite a lot of time with them while they did the actual writing," he remembered. "I gave them verbally much of the stuff they actually put in writing, and then I spent many hours going over their stuff. I suppose one might say I worked at 'editing' it."[35] He was being too modest; he did more than that. Certainly the ideas about love, sex, marriage, and the new hormonal contraceptives were pure Rock. He had been making many of these remarks to limited audiences since the 1950s, and more publicly, in speeches and magazine articles, since the approval of the pill in 1960.

Part of Rock's argument was that the pill's ingredients were manufactured versions of the natural hormones that governed ovulation. Since the Church did not prohibit sexual intercourse for married women at times when they did not ovulate or during early pregnancy when the dominance of progesterone prevented the release of another egg, he reasoned, it should not object to the pill, which produced the same situation throughout the month. Besides, the Church had already approved of the use of the pill to "regulate" the menstrual cycle so that couples could better practice rhythm. How was this any different? It was not, Rock concluded.

The Time Has Come also made Father Finnick famous. Finnick was the apocryphal priest who had urged John Rock in 1904, when the now-eminent doctor was just out of short pants and trying to navigate early adolescence, to "always stick to your conscience. Never let anyone else keep it for you." Pause for emphasis, then "And I mean *anyone* else."[36] Father Finnick was the star of the opening anecdote for *The Time Has Come* as well as resurfacing in numerous print interviews and on David Brinkley's hour-long television special on the pill.[37]

Widely reviewed, Rock's book was both praised and vilified. It served as a lightning rod for a battle not just over contraception, but over the meaning of sexuality and parenthood. It reignited religious antagonism between Catholics and non-Catholics and promoted divisiveness within the Church, galvanizing those Catholics who believed that the time *had* come for them to join their Protestant and Jewish counterparts in accepting birth control.

The Time Has Come unleashed a firestorm in large measure because the Catholic Church was itself at a critical turning point. Years earlier, Pope Pius XII had declared that the heart of the Church was its lay faithful in the parishes and dioceses of the world, and that the hierarchy existed to serve them. Of course, he did not expect the laity to take him literally, and they were wise enough not to do so. His successor, Pope John XXIII, took the idea further, calling for a Vatican Council (Vatican II) to revitalize the Church and to bring it into the modern era. The time-honored liturgy, the anonymity of the confessional, and the Church's refusal to recognize Protestantism as a legitimate form of Christianity were challenged. Each of them would be changed. Why should the opposition to birth control remain sacrosanct in the light of such questioning? Indeed, John XXIII, although he had expressed conventional views on the desirability of the large family, had begun quietly creating a committee to examine the Church's position on birth control in the months before his death. What would have happened had he lived will never be known, but Rock's ideas may have had a very different reception.

Among the reviewers of The Time Has Come were furious conservative Catholics (many, although not all, from the clergy), hopeful liberal Catholics (many, although not all, from the laity), and a number of wildly laudatory non-Catholics. The Christian Century, perhaps the nation's leading Protestant magazine, said that the book "began to shape history as soon as it was published." President Kennedy mentioned Rock and the book in a news conference, announcing his support for Rock's plea for more research on fertility regulation. Writer Michael Novak, soon to become a well-known voice on matters Catholic, insisted, without being much attended to by the clergy at this point, that "married laymen . . . are the Catholics in the best position to develop an accurate, realistic theory of personal sex," including the place that contraception would hold in such a theory.[38]

Conservative commentator Milton Himmelfarb may have been right when he said that underneath the praise for Rock among non-Catholics lurked "condescension and amusement," expressed only privately. He mocked the non-Catholic reviewers: What they really meant, he said, was this: "So there are, after all, enlightened spirits in Catholicism, and so a Catholic can, if he is brave enough, say things that will annoy the bishops and the Knights of Columbus; but how funny it is that someone should need so much courage and subtlety to plead for what everybody [non-Catholic "everybodies," that is] has long since known and does as a matter of course." Himmelfarb's assessment of non-Catholic opinion was not far off the mark. Anti-Catholicism was still an acceptable liberal pose, and Catholic patterns of fertility were not yet like those of Protestants and Jews.[39] Church leaders did fear the prospect of Catholic couples behaving in the same manner as their non-Catholic counterparts and would do their best to prevent it if they could.

While non-Catholics declared that "all of us have reason to be grateful that a man as devout and as professionally eminent as Dr. Rock has been raised up to point the way we should go," furious traditionalist Catholics denounced Rock's imperfect grasp, in their view, of moral theology. For several years

Rock had been advising Catholic couples, and telling the public, that since the pope had never spoken *ex cathedra* (i.e., infallibly) on the subject of birth control, contraception was a matter for each couple to square with their own consciences, after duly noting the pope's teaching on the matter.

That attitude drove the traditionalists crazy. They couldn't quite say "Nonsense!" since Rock was essentially correct. Instead, they insisted, in some variant of the line taken by one Jesuit reviewer, that "contraception is intrinsically evil and a violation of the 'law of God and of nature.'" For that reason, Catholics were obliged "to accept the official teaching of the Church even when promulgated by means of encyclicals and allocutions." (These are both instruments of papal teaching, but they do not have quite the same moral weight as an *ex cathedra* pronouncement.) Having disposed of the independence of conscience, the traditionalists insisted that since Pope Pius XII declared that the pill was "temporary sterilization" if used solely to prevent pregnancy, then temporary sterilization it was, and Rock had no business arguing the contrary. Furthermore, while the official Church surely agreed with Rock on "the general objective of keeping birth control out of politics," such an objective was "good . . . only to the extent that there is no formal approval of objectively immoral procedures."[40]

In short, keeping contraception out of the realm of public policy was good as long as public policy did not endorse anything that was "objectively immoral." Since contraception was, however, "intrinsically evil," then Catholics could not endorse laws that would support it. And yes, it was true that the pope had not spoken infallibly, but that did not matter. He was the pope, so what he said was binding on the faithful. No wonder Protestants (and many Catholics) were confused!

Most of the conservative Catholics concentrated their attacks on Rock's moral theology. Only one, Herbert Ratner, a physician and public health official in suburban Chicago, attacked his medical ethics. Ratner would go on to assail Rock and the pill again in future years, acting as a source for journalist Barbara Seaman later in the decade during her own war against the pill. In his review of *The Time Has Come*, he accused Rock of unethical conduct. "Dr. Rock," Ratner told the readers of *Commonweal*, "is a research physician most noted for his work on early human embryos. This work, which dates back to 1938, is referred to in his book. His embryos were recovered from *pregnant* women undergoing *elective* hysterectomies."

Ratner was the only reviewer to comment on Rock's discussion of his embryo studies, and not surprisingly, Ratner found the research horrifying.

"Those who recognize the human fetus to be a human being throughout development," he wrote, "and Catholics are numbered among them, will recognize these procedures to be a form of lethal human experimentation."[41] It was a telling example of what he saw as Rock's longstanding "intransigence to the teaching of his church." Not only longstanding, but also "deeper than one is led to believe by his present urbane speculations on the Church, the contraceptive pill, and birth control." Indeed, Ratner concluded, recent remarks by Rock "on the future acceptability of abortions leaves no doubt about his basic convictions."[42]

Ratner was correct as a conservative Catholic to mistrust Rock's doctrinal purity on abortion. Although Rock kept his views relatively private throughout most of his career, and in fact was never an advocate of or apologist for abortion, he did believe that there were times when abortions were acceptable. His unorthodox views on this matter were of long standing. One of his patients remembered with gratitude for the rest of her life that Rock had made it possible for her to have an abortion in the 1920s. When she was in her eighties, and he in his nineties, she once again expressed her thanks. One of the two sons born several years after the abortion appended his own note to his mother's letter to Rock, saying that his parents remained ever in his debt, and that they often talked of his understanding and compassion.[43]

In 1979, long after he had retired, Rock explained his attitude toward abortion to an interviewer from the Frontier Nursing Service Oral History Project. "I'm not opposed to abortion . . . as much as many people are because in the first few weeks of pregnancy, there isn't any human being in there anyway. It's just a conglomeration of cells that may turn into a human being . . . Just when the soul enters the body it would be a little difficult for me to stipulate." Rock's views were very much at variance with those of the Catholic Church, which opposed abortion in all instances (and still does), even to save the life of the mother.[44]

Ratner, who was neither a gynecologist nor an expert on fertility, declared the pill "the most dangerous contraceptive product now on the market." Rock's "candor and authority when it comes to the Pill," he contended, had "the same kind of value as the commercial advertisement of a drug manufacturer." Ratner was even more worried that the pill would overturn the "natural" order of gender relations. "The whole order of nature and of love is at stake," he claimed. Rock, he concluded, possessed "a poor grasp of the order of nature, . . . a poor grasp of function in nature." A woman's "nature . . . flows from her delicate and subtle psychohormonic [sic] harmony and lunar rhythms, that which keeps her in touch with the cosmos and her true self. The Pill . . . flattens her womanliness."45

The editors of Commonweal were probably surprised by Ratner's extremism, having already called Rock "one of the few Catholics in America who has had the nerve to say what is on his mind about a variety of matters where silence rather than talk is the rule." While regretting the "gleeful lionizing of the doctor by non-Catholics," Commonweal equally regretted the "indignant, trigger-quick Catholic reflex response." In the editors' view, Rock's book contained "distortions and oversimplifications" of Catholic moral teaching; nevertheless, they wondered rhetorically, "Is the matter of birth control and family planning such a closed issue that it can no longer be discussed in depth? . . . 'The time has come'—not to praise or condemn Dr. Rock's book, but for the church and its theologians to confront anew the issues which he raises."46

Ratner stood alone in his denunciation of Rock as a medical charlatan unworthy of belief even on medical matters. Except for Ratner, even the angriest detractors of Rock's book praised him as a clinician and researcher, contenting themselves with damning his views on moral theology and papal authority. Many Catholics who publicly disagreed with his advocacy of the pill went out of the way to praise his thoughtful assessment of public policy. Boston's own Richard Cardinal Cushing, for example, felt compelled to state that Rock's defense of contraceptives "does not meet the incisive arguments . . . which have been continually voiced by Catholic moral theologians," but then he made it a point to praise Rock for having "rightly criticized the excesses to which some Catholics have gone in this matter."47 Cushing was the head of Rock's diocese. His praise for Rock sent a message that did not fail to reach its audience.

Fueled both by his own conviction that his views on birth control were morally sound, and by the private support he received from Catholic priests whom he respected, Rock remained publicly unruffled by the criticism. He felt sure the Church would come around before too long. Increasingly, he became the world's most visible advocate for the pill. With Nan gone, he had less reason to stay at home, and his travel schedule picked up dramatically. He gave talks across the United States and in 1963 delivered the Oliver Bird Lecture in England, a major honor. His high-profile media appearances no doubt fueled his popularity. His still-handsome face continued to appear in nearly every news and women's magazine in the first half of the sixties.

Rock was profoundly gratified that The Time Has Come had influenced the views of a number of prominent Catholic theologians. Did John Rock single-handedly force his church to consider the issue of birth control? Of course not. In the United States, more and more Catholics were attending college and moving into the upper-middle class. The baby boom was winding down, and smaller families became more desirable. Throughout the Catholic world, the ecumenical movement ushered in by John XXIII encouraged the laity to speak out on issues heretofore reserved for the clergy. Several factors drove the change in Catholic attitudes. Rock was not alone.

But did he exert a major influence? Of course he did. His arguments, ridiculed by American theologians when *The Time Has Come* was published, were taken up seriously in Europe only a year later. All of a sudden, propelled by Rock's arguments and the promised openness of the Vatican Council, Catholics began to challenge the position of the Church regarding contraception. Rock was viewed, especially by European theologians, as a major force for change. They echoed his belief that the pill was as legitimate a birth-control method as rhythm, while other Catholics took up his contention that since Catholic teaching on birth control had never been expressed infallibly, it was open to revision.

In the spring of 1964, a Belgian Catholic journal, *Ephemerides Theologicae Lovanienses*, carried an essay by Father Louis Janssens, professor of moral theology at the University of Louvain. Father Janssens explained that his views had come directly from Rock's work. He went on to equate "periodic continence" (the rhythm method) with the use of the progestins. If the former was considered acceptable to the Church, he declared, then the latter should be equally acceptable. Directly countering Pope Pius XII's argument that the pill, when used for contraceptive purposes, was "direct sterilization," Janssens insisted that if that were so, then "periodic continence would also be a form of direct sterilization."[48]

The conservative wing of American Catholicism responded swiftly, in an article published in numerous diocesan newspapers, by saying that "no established Catholic theologian is on record as agreeing with [Janssens]." *Time* magazine begged to differ, reporting that "some of the keenest theological minds of Catholic Europe," at least privately, "wholeheartedly agree with Janssens."[49]

Time was correct. Within the next few months, it became clear that there was a major fault line within Catholicism on this issue, a fissure made visible by Rock's book. Surprisingly, the divide was not between the clergy and the laity. In favor of hewing to the longstanding Church position were several groups. The first included most of the American bishops, largely Irish American with ascetic views on marital sex. They were supported by men and women of the laity who believed that unrestricted marital sex was the proverbial camel's nose under the tent—if the Church approved the pill, then couples could have sex whenever they wanted, without consequences. Could approval of abortion, pre- and extra-marital sex, and divorce be far behind? They feared not.

Another group of opponents were American Jesuits, heirs to the legacy of St. Augustine, who argued that the natural law prohibited contraception, and therefore the argument was closed. *America*, edited by Jesuits, immediately and predictably editorialized against Janssens' article, and more heatedly against its coverage in *Time*, saying that Janssens' "argument will hardly convince anyone who is not already eager to be convinced."[50] The editors of *Time* responded quickly to *America*'s criticism, showing how important the issue was. One of the reporters for *Time* who covered the story went so far as to say of *America*'s editors that "in the new Open Church, it seems somewhat anachronistic for [them] to imply that thousands of priests around the world (who read *Time*) and hundreds of thousands of parents should be kept in the dark about new thinking on a vital issue."[51]

Ranged against these groups in support of a reexamination of the Church's position were other groups of clergy and laity, the laity emboldened by Vatican II and the clergy by the European bishops. Michael Novak wrote—more in hope than in prophecy—that the European theologians "regard themselves as teachers of the popes and bishops, as those who blaze the trail, 'rethinking the natural law' and also the past statements of the Pope."[52] Catholics eager for a change in Church thinking found *Commonweal*, with its lay editors, a receptive vehicle for their views. Those editors chided bishops and priests who told the laity that they did not belong in the debate about birth control. "Such an attitude no longer makes sense, if it ever did." A priest cautioned his fellows that "the theologian must trust the lay voice when it says that it finds theological formulae abstract and remote from married realities."

Pastors and parish priests could be found on both sides of the divide, but a number of them clearly wanted the Church to change. Father George Casey was not alone when he reminded his church that accepting as many children as one could have may be fine in the abstract, but what is a priest to tell a couple when the wife had borne "nine tiny monstrosities in a row, who lived but a few weeks each"? Or how was he to comfort a woman, who, after bearing "her fifth set of twins in as many years," found herself abandoned with ten children when the husband despaired of supporting them? Does he tell his parishioners, he asked, to abstain from sex? Why should they? When he looked to the Church for answers, Father Casey said, all he could find were "strictures and admonitions from bygone days." Did the conservative moralists care? It "makes me wonder. They seldom have [a] warm welcome for the physicians or scientists who come hopefully forward from their fields with proposed solutions . . . However, to my very inexpert eye, that is the direction from which relief will come."

The controversy soon roiled the Vatican. On June 23, 1964, Pope Paul VI informed his cardinals that the Church would study the birth-control question and would "soon" announce the study's findings. ("Soon" being a relative term; not until 1968 would the pope make a decision.) Rock was optimistic that his church would make the progressive choice. If he needed comfort, he might have found it in the words of Father Bernard Haring, who reminded Catholics everywhere of the importance of the individual conscience in making moral decisions. Haring advised his fellow Catholics to heed the words of Cardinal John Henry Newman, who said, "I have always believed that obedience to conscience, even to a conscience in error, is the best road to light."[53]

. . .

John Rock was now at the peak of his fame as a result of The Time Has Come. Leading European theologians commended him, and the pope had convened a commission to study the Church's position on birth control. Professional accolades and awards came his way, including the 1963 Ortho Medal from the American Society for the Study of Sterility. And Jack Searle, the president of the Searle Company, endowed a chair in his honor at Harvard. Searle gave $400,000 (about $2.5 million today) to fund the John Rock Chair in Population Studies at the Harvard School of Public Health. Its first occupant would be Roy Greep. Rock was both surprised and profoundly touched by Searle's generosity. Although Searle insisted the chair be endowed anonymously, Rock had helped the School of Public Health to solicit the gift, although he did not know until Searle and the dean met in his presence that the chair would be named for him. In 1966 Harvard also awarded him an honorary degree.[54]

In his campaign to change the mind of the Catholic Church on birth control, Rock was not looking for revolutionary change. He believed that the pill could help married couples create a satisfying sexual life and enable them to plan their families. As an observant Catholic, he was not looking for a revolution in sexual behavior. And he certainly did not expect that the pill would come under serious fire for medical reasons in the second half of the decade. He was seeking to settle one issue, and it became complicated by another, which called into question the entire future of the oral contraceptive.

Chapter 9

THE PILL FALLS FROM GRACE

Los Angeles, 1961. Two young women taking the oral contraceptive die of thromboembolic disease. This news shocks the Searle Company, whose scientists expected their research would have already uncovered the possibility of such a serious potential complication.

Castel Gandolfo, Italy, 1968. In his long-awaited pronouncement on birth control, Pope Paul condemns all methods of contraception, except the rhythm method, as against the will of God.

New York, 1969. Barbara Seaman's *The Doctors' Case Against the Pill* ignites a firestorm of controversy and leads to congressional hearings on the safety of oral contraceptives.

In 1964, John Rock expressed confidence that within a few years the pill would change the mind of the Catholic Church about the intrinsic evil of contraception, easing anxieties about unwanted pregnancies for millions of couples around the world. Once the Church liberalized its attitude toward birth control, he believed, the problem of global overpopulation could be addressed through various contraceptive practices.

The contraceptive landscape did change dramatically over the next several years. By the time the next decade opened, the pope had chosen to maintain traditional Catholic policies, and some women's liberationists had joined the Catholic hierarchy in opposition to the pill, although for very different reasons. For the church, opposition to the oral contraceptive arose from fear of the separation of sexuality and reproduction. For many feminists, the issue was medical malfeasance. Their opposition to the pill arose from the belief that doctors and the drug companies had conspired to keep from them information about what they believed were the pill's dangerous, and potentially lethal, side effects. Margaret Sanger, who died in 1966, and Katharine Dexter McCormick, who died the following year, would have been surprised to learn that what they saw as a force for women's liberation would come under attack from a new generation of feminists. Rock would be hit from both the left and the right. A heroic champion of a new and liberating technology in 1964, he had become a beleaguered defender of a suspect drug by 1970. What had happened?

The story is complex and begins, as does many a story of the 1960s, with the coming of age of the baby boomers. The men and women of the largest generation in American history were reaching adulthood in a world that was unprepared for them and coming of age just as the world of their parents was disappearing. Cracks in the foundation of America's international supremacy had widened, the Vietnam War provoked opposition and skepticism about cold war policies, glaring racial inequalities could no longer be suppressed in an era of rising expectations, colleges and universities were bursting at the seams, and increasingly, women were less willing to be content with the idea that their role in life was to marry and have children. We call this revolutionary era the sixties, but it really began at mid-decade. This is part of the context in which the pill controversy played out.

It's not that the kinds of behavior—unconventional sex, youthful rebellion—that would come to be seen as emblematic of the baby boomers had never occurred before. In fact, this sexual revolution wasn't even the first one that we had experienced. As long ago as 1913, a popular magazine claimed that "Sex O'Clock" had struck in America. Moralists in the days before World War I complained about an end to public reticence about matters best left in the bedroom. This earlier sexual revolution had been fueled by an urban working-class youth subculture that flaunted sexuality, by the glamorous bohemian lifestyles adopted by young (and some not so young) middle-class rebels, by feminism, and by an aggressive frankness on the part of the antivice movement. As a result, it seemed, everyone was talking about sex until they were forced to begin to talk about war.[1]

But the transformation that began in the mid-1960s was different, in part because the baby boom generation was so large, in part because higher education had become democratized, and in part because the civil rights movement among other forces had helped to broaden the "base of America's public culture," to borrow historian Beth Bailey's phrase.[2] This time around, the sexual revolution emerged from larger social movements—for racial equality, women's liberation, gay rights, and independence from constraints of various kinds.

By mid-decade the outline of the changes in sexual and reproductive behavior had become clear. Fertility patterns began to shift to one of later marriages and smaller families. By the 1970s the birth rate would plummet. (It
would rise again in the 1980s, but never again to baby boom rates.) The pill
was an important part of this shift.[3]

But there were other factors as well. Just as the baby boomers were about to
grow up, in the late 1960s and into the 1970s, with their expectations shaped
by postwar abundance, the economy was slowing. Their expectations would
collide with a period of recession and inflation, compounded, and to some
degree caused, by the continued turmoil over the war in Vietnam. The antiwar
movement, the sexual revolution, the explosion of a counterculture among
the country's more privileged and affluent youth, and the rise of feminism
all highlighted the ways in which the children of postwar affluence thumbed
their collective noses at the choices of their parents. Feminism encouraged
young women to reexamine and often to reject the wholehearted commitment to children and family to which many of their mothers had devoted their
lives.[4]

This is not to say that all of America's youth could fit neatly into one or
another of these categories. There were those among the young who supported the Vietnam War, married at twenty-two or younger, were shocked by the
behavior of the so-called Woodstock Nation, and would never even consider
dancing half-naked in the mud at a rock festival. And there were many young
men and women who buckled down to a serious life at an early age rather than
lengthening their youth beyond the age at which their parents had owned a
house and had already produced two or three children. Still, it was clear that a
cultural shift was under way, and the pill was a part of the nation's changing
cultural landscape.

· · ·

The Catholic Church—clergy, laity, and hierarchy—had begun its reassess-
ment of the matter of birth control early in the 1960s, when contraception
was still seen as family planning. But by 1965 or so, the hierarchy had become
nervous about both the growing power of the laity and the new sexual mo-
res. The pope, after a brief flirtation with the idea of revising the Church's
teaching about this issue, soon stepped away from what Church conservatives
viewed as the dangerous precedent of ceding too much power to the laity to
make moral decisions.

When the pill was developed, Margaret Sanger's feminist intentions notwithstanding, it was considered a tool for married couples to use as they planned their two, three, or four children. It posed no challenge to mainstream Protestant Americans, since it fit clearly into their own ethic of marital pleasure and devotion, but it played havoc with official Catholic teaching about the purpose of marriage and sex. Married Catholics, however, were beginning to adopt the views of their Protestant cousins, and many of them welcomed the pill as an alternative to the unreliable rhythm method. By 1968, when the pope decided to reinforce the ban on all forms of birth control except rhythm, he would be too late. His prohibition would make little difference to the contraceptive practice of Catholics in the United States and Western Europe, because lay Catholics and many of their own confessors had already decided that whatever the pope said, the most they were prepared to do was take his words under advisement.

Lay Catholics and many of their priests were not alone in their mistrust of authority in these years. The civil rights movement challenged the racial divide. Antiwar activists rose up in protest against the war in Vietnam, no longer believing their political leaders who justified it in cold war terms. College and university students rejected the paternalism, known as in loco parentis, practiced by nearly every institution of higher education well into the decade. The scientific and medical establishments came under attack as skepticism replaced confidence about the many new inventions, including drugs, that were supposed to have made people's lives healthier and more secure. Blind opposition replaced blind faith in better living through legal drugs, while the use of illegal ones flourished. Experts in all fields came under increasing attack.

The story of the backlash against the pill brings together many of these threads. Several prominent Catholic doctors, furious with Rock over his role in developing and then advocating the oral contraceptive, did their best to take advantage of feminist perceptions that there was a conspiracy within the medical establishment to cover up the health risks of the pill. Other doctors, with their own future profits in mind from the development of competing technologies, also attempted to exploit feminist pill opponents. The media covered every claim and counterclaim; journalists who specialized in science and medicine tried valiantly to keep up with the articles in the medical literature. Through it all, John Rock would continue to make the same argument: The oral contraceptive was as natural as the rhythm method. And it was as safe a drug as any, surely safer than a pregnancy. Rock, as did many physicians among his generation, relied far more on his own clinical experience prescribing the hormones than he did on epidemiological data. For him, whether a woman should take the pill depended on her own particular medical history, evaluated, as he always said, by "a competent physician."[5]

Rock's 1965 article in the *Journal of the American Medical Association* was called "Let's Be Honest About the Pill!" The exclamation point was his own. Rock believed that the moral and medical opposition to the pill were linked and that both were equally wrongheaded. Those who objected to the pill on moral grounds, he said, were victimized by "fond but false" theories about the pill's mode of action. A moralist could object to a method of birth control that prevented the sperm from meeting the egg, he supposed, but since the pill prevented the release of an ovum, the egg had no chance to meet the sperm and therefore there could be no real objection. (If the reasoning seems a bit Jesuitical to a twenty-first-century reader, perhaps it was because he was being both advised and attacked by too many Jesuits.)

Rock was just as dismissive of medical objections. Concerns that the pill might cause cancer, or might artificially extend a woman's reproductive years beyond the usual age of menopause, had been raised during the pill's approval process. Reports of thromboembolism were new and of even more worry. Rock was utterly convinced that the pill did not cause cancer and might even be protective against it. He believed that any association between the pill and thromboembolic disease, if it existed, was caused by the fact that the hormones in the pill simulated early pregnancy. He did advise women who had trouble from varicose veins not to take the pill. And in the years to come, he would routinely insist that "pill medication everywhere requires . . . medical supervision." But as long as women and their physicians took appropriate care, he argued, the drug was safe.[6]

· · ·

When writing about the supposed irony of a Catholic developing a new method of birth control, journalists often called Rock "devout." Sometimes he used that word about himself. But in fact, although he remained sincerely observant, Rock had stopped being devout in the accepted sense of the word by the end of his high school years. He poked gentle fun of his religious daughter Ellen, and most of his long-held views about reproductive sexuality were in direct contravention to conventional Catholic teaching. He did believe that couples should have as many children as they could properly raise and educate, but he refused to glorify the large family as such. He continued to hold less-than-orthodox views on abortion, even if he rarely publicized them.[7]

In the two years following the publication of *The Time Has Come*, his cause was taken up by several prominent theologians. Books written by lay American Catholics supporting a change in Catholic teaching on birth control generated even more pressure on the Church. Two of the most widely read were Michael Novak's *The Experience of Marriage*, published in 1964, and John Noonan's influential *Contraception: A History of Its Treatment by Catholic Theologians and Canonists*, which appeared in 1965. Noonan, an attorney turned law professor and an expert on the history of usury (a practice on which the Church had centuries earlier made a major about-face), argued that the Church's teaching on contraception, like its teaching on the legitimacy of interest, had evolved historically and could continue to evolve. His readers could conclude that a change in the Church's attitude to allow contraception would not violate any fundamental Catholic principle any more than its change in teaching regarding the morality of charging interest had. Indeed, as Noonan told a reporter for *Time* magazine shortly after his book appeared, it would be a mistake "to confuse repetition of old formulas with the living law of the church. The church, on its pilgrim's path, has grown in grace and wisdom." And, the reporter added, Noonan's book "suggests that [it] will continue to grow."[8]

Rock was clearly not alone in his argument for a change in Church policy. But he did hold a unique position as one of the most prominent medical experts on human fertility in the country and perhaps its most recognizable Catholic physician, not to mention his role in developing the technology that he hoped would allow the Church to change its mind. After Nan's death he had become a near-daily communicant. He counted priests among his close friends, among them Monsignor Francis Lally, the official spokesman of Richard Cardinal Cushing of Boston. Cardinal Cushing himself was an acquaintance, although Rock would not have claimed him as a close friend. When the intra-Church conflict grew ever more heated, Cushing would decline to reprimand his own diocesan priests who supported contraception.[9]

At mid-decade Rock was spending most of his time on the road, promoting the pill to lay and medical audiences alike. He remained in the headlines and was in constant demand as a speaker. From Planned Parenthood events in suburban Philadelphia to named lectures in London, from lecture series in Mexico, Chile, and Peru to addresses at national professional meetings, he seemed to be on the road more than he was at home. In public he seemed indestructible—courtly, energetic, and looking much younger than his actual age. Only his diary bears witness to his fatigue. In April 1966, just after he turned seventy-six, he noted, "No pain, no untoward symptoms—just darned weak and tired." No wonder, with his schedule! Within a few weeks after that entry, he would be hospitalized for what he called a "slight infarct" in Washington, where he had gone for a speaking engagement. But even his chronic heart disease did not slow him down much.[10] He continued to respond to a stream of letters from admirers, detractors, and ordinary men and women who simply wanted advice.

Conservative Catholic journalist William Buckley wrote about Rock, "Although he has been perfunctorily disavowed by the hierarchy, he has not been exactly anathematized—precisely because the problem [of birth control] is undergoing a most intensive examination." And, Buckley continued, "The fact of the matter is that a solution must be found."[11] The pope knew that he could not duck the issue forever. In 1965 Paul VI convened a closed meeting of his advisory commission on birth control, which he had appointed the previous June. Addressing them on March 27, the pope pressed for a set of recommendations soon. "We ask you, with insistence," he said, "not to ignore the urgency of a situation which requires from the Church and its supreme authority indications which are extremely plain." But it was pretty clear that no "extremely plain" recommendations would be immediately forthcoming. His committee was a divided group, although reformers suspected, according to *Time* magazine, "that the membership has been stacked in favor of the status quo."[12]

By the end of the year, speculation grew that the report was being readied, with the Jesuit magazine *America* stating that "Unless [the pope] has a radical change of mind . . . contraception will not be approved." *Commonweal* also feared that the pope would choose the status quo, but its editors were not prepared to leave the matter there. "Even if one assumes that the Pope will in the end reaffirm the teachings of Pope Pius XI and XII (and we make no such assumption) would this lay the matter to rest? How could it?" In other words, if the pope decided against birth control, Catholics might just ignore him. The University of Toronto's Father Gregory Baum, who served as a theological advisor to the recently concluded meeting of the Council of Fathers, certainly believed they would. "Since the conscience of the Church is so deeply divided over this issue, and since the solution is in no way contained in divine revelation, the authoritative norms which the Pope . . . will propose in due time shall not be a definitive interpretation of divine law, binding under all circumstances, but rather offer an indispensable and precious guide for the Christian conscience."[13]

Catholic couples, however, were no longer willing to wait for the pope's guidance. Even in 1963, when Rock's book was published, 53 percent of Catholics believed that birth control should be available to anyone who asked for it. By 1965, the percentage was up to 78 percent. While such a response did not mean that nearly 80 percent of Catholics were themselves willing to use birth control, studies of contraceptive use also showed a change in Catholic habits. Whereas in 1955 only 30 percent of Catholic wives in the United States had ever used contraceptive measures other than rhythm, by 1965 the figure was 51 percent. In other countries the figures for Catholic wives were even higher—78 percent in Great Britain, for example, and 82 percent in Canada. Studies continued to show, however, that Catholics used birth control somewhat differently from their Protestant and Jewish counterparts. While the latter used contraceptives to space their pregnancies, Catholics did not tend to begin contraceptive use until they decided that they had as many children as they wanted.[14]

While its advisory commission debated, the Church lost more and more control over the issue. Rock insisted that his faith led him to believe that the pope would make the "right" decision—that oral contraceptives, at the least, would be approved as a legitimate offshoot of the rhythm method. Parish priests authorized the faithful to use birth control and wrote letters of permission to Catholic doctors allowing them to prescribe the pill; notable theologians among the clergy and Catholic laity alike insisted that because there was "no Catholic consensus on contraception," in the words of one of them, "the Catholic must follow his conscience." Or, as Newsweek translated for the dense of mind, "In plain words, this means a conscientious Catholic can use contraceptives without sinning."[15]

Soon, leaks from the commission suggested that a majority of its members favored a change in the teachings of the Church on birth control. By the summer of 1966, the commission had made its reports. According to Time, at least four-fifths of the members concluded that the pill was an acceptable alternative to the rhythm method, and a majority believed that all forms of birth control should be allowed. However, there was strong dissent from a minority of the committee, which believed that Church teaching should remain intact and that the only legitimate function of the oral contraceptive was its short-term use to regulate the menstrual cycle. It was now up to the pope to decide. But apparently he had difficulty making up his mind, telling a Milanese journalist, "Deciding is not as easy as studying. Well, we must say something. But what? Really, God's light is needed here." He told the faithful to abide by the old norms while he waited for that light.[16]

In October of that year, in an address to the Italian Society of Obstetricians and Gynecologists, the pope once again announced a delay. "We know the people are waiting for us to give a decisive pronouncement," he said, but he had not yet given the matter enough study. Perhaps to hasten his decision, in spring 1967, one or more commission members leaked the entire report to the *National Catholic Reporter* in the United States and the French newspaper *Le Monde*. The report revealed that a substantial majority of the commission agreed that Catholics could use artificial birth control. This group included sixty of the sixty-four theologians and nine of the fifteen cardinals. The minority, apparently led by the American Jesuit John Ford, issued its own report, calling contraception "intrinsically against nature." *Commonweal*'s editors, not surprisingly, announced that they "accept the majority report and reject the thinking of the minority." And, the editors made clear, while they were willing to consider the teaching of the pope with all seriousness, in the matter of contraception they were by no means willing to substitute the pope's authority for their own consciences.[17]

And there matters stood for yet one more year. *Time* reported in June 1968 that the pope had decided to affirm the ban on birth control, and to do so through a *motu proprio* (translated as "on his own initiative"), a less formal pronouncement than an encyclical. According to *Time*, the motu proprio was "already rolling off the presses" at the Vatican printing office. Then, apparently, the pope withdrew it on objections from European prelates who favored change.[18]

Shortly thereafter, in the middle of his annual summer retreat to Castel Gandolfo in the Alban Hills, Pope Paul VI pronounced on the subject of contraception, and reaffirmed all the old prohibitions against it in a formal encyclical, called *Humanae Vitae* (*Of Human Life*). He condemned all methods of contraception except for rhythm. They were, he said, against the will of God. The news was unexpected. Even many members of his commission were shocked. The *National Review*'s editors said that the Church would come to regret this decision. John Noonan told the *New Yorker* that the encyclical "is not an infallible statement. It is a fallible document written by a fallible man in the fallible exercise of his office." Noonan was hardly a radical—he would go on to become a chief architect of the Catholic wing of the antiabortion movement—but on this issue he was convinced that the pope was wrong. More predictable opposition came from Catholic reformers—and from John Rock.[19]

When interviewed for the *New York Times* several days after the publication of the encyclical, Rock reacted with surprise and dismay. He expressed his opinion that the encyclical would cause "defections" from the Church and a crisis within the priesthood that would put "younger members of the clergy ... in conflict with their elders." But he did not believe that Catholics, having already made up their minds that contraception was not in contravention of Catholic faith or practice, would stop using birth control. He refused to call himself "embittered." He preferred the word "saddened," he said, telling one reporter that "the Church did this with Galileo, remember, delaying application of his scientific insights for human benefit. But the delay was slight, really, and the truth eventually triumphed." He had no plans to abandon his religion, he continued. "I regard myself as a Catholic and I don't think I'm going to be kicked out."[20]

Rock's views were in line with those of much of the American clergy and laity. Neither the editors of *America* nor of *Commonweal* thought of themselves as repudiating the Church in disagreeing with the pope. Rather, the editorial staffs of these journals tried to be both respectful of Paul VI and clear about the independent role of the informed Catholic conscience. Most married Catholics, said the editors of *Commonweal*, had already consulted their consciences and found birth control acceptable. Still, they insisted, "As a solemn although not infallible statement, the new encyclical must be taken seriously and weighed soberly." After all that, however, "it will fail the test of history." *America's* editors, though more measured and reverent, came to much the same conclusion. While declaring that the pope's authoritative pronouncements deserve "respect," and urging all Catholics to engage in "prayerful study and reflection on the pope's judgment," they considered it likely, and reasonable, that many would reject it.[21]

The battle over birth control, as John Rock had framed it, did not destroy the Church, but along with the changes that had been sanctioned by Vatican II, it did change the American Church in significant ways. Shortly after the encyclical's release, two hundred American theologians, in a widely circulated statement, declared that it was "common teaching in the Church that Catholics may dissent from authoritative, non-infallible teachings of the magisterium when sufficient reasons for so doing exist." (An encyclical, remember, is by definition "non-infallible.") In consequence, "as Roman Catholic theologians," they concluded that "spouses may responsibly decide according to their conscience that artificial contraception in some circumstances is permissible and indeed necessary to preserve and foster the values and sacredness of marriage."

Other theologians in the United States signed on as well, bringing the number to about four hundred by September. Many members of the clergy agreed, either publicly or privately. Although Patrick Cardinal O'Boyle of Washington threatened to suspend any priest who did not recant his opposition to the encyclical, and later did so, his response was unusually harsh. Nearly all the other American bishops, while careful to acknowledge the pope's teaching authority, gave couples and their priests the right to rely on their own consciences. According to Time magazine, most of the bishops in the United States and Western Europe "have said, in effect, that Catholic couples who feel duty-bound to practice contraception may do so and still remain in the Church." Most American bishops did not wish either to disagree with the pope or to alienate the faithful on this matter. As a result, when the National Conference of Catholic Bishops issued its own pastoral letter, it endorsed the encyclical while urging those who chose to use contraceptives anyway to continue to attend church and take the sacraments. While at least one bishop seemed to believe that contraceptive use required confession before taking communion, the document did not mention any need to do so.[22]

Although the controversy among theologians would continue for several years, in a strange way the encyclical did settle the matter for most American Catholics. They learned of it, and they also learned that most American theologians did not believe it to be binding. Contraceptive use, for Catholics, would in a few short years mirror that of contraceptive use for other Americans. No wonder Rock, while upset, did not proclaim the encyclical to be a major setback for the pill. He had in fact predicted in 1961 that the pill might win de facto acceptance by the Church without official sanction. Writing to fellow physician (and fellow birth-control advocate) Curtis Wood, he said that he was "still optimistic about Catholic acceptance of the 'pill.'" He added, "When I say accept, I do not imply that they will come out clearly that this and that is OK; but, by default, many things have been approved by lay Catholics and their confessors that had suffered vigorous official rejection in the past."[23] The behavior of American Catholics after the encyclical certainly bore out his prediction.

• • •

A more serious challenge to the acceptability of the pill came in the form of claims that it was a dangerous drug. Although he was as confident of the safety of the pill as he was about its morality, Rock would take the attacks on the drug's safety far more personally than he would the attacks of some Catholics on his moral character.

When oral contraceptives first came on the market, most of the concerns about side effects revolved around such issues as the pill's effect on later fertility and its possible implication in cancer of the breast, ovary, cervix, and endometrium. Rock was most concerned about the fertility issue and believed a larger-scale study of "treated ovaries" than he and others had conducted for the drug's approval should be done. In the early 1960s he was also quite concerned about several cases of hemorrhaging (none fatal, he was grateful to note) among Enovid patients.[24] But no one was prepared when the pill became implicated in fatal thromboembolic disease. Rock, for one, refused to believe in a cause-and-effect relationship.

As he traveled the country promoting the pill, Rock was often asked about its safety. His answer was invariable—the pill produced a condition much like early pregnancy. He said it in the Journal of the American Medical Association. He said it on television. He said it in Family Circle magazine. Women prone to certain conditions in early pregnancy would be liable to experience similar conditions on the pill. But the pill, he said, was safer than pregnancy. He did not expect women to be on the pill for fifteen or twenty consecutive years, however, so it did not occur to him to address issues surrounding very long-term use. And he did not say that the pill was safer than a condom or the diaphragm. After all, when they work, both are safer than anything else.

But then came reports of thromboembolic disease in Enovid users, both in Great Britain and in the United States. (In the 1960s the condition was often referred to as thrombophlebitis, a term less commonly used today.)[25] In the United States in 1961, two women died in Los Angeles. One had been taking Enovid for contraception for two months, the other for an unspecified "medical indication" for ten days. Searle's I. C. Winter, when reporting the deaths to the FDA, insisted that "there is nothing in the record of either case to suggest that Enovid had anything to do with the onset of the disease." The Searle Company was taken by surprise. Because critics had been raising the question of cancer for several years now, Winter had expected that the pill would soon face indictments—in his view, completely unwarranted ones—for causing cancer. "We had not," he told one physician, "anticipated thrombophlebitis." Winter expected that he would have known already if thromboembolic disease could be caused by the pill, but Searle would now have to consider the possibility, and Winter informed the FDA that two studies were already under way to try to determine if "some obscure variation in the enormously complex mechanism of blood coagulation might be rarely affected by Enovid administration."[26]

Of course Winter did not want Enovid to be found to cause thromboembolic disease, which was rare in otherwise healthy young women, just as he did not want the pill to be found to cause cancer. Searle executives were worried. Winter, Crosson, and members of Crosson's staff kept in close touch with Rock as they formulated their response to the FDA and the public. Once the issue was raised, critics, opponents, pill users, and physicians who needed to know what to advise their patients all wanted to have answers.

The fact that the problem had been completely unforeseen complicated matters. Mary Calderone, medical director for the Planned Parenthood Federation of America, responded by conducting a survey of Planned Parenthood affiliates in the summer of 1962 to discover the incidence of thromboembolism among its oral contraceptive patients. In more than thirty-five thousand patients, three cases of "mild thrombophlebitis" were reported, and that was it. No cases had been reported in the Puerto Rican study. Calderone also discovered that "to judge by current medical literature, thromboembolic disease is poorly studied and even more poorly understood . . . It would be a disservice to the future of medical practice if the opportunity were lost for a thorough examination by . . . experts [in gynecology, vascular disease, pharmacology, pathology, and statistics] of Enovid and thromboembolism." Meanwhile, she urged everyone involved not to panic. Instead, she entreated "responsible officials of the public and voluntary agencies, as well as the manufacturers, to do everything reasonable and possible to avoid a reaction of panic among the million women who are successfully taking the oral contraceptive."[27]

Throughout the long controversy, Rock would never waver from his first position, expressed in a letter to Searle's I. C. Winter in October 1962. His "quite unprejudiced judgement . . . derived from 30 years in obstetrical practice and 40 years in gynecology" was that "thrombophlebitis or embolism is in no way related to Enovid medication."[28] Maybe so, but Rock did not prescribe the pill to women with histories of clotting disorders, and once a partial thromboplastin time test became available at the Free Hospital for Women in early 1963, Rock annually tested all women taking hormones for birth control or any other reasons.[29]

By that year, the Ortho Division of Johnson and Johnson had joined Searle in marketing an oral contraceptive. Within another year, Parke-Davis, Mead Johnson, Upjohn, and Eli Lilly companies were all marketing one or another pill variety, and most of them were using compounds developed and manufactured by Syntex. Searle had taken the initial step, but it did not remain alone in this business for long. By mid-decade, it had lost its lead in the market, and would not regain it.[30] In defending the pill, Rock was not exhibiting any special loyalty to the company that had first developed it.

How well did Rock's views hold up during the course of the decade? During the next three years or so, the research seemed to support him, but then for the rest of the decade, the weight of the evidence began to go the other way. The issue would remain contested.[31] At the close of the 1960s, Harvard reproductive expert Robert Kistner listed in his book The Use of Progestins in Obstetrics and Gynecology, in a category called "Cause and Effect Not Definitely Established," the conditions of thrombophlebitis and pulmonary embolism, referring to them as possible but not proven side effects of oral contraception.[32]

Once the Los Angeles and British cases came to light in 1961, there was a need for immediate research to learn if it could be determined whether a cause-and-effect relationship between the pill and thromboembolism existed. Clinical trials of new contraceptives now looked for the condition. One study in the early 1960s, funded by the pharmaceutical company Upjohn, found no cases in 843 accumulated cycles, but women refused to continue the trials after news reports of fatalities from thrombophlebitis appeared.[33]

The law required doctors to report to Searle, and Searle to report to the FDA, any cases of illness or death that could be related to Enovid, which at the time was still the only brand of birth-control pill on the market. By the end of 1961, when more than three million new prescriptions for Enovid had been written and filled, Searle said it had received 272 reports of thromboembolic disease, including thirty-one fatalities. Searle concluded, "Thus far the evidence does not indicate to us nor to our medical consultants that there is a causal relationship between Enovid administration and the occurrence of thrombophlebitis, but caution continues to require the constant consideration of this possibility."[34]

Searle presented more than a hundred of the cases to an FDA review panel, and the FDA in turn commissioned an ad hoc committee to investigate the possible relationship between Enovid and thromboembolic disease. Led by Irving S. Wright of Cornell, the committee concluded in 1963 that there was no increased risk of death in Enovid users. But it did recommend the creation of "carefully planned, prospective studies" to study the matter further. Many fertility experts, including Edward Tyler, also urged this course.[35] Two years later, a retrospective Planned Parenthood Federation of America study of almost twelve thousand patients using any brand of oral contraceptive concluded that the "incidence of thrombophlebitis . . . in the women being studied seemed to approximate that of the normal population."[36]

But by the summer of 1966, a new note of caution had seeped into official language. At the time, the FDA was still mopping its collective brow after its near escape from blame in the thalidomide disaster. In 1962, thalidomide, a sedative and antinausea drug considered so safe by Europeans that in some countries people could buy it over the counter, was discovered to cause severe limb deformities in babies born to pregnant women who took it for morning sickness during pregnancy. Although the FDA had not yet approved the drug when these terrible complications were discovered, it had been considering it. The thalidomide tragedies made everyone more cautious, and Congress mandated tougher standards for the drug approval process.

The FDA became much more wary. When its new Committee on Obstetrics and Gynecology concluded a nine-month study of all the pill's reported side effects, its statement of approval was carefully worded. The committee found no evidence to connect the pill with breast or endometrial cancer or with diabetes, and found no statistically significant connection between thromboembolic disease and pill use. But in the end, recommending continued study, the most the committee would say was that it had found "no adequate scientific data, at this time, proving that the compounds are unsafe for human use."[37]

The medical reports on the pill were reported in the press and on television. Still, at least through 1966, the public maintained its enthusiasm for the oral contraceptive. In 1965 *Good Housekeeping*, in one of its periodic updates on the pill, reminded its readers that while the pill could produce some "unpleasant reactions," it was nevertheless safe for young women to take for up to the three-to-four-year time limit indicated by the FDA. "Evidence has not been produced," the magazine's editors noted, "that establishes the pills as a cause of any disease."[38]

Physicians writing for a popular audience, including Rock's friend Anna Southam, sang the same refrain. Southam, citing Rock as her authority, reassured readers in *Parents* magazine in 1965 that the pill was safe. The following year, when *Newsweek* covered the cautious endorsement of the pill by the FDA's Ob/Gyn Advisory Committee, its headline read, "Popular, Effective, Safe."[39] An article that same year in the *New York Times Magazine*, lionizing Pincus, Worcester Foundation laboratory scientist M. C. Chang, and Rock as "Three Men Who Made a Revolution," also emphasized the pill's safety. By then, more than 6.5 million American wives were "on the pill," along with hundreds of thousands of unmarried women. More than two-thirds of the new Planned Parenthood patients were using it. Worldwide, more than 12 million women used oral contraceptives. The *New York Times* was right—it was a revolution.[40]

· · ·

The enthusiasm, however, was not universal. Traditionally minded Catholics, whether priests, physicians, or members of the laity, remained adamantly opposed to the pill. Among them was Herbert Ratner, director of Public Health in the Chicago suburb of Oak Park, the devout Catholic physician who had denounced Rock as an unethical researcher. As editor of a journal that promoted traditional family life, he wasted no opportunity to denounce the pill throughout the 1960s. He also made himself available as an expert witness to plaintiffs in lawsuits against the pill's manufacturers. So did John Hillabrand, a Catholic gynecologist at St. Vincent's Hospital in Toledo, Ohio, who headed a national anticontraception organization that endorsed only the use of rhythm. Neither of the men were researchers or board-certified gynecologists, and Ratner, although trained as a general practitioner, had not treated patients for years. Both men, in addition to being religious conservatives whose moral views determined their medical ones, harbored considerable resentment and unsuppressed envy of their board-certified and university-based research colleagues.[41]

It may seem easy in retrospect to criticize the doctors who used their medical credentials to criticize the pill when their real reason for opposing contraception was religious. But the fact that some observers viewed their lack of board certification as a plus indicates that trust in experts was coming under siege. This was an era that was coming to celebrate the outsider, and there were those who saw men like Ratner and Hillabrand as doctors of the people who were therefore more credible than the elite physicians affiliated, say, with Harvard or Cornell. One trial directly pitted Robert Kistner, a Harvard Medical School faculty member who was one of the leading experts on the oral contraceptive in the late twentieth century, against Ratner and Hillabrand. Kistner was an expert witness for Searle, which was being sued by a man whose wife died of thromboembolic disease in 1965. In his own testimony, Ratner claimed that Kistner's very expertise made him a "biased person." Kistner could not be viewed as "authoritative," claimed Ratner, because he defended the safety of the pill.

At least one reporter who covered the trial found Ratner's reasoning—that research expertise is not to be trusted—to be persuasive. Hillabrand, who also testified for the plaintiff, claimed in his testimony that board-certified physicians in his city were often incompetent and yet they "drove Cadillacs." Highly trained physicians, such as Kistner, were not too long ago valued for their expertise. Now, that expertise was considered suspect.[42]

Ratner and Hillabrand may have been using medicine as a screen for their moral views. And yet, until research could determine one way or another what risks the pill actually posed, how could ordinary people know how to respond to the headlines? It was essential that medical researchers conduct data-driven studies that would determine, if at all possible, how risky the pill actually was, and these studies became a high priority during the second half of the decade. Some of the most important of them were being conducted in Great Britain, where the incidence of thromboembolism among pill users was almost twice as high as in the United States.

The problem was difficult. The British reports were all retrospective case-control studies, which meant they were observational and backward looking.[43] So were most of the American studies. It was difficult to conduct a prospective study, since thromboembolic disease among young women was so rare, in pill takers and non–pill takers alike. Determining a causal relationship, or lack thereof, was a daunting task. Edward Tyler expressed the frustration of many when he noted that while researchers could find data indicating that blood-clotting factors among pill users sometimes changed during use, no one knew whether the changes were significant.[44]

The controversy continued with no clear answers. By the end of the decade, nevertheless, many researchers had concluded that however little they understood the reasons for it, there was an association between thromboembolic disease and the use of oral contraceptives, at least for some women, especially women over thirty-five and those who smoked. Furthermore, the risks seemed to be higher for women taking pills with the highest estrogen content.[45]

But they still did not know why. Today we can say that it was no wonder researchers disagreed on this issue in the 1960s. Even now, the relationship between hormonal contraceptive use and thromboembolic disease is still being evaluated.[46] Was the culprit the higher doses of estrogen in the earlier pill formulations? What about smoking as a contributing factor? And then there are the inherited predispositions to clotting disorders, such as the Factor V Leiden mutation, which predisposes individuals to deep vein thrombosis. Fifty years ago, doctors would have had no way of knowing that certain women had a special predisposition to develop blood clots. The exact nature of the relationship between oral contraceptive use and clotting-factor changes is still under discussion fifty years after the pill came on the market.

As for claims that the pill was a cause of breast, cervical, or endometrial cancer, which had been around since the early days of pill testing but would become the subject of much speculation by the end of the 1960s, these too would have been difficult to affirm or refute in any immediate sense. It might easily take a decade or more after a woman had stopped taking the pills for cancer to appear. Although by the early twenty-first century, scientists had learned that cervical cancer is caused by a virus, low-dose pills do not cause breast cancer, and that the pill protects against ovarian cancer, none of that was known in the 1960s. The medical opinion about any relationship between the pill and cancer in that decade was indeed just that—opinion.

And Rock was invariably asked for his. He continued to engage in a robust correspondence with the scientists from Searle, offering advice to the company on its response to pill critics, commenting on drafts of letters to physicians about the oral contraceptive, and preparing a film for Searle on the physiology of menstruation.[47] And every week, it seemed, he responded to journalists who called him for interviews or quotes for their newspaper and magazine articles.

. . .

Rock's public life in the mid-1960s was making it extraordinarily difficult for him to remain a personally engaged, practicing physician and researcher. The Rock Reproductive Clinic (RRC) suffered as a result. His travel and lecture obligations left him little time to tend to patients. The clinic's existence now depended on the relatively small grants Rock received from Searle and other pharmaceutical companies for testing new compounds and the $5,000 the Searle Foundation provided him each year in support of the clinic operations.[48] Finances became ever tighter.

Rock obviously wanted to save the RRC, but even as the situation grew dire, he didn't know what to do. He couldn't seem to help subverting his budget manager's attempts to collect from patients. Without adequate funds, the entire enterprise faltered. The Free Hospital, had it wished to do so, perhaps could have stepped in to help, but neither the managers nor the board of trustees had any interest in keeping Rock around. Quite the contrary. In the decade since his retirement and removal from his position as director of the Fertility and Endocrine Clinic, they had come to resent even more the fact that his famous name drew patients to the Rock Clinic instead of to the Free Hospital.

Bluntly stated, Rock was convinced that the hospital now really wanted to eliminate him as a competitor. The younger generation of managers and administrators viewed Rock as an impediment to their own ambitious plans. Here was one of the most famous infertility specialists in the world, with his own clinic literally in the shadow of their own, competing for the same pool of patients. The hospital was trying various strategies to dislodge him, including, in the mid-1960s, denial of Harvard affiliation and privileges at the Free Hospital to Rock's junior associates. Not being able to offer these perquisites made it much more difficult for him to attract the best among the younger physicians. As one consultant to the clinic observed in rhetorical puzzlement, how could it be that "in one of the great teaching universities of the world . . . the staff of a small Clinic, whose Director is a revered Emeritus Professor on . . . [its] faculty, is unable to obtain privileges of the Hospital connected with the University."[49]

The strain was becoming too much, and the meaningful clinical research conducted at the RRC dwindled almost to nothing. But there were other reasons for the decline in research besides Rock's arduous schedule and his inability to manage his clinic. Medical research now required battalions of talented research assistants, residents, and medical students, as well as major grants from the National Science Foundation or the National Institutes of Health. Those in turn required budget managers and grants accountants. There were some successful independent research institutes, such as Pincus's Worcester Foundation, but they conducted animal and not human research, and they had matured into the kinds of institutions that provided all the ancillary services that the new research bureaucracy required.

Rock's shrinking enterprise couldn't compete in such a world. The three physicians on Rock's staff, and Rock when he was there, were by 1965 seeing an average of only eighteen patients a day. The clinic treated patients and tested new fertility compounds, such as Pergonal and clomiphene citrate (Clomid), the major breakthrough drugs of the era for treating the failure to ovulate.[50] Rock may have been correct that a male pill ought to be the next contraceptive priority, but his age, his lack of facility with all things financial, and his clear inability to pull together the kind of research team necessary for such work, would ensure that he would never have a chance to participate in such a breakthrough, regardless of the attitude of Harvard or the Free Hospital.

In 1965, he and Bill Mulligan considered joining forces at the RRC, with Mulligan taking over as director and Rock serving under him as director of research. Mulligan was interested in helping to save Rock's legacy, but before making a final decision about a partnership, Rock and Mulligan hired a medical consulting firm to help them work their way through the issues involved in the proposed venture. The consultant believed that if the organizational and management issues of the clinic could be solved, and an arrangement could be reached for "some logical and acceptable University affiliation to which highly qualified clinical and research fellows can be attracted," the RRC's future could be assured. It would be essential, however, that "Dr. Rock continue to lend the weight of his prestige, ability and charm" to the enterprise, the consultant tactfully stated.[51]

What this meant was that Rock would have to give up control of the enterprise. For someone like him, long accustomed to having things his own way, this would not have been easy. In order for the new venture to work, everyone agreed, Mulligan would have to take complete charge of the clinic's operation, serve as director, and choose his own board of directors. Rock would be the inspirational force, but Mulligan would call the shots. At fifty-four, Mulligan was ready for a new challenge. His ideas for the clinic included the integration of Harvard medical students as well as the house staffs of both the Free Hospital and the Boston Lying-In Hospital into the new operation, plus the hiring of a professional administrator.

Rock knew, to put it mildly, that management was not his strength. He hated to deal with finances. He was unable to fire anyone, and the consultant told him pointedly that never had he seen so many employees do so little work. Miriam Menkin, at sixty-three, was singled out as a particular problem. She seemed by now mostly to spend her time clipping articles and making lengthy notes that resulted in little finished product, but Rock would never agree to let her go. She had been with him too long, she had served him devotedly, and she'd had a very hard life. He remained loyal to her.[52] But the whole staff, with a few exceptions, seemed almost equally aimless, lacking clearly defined duties. Mulligan recognized that administration was not really his strong suit, either. If he took over, he agreed to hire a full-time manager who would reorganize what was then still called the lay staff, reducing their numbers, more clearly defining their duties, and supervising them appropriately. The consultant believed in Rock's work and his legacy. "During the length of time (and it has now been a very long time indeed)," he wrote, "that I have been considering and puzzling over this proposition, I have become convinced that there is an enormous value here that must be preserved and enhanced at nearly any cost."[53]

In the end, however, it all came to nothing. Mulligan chose not to take over the clinic. Perhaps the challenges were simply too daunting, but our best guess is that the stumbling blocks were Harvard and the Free Hospital Board. Mulligan's proposed alliance of the clinic with Harvard and its teaching hospitals was essential to make the plan succeed. It proved impossible to negotiate, so Mulligan stayed where he was, as director of the Fertility and Endocrine Clinic, until his retirement in 1973.[54]

This plan having failed, by 1966 the RRC was living on borrowed time. And so, in its own way, was the Free Hospital. Small specialized hospitals, like the Free and its obstetrical counterpart, the Boston Lying-In, were relics of the nineteenth century. Harvard had long ago pulled them into the orbit of its medical school, but they remained independent entities. In 1964 the medical school, attempting to streamline its operations and eliminate competition for patients among its own facilities, persuaded the boards of the two hospitals to consolidate.[55] By 1968 they had done so, becoming the Boston Hospital for Women. (Later the two Brigham hospitals—Peter Bent and Robert Breck—were added, and the consolidated hospitals became Brigham and Women's Hospital.)

In early 1968 Rock and his clinic were evicted from the building that McCormick had long ago dubbed the "hovel," and which she had renovated for him in the 1950s at great expense. He was almost seventy-eight years old, his clinic was being taken from him, and he was close to going broke. He had worried so much about his clinic's survival, and about the welfare of his employees, that for several years he had foregone much of his own income to support the clinic and its staff. As he did so, his financial situation became increasingly precarious. He had virtually no Harvard pension, and he had chosen not to invest in (or keep) Searle stock when it might have been of great profit to him. Some of his wealthy supporters had given gifts to the clinic, upon which he could have drawn for his own use, but he generally didn't do so. Jack Searle, recognizing Rock's role in Enovid's success, had since 1962 provided him with a no-strings-attached salary supplement. More often than not, Rock turned that over to the clinic also.[56] As time went on, Rock simply lived on less and less. Journalist Loretta McLaughlin reported that no one outside his family knew how poor he really was. It had gotten to the point where he had moved out of his house, and when he wasn't traveling, he was living in a single room above the clinic.[57]

The original terms the hospital offered Rock for his agreement to turn over the clinic included a new position for him as senior consultant in fertility and endocrinology with a stipend of $1,000 per month ($5,800 today) and an office. The Searle Company had pledged to pay the stipend. But he would have no examining rooms, and the office was in an out-of-the-way corner. His daughter Rachel, who went with him to look at the facilities, was shocked when she saw them.[58] In addition, all his staff, including Menkin, would lose their jobs. Perhaps the trustees persuaded themselves that by giving Rock a title and an office, they were treating him with the respect his long career deserved. But for him, it would mean that the Rock name—and with it, perhaps, his legacy—would be erased from the entity he had founded. In the end, the hospital and Rock did not come to an agreement. By March 1968 Rock was forced to lease quarters elsewhere for his practice and whatever clinical studies he would be able to conduct.[59]

To doctors at the newly formed Boston Hospital for Women, Rock must have seemed like an aging lion who would not make way for the next generation. And we know what happens to aging lions. For Rock, letting the hospital shunt him off to a little spot in the new enterprise, with a title but no ability to do any work, was not acceptable. This would be his last effort at maintaining a medical practice. By 1968, he had cut down on his patient load. He was also spending more time at his house in Temple, New Hampshire, which he had bought in 1964 from his daughter Ellie and her husband. They had found it too remote to raise their family. Here he wrote, read, and gathered his strength to keep up the battle for birth control.

He would need that strength. In 1968 and 1969 he was still lecturing throughout the country, with talks to lay and medical groups in Chicago, Baton Rouge, and Cleveland, as well as closer to home in various New England states. Aging lion or not, Rock remained a force to be reckoned with throughout what we might call the great pill controversy of the late 1960s.

By 1967 nearly 13 million women worldwide were on the pill. Six and a half million of them were Americans, and nearly 2 million more were in Great Britain and Europe. Canada and Brazil each accounted for about 750,000. The rest were scattered throughout the world. While the pill clearly had not become the panacea for overpopulation in developing nations, women in the Western Hemisphere and in Western Europe had made it a popular contraceptive option. In the United States it had displaced the condom as the dominant form of contraception by 1963, and by 1968 Americans, according to historian Andrea Tone, were twice as likely to use the pill as the condom.[60]

Newcomers to contraception were ever more likely to choose the pill, and Planned Parenthood was particularly influential in promoting its use. In 1961 about 14 percent of new Planned Parenthood clients selected the pill; by 1966 70 percent of new clients were doing so. Mary Steichen Calderone, Planned Parenthood's medical director, believed in both its effectiveness and its safety. John Rock gave lectures on the pill to regional Planned Parenthood affiliates.

The organization by mid-decade had fully overcome its earlier reservations about oral contraceptives.[61] And the media still considered Rock's opinions important. Gregory Pincus had been the driving force behind the pill, but even before his sudden death in 1967, both print and broadcast journalists had gravitated to the photogenic visage and reassuring voice of Rock. After Pincus succumbed at the age of sixty-four to a rare blood disorder caused by years of exposure to toxic laboratory chemicals, reporters didn't have a choice: Rock was called on to speak for the fathers of the pill whenever an issue arose about its safety.

But now, when he was called on for his opinion, some of his questioners were less deferential than they would have been a few years earlier. Others even tried to put him on the defensive. Rock, who had spent most of his media life being acclaimed as a friend to women—whether in helping them to overcome infertility or making it possible for them to prevent conception—now found himself attacked as a visible symbol of a patriarchal medical profession that felt little concern for the opinions of the women to whom it provided care.

. . .

One of the oldest clichés in history is that politics makes for strange bedfellows. The same might be said for causes. So we should not be surprised to see that the most influential feminist indictment against the pill, Barbara Seaman's *The Doctors' Case Against the Pill*, included among its experts some of those who opposed the pill for religious or conservative social reasons rather than on medical grounds. Seaman had already decided the pill was dangerous before she went looking for medical support for her belief, and her data-gathering method was simply to include all criticism of the pill from any source.

What this meant in practice was that antifeminists, religious zealots, and at least one downright dissembler ended up, side by side with the true medical skeptics, on her list of voices against the pill. Among the religiously motivated was Rock's old nemesis Herbert Ratner, who opposed all types of birth control except rhythm and was a powerful voice for traditional family values. More unfortunately for the women who had faith in the doctors who appeared in the book, however, Seaman was also duped by a doctor pushing a more dangerous hidden agenda.

In the course of denouncing one new medical technology, Seaman inadvertently provided a platform for the developer of another, more dangerous one. One of the pill's most vocal young opponents, prominently featured in

Seaman's book, was Hugh Davis. A gynecologist at Johns Hopkins Medical School who was not board certified, Davis claimed to be an independent researcher testing a remarkable new intrauterine device that, unlike existing IUDs, was effective in women who had never had children. In addition, he proclaimed, this new device was remarkably safe. Davis and his IUD, soon to be marketed as the later infamous Dalkon Shield, were prominently featured in Seaman's book. Sure that the pill was dangerous, she did not question Davis's assertions about this new IUD. Within the medical community, there was some skepticism of his claims, but it was not revealed until several years later that Davis not only held more than a one-third share in the company that owned the Dalkon Shield, but also that he had falsified the data used in his studies.[62]

The Doctors' Case Against the Pill, with an introduction, entitled "A Public Scandal," by Hugh Davis, appeared in 1969. Seaman mined the literature on the oral contraceptives for sometimes serious and occasionally lethal side effects. She believed that the pill was a danger to women's health, and her book was a call to arms.[63] Having decided that the pill was a potentially lethal drug, she was convinced that the gynecological establishment was at fault for unleashing it on the world. Worse yet, as she saw it, pill proponents refused to acknowledge the drug's terrible effects. Although she carefully worded her indictments so that most of them came from the mouths of the doctors and women she interviewed, the message was clear: In addition to thromboembolic disease, the pill caused cancer, heart disease, strokes, sterility, gum disease, hair loss, abnormal hair growth, and depression, not to mention loss of sex drive and its converse, "pill-induced nymphomania."[64]

Seaman selected certain groups of medical practitioners and enabled them to skewer other groups. Although a few of her experts practiced obstetrics and gynecology, gynecologists were mostly her targets, not her sources. She was particularly suspicious of the board-certified specialists, whose professional organization was the American College of Obstetricians and Gynecologists, and the Planned Parenthood Federation, then as now the leading provider of reproductive medical services to the poor and near poor in the United States.[65] Most gynecologists, she believed, were too much in thrall to the pro-pill forces. The medical and scientific voices heard in The Doctors' Case Against the Pill included general practitioners, internists, psychiatrists, and neurologists, as well as the cancer specialist Roy Hertz of the National Cancer Institute.

Among the few gynecologists was Davis, then an assistant professor at Johns Hopkins. There was, he argued, "evidence that the pill isn't safe," and he was grateful to Seaman for making the public aware of that evidence.[66] His condemnation of the pill was absolute: "I think that anyone is entitled to the right of selective suicide whether by the cigarette or the pill or any other means," but doctors were misleading their patients if they didn't tell them that taking the pill could endanger their lives.

Davis, let us remember, was promoting the IUD; specifically, he was promoting the new Dalkon Shield. He told Seaman that "the newest 'safe' contraceptive is the . . . IUD, [which] has many virtues, not the least being the fact that it is not directly connected with the timing of the sex act. No preparations are necessary before intercourse. Nothing needs to interrupt the spontaneity of foreplay or love-making." And while many women report "cramps and spotting, . . . in most cases the discomfort disappears within a few weeks." Readers of this book who ponder these words will not fail to note the echo of claims for the first generation of birth-control pills. IUDs, Seaman reported, heretofore were not suitable for women who had not yet given birth, but she seems to have accepted uncritically Hugh Davis's reports of "a number of happy brides" who had been fitted with "new intrauterine devices, including one they call the Dalkon."[67]

One of Seaman's most serious assertions was that the pill had not been adequately tested. Claiming to have seen the evidence herself, in the papers of Gregory Pincus, that the researchers falsified controls and did not adequately report side effects, she attacked the FDA approval process in a way that could not have failed to resonate in the wake of the thalidomide disaster. Our own careful review of the same papers, however, has failed to turn up any such evidence. More important, the recent scholarly analysis of the FDA's review process by historians Suzanne Junod and Lara Marks has revealed that there was no perfidy or incompetence. Junod and Marks demonstrate definitively that the data provided by the drug company were fully in line with contemporary standards, and that the FDA was much more careful in its review of the evidence for the approval of the pill than it had been for almost any new drug heretofore. This is not to say that their data would pass muster by early twenty-first-century standards; but by the standards of the time, the pill was seriously scrutinized.[68]

Seaman employed the voices of medical experts to express her disenchantment with medical expertise. Her criticism was fully in tune with the times, embodying a major shift in popular attitudes toward medicine and its practitioners. The disenchantment was widespread, and Seaman's book found a large audience. Americans in the late 1960s had begun to display a much more

critical attitude toward science and technology than had the previous generation. The cold war consensus that had viewed almost all scientific and medical
developments as invariably positive and progressive was ending. From now
on researchers would no longer enjoy immunity from cultural challenges to
the moral and ethical validity of their findings and applications. Some of the
strongest resistance to medical science came from the left, and Seaman and
her supporters were exemplars of this new trend.

Seaman's challenge to the medical establishment was an important challenge to the previous age of uncritical celebration of medical progress. As sociologist Paul Starr has observed, the 1970s witnessed a new "health rights
movement" that "challenged the distribution of power and expertise" between
doctor and patient. The feminist attempt to "demedicalize" childbirth—for
which Seaman was also an advocate—was only one example of a pervasive
distrust of the methods as well as the motives of the medical specialists who
treated women. Indeed, Starr views the feminist challenge to medicine as a
significant part of "a broader revival of a therapeutic counterculture with political overtones," in which "the content of medical practice was imbued with
political meaning."[69]

Seaman was an important leader of what Starr has called the "therapeutic
counterculture," but in her eagerness to debunk the pill, she unfortunately
fell for the claims of physicians like Davis, with considerably more flawed
technologies to sell, and Ratner, with a religious ax to grind. Perhaps she was
too invested in her anger to see what seemed so evident in hindsight to historian Elizabeth Siegel Watkins. Women demanded the pill. They were active
consumers of this product. Indeed, Watkins has convincingly argued that the
pill was largely responsible for the "empowerment of women in the doctor-
patient relationship."[70]

Rock was not the principal target of Seaman's fiery denunciation, although
he did come in for criticism. She dismissed his claim that "the pills, when
properly taken, are not at all likely to disturb menstruation, nor do they mu-
tilate any organ of the body, nor damage any natural process." And she expressed incredulity when Rock argued that a *competent* physician would not
prescribe the pill to women with family histories "indicating that they never
should have taken the pill in the first place." Rock, she said, was either "over-
estimating the thoroughness of some of his colleagues" or—in a not-at-all
veiled slam at his age—living in the past. He must have, she argued, been
"thinking of medicine as it was practiced in the old days." Of course, in "the
old days," women never saw a doctor unless they were sick. Another "side ef-

fect" of the pill and other new drugs that required medical supervision was that they surely hastened the modern trend toward the annual office visit to the gynecologist.

. . .

Seaman's book had a major impact, inspiring Senator Gaylord Nelson, long suspicious of big business in general and the pharmaceutical industry in particular, to schedule hearings on the safety of the oral contraceptive. The hearings, begun in January 1970, called even more attention to the oral contraceptives and to contentions that they were unsafe. Nelson led off with Hugh Davis, whom *Time* magazine called a specialist in "IUDs and one of the inventors" of a device not yet on the market. Davis, who asserted that "the widespread use of oral contraceptives . . . has given rise to health hazards on a scale previously unknown to medicine," also questioned their effectiveness, which, he said, "has been greatly overrated."[71]

Davis took every opportunity during his testimony to promote his IUD, at the same time concealing his own financial stake in it. When one senator said he understood that "you yourself have devised an intrauterine device that is extremely good?" Davis hastily responded, "This is not a development of mine, . . . [but] the particular device [the Dalkon Shield] that we have been using . . . has proven quite effective." When asked directly whether he had any "commercial interest" in any IUD, he said he did not. He was lying.[72]

Also on the roster was Herbert Ratner, whose testimony was a litany of dangers from the pill, to which he added a new allegation of "child poisoning." Birth control was not the answer to society's ills, Ratner told the senators. Rather, "the road to social maturity is wanting the unwanted child and the road to responsible parenthood is not technology but the inculcation of responsible attitudes." His remarks elicited some skepticism from the acerbic Senator Robert Dole, who asked Ratner whether he actually treated patients or conducted any research, and wondered whether he was board certified. Ratner tried to dodge the board-certification question by saying he was qualified by the state. He had to answer "no" to the questions about research and patient care, but, he said, he kept up in the literature. With his trademark rapier style, Dole retorted, "You do not do research; you do not have any patients; you read articles; is that the basis of your expertise?"[73]

Ratner and Davis were joined by a roster of pill opponents. "Adamant critics outnumbered defenders by seven to one," *Time* reported, and "most conspicuously missing from the roster was Harvard's Dr. John Rock," mischaracterized by Time as a "thoughtful advocate of research to reduce the Pill's admitted and harmful side effects."[74] Nelson's decision to lead off with the pill's critics was a deliberate one; he already had his own misgivings about the pill. Historian Andrea Tone reports that as a consumer advocate, he was "worried that it had been inadequately tested, that its long-term effects were unknown, and that women were inadequately informed about the drug's risks." Strangely (or perhaps not so strangely given the tenor of the times), he refused to call as witnesses any women who had taken the pill, or any of the feminist activists. He had been influenced by Seaman but never called her as a witness. As a result, a feminist group called D. C. Women's Liberation disrupted the hearings, and television viewers throughout the nation were riveted during the evening news by their demonstration.[75]

The protesters were angry that women's voices were not being heard, but the demonstration did not result in the women being called to testify. In fact, during the first phase of the hearings, not a single woman spoke to the committee. Later, four women spoke or provided written statements, but none of them were feminist activists. There were two women physicians, one of them Columbia University gynecologist Elizabeth Connell, who testified, and another Columbia gynecologist, Rock's longtime friend Anna Southam, who provided a written statement. Not only did John Rock not appear, but neither did Celso-Ramon Garcia, who had overseen the pill's first field trials.

When reporters called on Rock for his views of the testimony given by pill opponents at the hearings, he reiterated what he had been saying for the past decade, that taking the pill was safer than pregnancy and that contraceptive studies based on animal research did not convince him otherwise, since the "effects [that] contraceptive materials have on laboratory animals are not at all indicative of how they work in humans." He told the Boston Globe that when properly monitored by a physician, as many as 90 percent of women of reproductive age could safely use the pill. However, the pill should never, he emphasized, become "an over-the-counter item." In countering critics who claimed that the pill caused breast or endometrial cancer, he insisted "that if the progestational steroids . . . in the approved pill have any effect on cancer of the breast or uterus, 'it is one of prevention, retardation, or suppression.'"[76]

Rock, as a longtime critic of facile animal-human analogies in drug testing, didn't consider animal studies useless, just not foolproof. As Carl Djerassi, who invented one of the two compounds on which the oral contraceptives of the 1960s were based, put it, "In order to gain as much knowledge as possible from animal studies, a species should be selected which most resembles man in its metabolic handling of the drug in question." That could mean different animals for different drugs, and in 1970, when Djerassi was writing, he claimed that scientists still did not know enough to make accurate choices.[77] Rock came to the same conclusion as Djerassi but from a different starting point: Djerassi, a scientist, had long experience with animals. Rock, a clinician, based his judgment on his long experience of having the animal analogy prove misleading.

. . .

An astounding 87 percent of American women paid attention to the Nelson hearings. They did not like what they heard, and oral contraceptive use declined over the next three months. Senator Dole, on learning that women were going off the pill, said that he "hoped the resulting babies [would] not all be named for subcommittee members." History does not record how many little Gaylord Nelsons and Robert Doles were born in the waning months of 1970, but women's use of the pill declined only in the short run. A *Newsweek* poll conducted in February found that 18 percent of pill users had stopped taking the oral contraceptive and another 23 percent were considering doing so. But the pill rebounded in short order. By April, a Gallup poll found that pill use had come back up sharply. Sales dropped, but then they rebounded. They would reach a peak of ten million three years later.[78]

But some women, taking seriously their new role as educated consumers, decided that oral contraceptives were unsafe. Many of them turned to the IUDs so heavily praised by Hugh Davis. He seemed trustworthy, having written the foreword to Seaman's book and testified to the IUDs' safety at the Senate hearings. By January 1971 the particular IUD touted by Davis—the Dalkon Shield—was ready for mass use. From that date until May 1974, just before its manufacturer withdrew it from the American market because of safety complaints, the Dalkon Shield had outpaced the sales—taken together—of all other IUDs. About 2.2 million women in the United States had been fitted with one.

These women had been misled, intentionally so or not. At least eighteen women died from infections caused by the device. More than two hundred thousand cases of complications resulting in infections, hysterectomies, miscarriages, other gynecological disorders, and birth defects were documented by 1974. In 1985, the A. H. Robins company would go bankrupt, and before the deadline for claims against the company would pass in 1986, more than 325,000 claims would be filed.[79] In their search for something better than the pill, American women had been duped by a dishonest doctor, who lied to the press, to Congress, and to the manufacturer who bought the device he and his partners invented. Many women would have been far better off if they had stayed with the pill or had returned to the tried-and-true barrier methods that pre-dated it.

The most important and longest-lasting outcome of the pill hearings was a new regulation requiring patient package inserts for oral contraceptives. Seaman and her supporters rightly deserve the credit for making such medical information available to patients. The first proposed draft of the insert, which warned of potential side effects ranging from blood clots to depression, raised an outcry among physicians, pharmaceutical companies, and government officials. In the end, the patient insert did not discuss specific potential complications but directed women who wanted more information to request a booklet, authorized by the American Medical Association (AMA), from their physicians. Although the AMA distributed four million booklets over the next five years, most pill users probably did not see them.[80]

Senator Nelson wanted to be able to guarantee the safety of the pill. If it were not safe, then he wanted women to be fully informed of its dangers. Women in turn wanted to know definitively: Could they take the pills safely or not? Was a "yes or no" answer possible? Probably not, said Carl Djerassi in an essay for *Science* later that year. "No drug can be *totally* effective and *completely* safe," he wrote, and the "consumer suffers from the delusion that drug safety and drug efficacy are all-or-none propositions. The fact that people experience side effects from 'safe' drugs should be no more surprising than the fact that occasionally some people die when 'safe' airplanes crash."

We can disagree with the conclusion that Djerassi drew from such an observation, which was that provisional approval should be given to new drugs with high potential even if the question of "low incidence toxicity" remained. Still, he had a point about our desire for absolute answers.[81] More than forty years into the health rights movement, when we are all expected to be partners with our physicians in making decisions about our health care and medications, many of us are still seeking yes and no answers when the truest answer is likely to be, "It depends."

. . .

John Rock briefly appeared in the limelight as a result of the Nelson hearings. He had for so long been identified with the pill that it was natural for journalists to seek him out for comment. But by now, at the age of eighty, he was beginning to slow down. In November 1969 he had been laid low by an attack of viral pneumonia. Hospitalized for ten days, he recovered slowly. He spent the Christmas holidays in Florida, where, as he told a colleague, he slept most of the time. By now, he was beginning to let much of his practice drift, he admitted, hiring an assistant to see many of his patients. He remained an active lecturer, however, with plans to crisscross the country on a lecture tour in the early part of 1970.[82] He began to spend more long weekends in Temple. In 1972, at the age of eighty-two, he would retire from practice and make his permanent home in that New Hampshire town.

Chapter 10

A TRUE VISIONARY

Boston, Massachusetts, 1972. John Rock closes his medical practice and retires to Temple, New Hampshire.

Lancashire, England, 1978. Robert Edwards and Patrick Steptoe announce the birth of the world's first test tube baby, Louise Brown, on July 25, 1978. Her entry into the world by cesarean section, filmed by a professional television crew, was irrefutable proof that in vitro fertilization could produce a healthy baby.

Temple, New Hampshire, 1984. John Rock dies on December 4, a bit more than three months shy of his ninety-fifth birthday.

It was the summer of 1971. John Rock was at his house in Temple, New Hampshire, a tiny town about fifty miles southwest of Concord. He was marking the tenth anniversary of Nan's death and contemplating his own mortality. He now felt more at home in his wooded retreat than he did in Boston. Rock had been summering and spending long weekends here whenever he could get away, since the middle of the 1960s. He used the house, "nestle[d] among the hills of southern New Hampshire," as an escape from his hectic life.

John and Nan had both taken considerable pleasure in the natural world. Now, he treasured his time in the woods, bird-watching, reading, relaxing from his travels, and trying to quell the anxieties attendant on his unraveling relationship with Harvard and its newly consolidated hospitals. Rock came to fancy that here he led a rather Thoreau-esque existence, with few "companions [other than the] flocks of varicolored birds, two red squirrels and ten chipmunks."[1] Well, maybe. As anybody who ever read Thoreau knows, the nineteenth-century author of *Walden* was a bit less isolated than he claimed. And so was Rock. John's friends—plus his children, grandchildren, and their friends—were constantly driving up and down the dirt road that led to his house. Temple was only about two hours from Boston and a bit less from Boxford, Massachusetts, where his daughter Rachel and her family lived. Rock had a car and made frequent trips into Boston for club meetings and dinner with friends.

Still, although he did not feel disconnected from his friends and family, he was becoming increasingly disengaged from his profession. A few weeks before his eighty-second birthday in March 1972, he confided to his diary that he had no energy left for the practice of medicine.[2] He could no longer conduct serious research, found no satisfaction in the practice of general gynecology, and was bruised from his lost battle to secure the permanent existence of the Rock Reproductive Clinic. Nevertheless, the decision to leave his professional life did not come easily. Rock had practiced medicine for more than half a century and had enjoyed international prominence for the past three decades. But he was bewildered by the virulence of the criticism of the pill, and in any case, the spotlight had moved on to younger men and women.

The debate over human in vitro fertilization was raging once again in the 1970s as it had in the early 1950s, but this time Rock's voice would be absent. That was partly because the real action in IVF research had shifted away from the United States; here, the vocal "right to life" movement had virtually shut down American IVF experimentation. Inflamed by the Supreme Court decision in 1973 legalizing abortion, antiabortion activists paralyzed research on IVF and related technologies in this country. In response to antiabortion sentiment, several states soon imposed bans on fetal research; in 1975 the Department of Health, Education, and Welfare suspended any funding of human IVF research until it could convene a National Ethics Advisory Board. But even the creation of such a board engendered controversy. It was not created until January 1978, six months before the birth—outside the United States—of the world's first IVF baby.[3]

The American government's deliberate inaction left the field to scientists in other nations—Australia, India, and England. In 1973, Carl Wood and John Leetong of Queen Victoria Hospital in Melbourne reported that they had implanted a fertilized egg, although it survived in the woman's uterus less than two weeks. In India, scientists conducted their research quietly and without fanfare. And in England, Robert Edwards and Patrick Steptoe made no secret of their determination to bring into the world its first IVF baby. The two men performed more than eighty in vitro fertilizations before they achieved a successful implantation. However, even though achieving the implantation took many attempts, their record of consistent fertilization seemed to predict their ultimate success.[4]

As Steptoe and Edwards made progress, American researchers remained effectively barred from work on humans, reluctant to jeopardize their funding for other projects by ignoring the federal research moratorium. The British government disapproved of IVF, too, but Steptoe and Edwards were able to circumvent official national disapproval by funding the research themselves and by enjoying strong support from the Oldham hospital administration and board, where Steptoe practiced. Steptoe funded the research from his fees for the performance of legal abortions that were not covered by National Health Insurance. Access to patients was guaranteed by his hospital. Thus supported, the two men pressed ahead.[5]

Until 1975, they were unable to get a single woman pregnant. Frustrated, Steptoe and Edwards decided to use fertility drugs to induce ovulation. But when the first patient to conceive in this manner experienced an ectopic pregnancy and required surgery, and no other pregnancies occurred, they discontinued the fertility drugs and returned to single egg retrieval. This method, combined with implantation at an earlier stage, took three years to succeed. In late 1977 Lesley Brown, a thirty-one-year-old Bristol homemaker, became pregnant.[6]

Louise Brown's birth on July 25, 1978, was irrefutable proof that in vitro fertilization could produce a healthy baby. Her entry into the world by cesarean section was filmed by a professional television crew so that the researchers could show both that Lesley did indeed deliver the baby and that her fallopian tubes had been severed (proving that she could not have become pregnant naturally). The day after the birth, a triumphant Steptoe and Edwards told the world that the baby was absolutely normal. By having the birth filmed, they brought about the first documentable IVF birth.[7]

One might have expected Steptoe and Edwards's success to embolden American researchers to defy the federal moratorium, but the leading academic medical centers remained skittish, making it possible for a little known institution to claim the first American IVF birth. The Eastern Virginia Medical School had just hired celebrated fertility experts Georgeanna Segar Jones and her husband Howard Jones, who had reached the age of mandatory retirement at Johns Hopkins. The two researchers had worked together for most of their careers. Georgeanna Jones was a leading reproductive endocrinologist who had been president of the American Fertility Society (now the American Society for Reproductive Medicine), the successor organization to the American Society for the Study of Sterility. When the medical school promised the couple that they could pursue whatever research they chose, that clinched the deal for the Joneses.

Arriving in Norfolk just after the announcement of the birth of Louise Brown, the couple decided to focus on human IVF. While abortion foes vocally despaired over the embryos that would be lost in the transfer process, and newspaper columnists with their own biological children wondered in print why the infertile did not simply adopt, and commentators worried about where the technology might ultimately lead, the Joneses calmly persevered.[8] In December 1981, three days after Christmas, Elizabeth Jordan Carr came into the world. The daughter of a teacher and engineer, she became the first American IVF baby. She was the fifteenth in the world.[9]

Soon other medical centers, emboldened by the Joneses' success, opened their own IVF centers. Meanwhile, the federal government remained determined to hew to a hard line. Not only did it continue to refuse to allow funding for IVF research, it even went so far as to prevent a government embryologist from even speaking at an IVF conference in 1982 on the grounds that it might violate the federal funding ban. However, private medical schools, and increasingly private practices, now simply decided to bypass the government. By fall 1982, Rock protégés Luigi Mastroianni and Celso-Ramon Garcia had created an IVF center at the University of Pennsylvania Medical School. So had researchers at Yale, the University of Texas, the University of Southern California, and Vanderbilt. All but the Texas universities were private institutions. Test tube babies were now a reality, and these researchers did not want Eastern Virginia to leave them in the dust.[10]

With both foolproof birth control in the oral contraceptive and now successful IVF births, modern medicine had made possible the complete separation of sex from reproduction. Like the pill, IVF drew fire across the political spectrum. Feminists were divided, just as they had been over the pill. Some radical feminists had looked forward to the new fertility technology as a step toward women's ultimate liberation from their biology. Shulamith Firestone, in her now classic book, The Dialectic of Sex, declared that she eagerly anticipated the day when babies would be not only conceived in vitro, but nurtured in an artificial uterus. "Pregnancy is Barbaric," she declared in capital letters. "Childbirth is at best necessary and tolerable. It is not fun." If humans could accomplish not only in vitro fertilization, but also in vitro birth, then "the tyranny of the biological family would be broken." But other feminists were appalled: The equally radical Renate D. Klein did not speak only for herself when she declared bitterly, "Reproductive Technology Fails Women: It's a Con."[11]

Rock probably never heard of Firestone and would have surely condemned her exultant forecast of the demise of the conventional family. He did of course know about the work of Steptoe and Edwards, and had long known Georgeanna and Howard Jones. But few reporters in the 1970s sought his opinion about IVF anymore. Journalism may be the raw material of history, but by its nature it has a short shelf life. Reporters in the 1970s rarely recollected the earlier John Rock. Their memories stretched back only to the pill. They did continue to seek out Rock for his views on oral contraception and the ongoing controversies surrounding it, but they did not ask him what he thought about the success of IVF, three decades after he and Menkin had been the first to fertilize a human egg outside the uterus.

· · ·

But as Rock contemplated retirement in 1971, although IVF was in the news, these milestones were still several years away. And right now he was thinking less of his legacy than about how he would manage to support himself in retirement. With no pension, no life savings, and with an annual income in the past couple of years of only around $16,000 (about $79,000 today), he would not be well off. Even in the structured environment of the Free Hospital, he had found it difficult to pay attention to the financial aspects of his career. Once Katharine McCormick stopped funding his research in 1960, things had only gotten worse. And then, in the late 1960s, his inability to come to terms with Harvard and the new Women's Hospital for the use of his name on its reproductive clinic meant his income only declined further. By the time he reached his late seventies, he was in a precarious situation. In 1972 he would sell his private practice for $7,500, but he wouldn't see most of that money for several more years.

On the other hand, by retiring he didn't seem to be losing much, given that he had retained so little of his income anyway. He would continue to have the $12,000 a year that the Searle Company had been paying him for several years. Jack Searle, who knew of Rock's precarious financial situation, now arranged to have those funds continue for the rest of Rock's life. In addition to what amounted to a Searle pension, he would also have about $300 a month in social security income. He concluded that he would have to be content with that. He closed the door on his practice and said good-bye to the life that had first captured his imagination when he had been adrift in Guatemala, learning his way around an operating room out of a lack of anything better to do. He would live another dozen years.

Retirement allowed Rock to spend more time with his daughters and their families. He also kept up with many of his old friends and many of his former protégés, who regularly visited him or invited him to come to them. Every winter he would spend several weeks in Florida with Tip Martin, Nan's close friend since her days at Bryn Mawr and the widow of Milward "Pidge" Martin, the former treasurer of Pepsi Cola. Tip's wealth and social position made it possible for Rock to winter in grand style in spite of his own lack of means. And for the next few years, he still enjoyed occasional times in the public eye, thanks to the journalists who came to hear him reminisce about his battle over birth control. He also remained in demand as a member of honorary committees through the middle of the 1970s, gracing fundraisers for Planned Parenthood and similar organizations. And he frequently drove back and forth to Boston for dinners and events at the Tavern Club and the Medical Exchange Club. In 1974, the American College of Obstetricians and Gynecologists presented him with its Distinguished Service Award, and later that year the Worcester Foundation for Experimental Biology also honored him at a memorial symposium commemorating Gregory Pincus.[12]

In spite of these activities and events, by mid-decade he was beginning to feel more and more detached from the field he had done so much to develop. Politely but firmly he turned down offers to write chapters and essays, offending Celso-Ramon Garcia by declining to write a foreword to Garcia's new textbook on contraception. Garcia simply could not accept Rock's view of himself as "almost brainless" and was unwilling to believe Rock's insistence that while "I can still indulge in persiflage and throw words around, . . . when it comes to substantial exposition, I'm quite incompetent."[13]

Journalists who came to visit him in these years produced articles that leaned toward the elegiac. In a 1973 report that was picked up by news services from New Hampshire to Cedar Rapids and from Philadelphia to Brussels, readers saw Rock's ever-handsome face and read that he was still "tall and slender, still standing erect, [his] blue eyes . . . bright."[14] He continued to charm his interviewers, whose prose remained flattering and deferential in spite of the pill's bad press in the aftermath of the Nelson hearings. He enjoyed the attention. It made him feel, as sometimes he was inclined to doubt, that he had truly made important contributions to human welfare.

In 1975 Richard McDonough, an editor at Little, Brown, and Company, invited him to write a memoir. He declined, but when McDonough offered to find an author to write his biography, Rock was both flattered and pleased. The editor now set out to find an appropriate writer, and Rock took great pleasure in the ensuing correspondence. Why do you care about my life? Rock often asked, probably just to hear McDonough say once more that in his view

Rock's work had "change[d] the rules of the biological game." When the editor put him in the same category as Freud, Einstein, and J. Robert Oppenheimer, naming him as one of "the handful of names from this century that will have made a real difference in the world," Rock *believed* it was an exaggeration, but secretly hoped that it was not too much of one.[15]

McDonough, principally interested in Rock's work on the pill, regularly updated him on the search for a writer. John McPhee declined, as did one or two others, but the editor remained encouraged. Rock was openly delighted, reporting to his friends and family whenever the "avid editor . . . who thinks I have a biography or autobiography . . . tucked inside of me which he intends to extract" called or visited. To McDonough, Rock wrote, "Sometime when you have a minute, send me a few words about this fellow Rock, whom you think has done something worth writing about . . . I've known him for some 60-odd years and I have difficulty wondering why anybody would want to perpetuate his memory." Rock was thrilled to think that his life's work was considered to be of such major significance. In addition to the persistent McDonough, Rock continued to receive a gratifying amount of media attention, almost all of it related to the pill. *Time* did a story on him in 1976. So did the *Boston Globe.*[16]

But 1976 turned out to be something of a watershed for his health. He had surgery to remove his enlarged prostate; after that, he began to weaken. Still, despite his constant complaints that he could no longer "cerebrate," he kept up a lively correspondence, continued to spend several winter weeks in Florida with Tip Martin, and enjoyed what looks from this distance to be a near-constant stream of family and friends.

Rock had always argued that the pill did not cause the sexual revolution, and of course he was right. However, as the first truly foolproof method of birth control, it did have an effect. Women who took the pill knew they wouldn't get pregnant. They could postpone marriage without foregoing sex. They could have an extra-marital affair. They could choose not to have children in order to pursue a career. In the last decade of his life, Rock seemed to have become a bit more philosophical about what for him were some unintended consequences of the pill.

Rock had long had an interest in sexuality as an area of study. He knew Alfred Kinsey. He knew that people had sex before marriage and often outside of it. But in the past he had always been publicly reticent about his own views. Now, when reporters asked him about the pill and nonmarital sex, he would still say that "the opening up of sexuality was already on its way" when the pill was developed, and history does bear him out. But now, he would sometimes add that he was happy that the pill had made sex "safer and easier for some people"—and not only for married couples. After all, he would add with a chuckle, "I thoroughly approve of safety—even in illicit intercourse." When a journalist asked him whether he approved of teenagers taking the pill, he could only say, "It's better than exposing themselves to a pregnancy. If they are going to play around, they might as well play safely."[17]

He had less to say about the pill as a vehicle for world population control. In the 1970s, many of those who cared about this issue were turning their gaze toward the United States rather than blaming the rest of the world for the problem. In the 1950s and 1960s, demographers, birth-control advocates, and population-control scientists had spent most of their energy worrying about the developing world. Some environmentalists began to attack the values that had contributed to the American baby boom, blaming those ideas, at least in part, for the deterioration of the world's environment. Paul Ehrlich, one of the most powerful voices of American environmentalism, argued that saving the planet required a direct attack on the large family. As historian James Reed declared in 1978, "The deterioration of the American habitat provided a focus for criticism of the quality of life in a mass society. Social order everywhere suddenly seemed threatened by human fertility."[18]

Rock probably never read the 1970 Look magazine article entitled "Motherhood—Who Needs It?" If he had, he would likely have been shocked, perhaps even scandalized, by its subtitle—"A Provocative Report on What May Be History's Biggest Fallacy: The Motherhood Myth." He believed strongly that children (as long as there weren't more of them than a couple wanted or could afford) brought profound joy in marriage. He would never have countenanced the magazine's blithe attack on the joy of parenthood. "Often when the stork flies in, sexuality flies out," Look declared. "It doesn't make sense any more to pretend that women need babies, when what they really need is themselves. If God were still speaking to us in a voice we could hear, even He would probably say, 'Be fruitful. Don't multiply.'" Look was not alone. By the middle of the decade, survey research and letters to advice columnist Ann Landers showed that many Americans held an equally negative view of parenting.[19]

Americans are joiners, and in 1972 the new mood was captured nationally by a new organization, the National Association of NonParents (NON). NON's organizers committed themselves to advocating childlessness in order "to conserve planetary resources, beat the high cost of living and free husbands and wives for political activism and the pursuit of free life-styles." For such a small organization—it started out with only two hundred members and never passed the two thousand mark before it faltered and collapsed in the early 1980s—NON got a lot of press. Time and Newsweek covered its events and meetings. Its very existence provoked a flurry of popular and scholarly articles on voluntary childlessness in the 1970s. That such a small group could make such a big media splash suggests that in spite of the insistence of NON cofounders Ellen and William Peck that "pronatalist pressure [was] everywhere," the "childfree" were enjoying a very good decade.[20]

Aggressive antichild sentiment among the voluntarily childless, a growing belief in the existence of a worldwide population crisis, and the heady confidence among young women that the pill would make it possible for them to delay childbearing as long as they desired all made the decision not to have children—or at least not have them right now—a respectable choice for larger numbers of young Americans. That was not a bad thing. The baby boom consensus had been both dogmatic and oppressive, damning those who did not have children as selfish and neurotic and unrealistically extolling the joys of parenthood. NON was a healthy challenge to this older consensus that helped to empower the voluntarily childless.[21]

The "childless by choice" movement, however, also provided women with a false sense of security. The corollary to the idea that women could choose not to become pregnant was the idea that once they threw away their prescription for the pill, they could choose just as easily to conceive. And that would not always be the case. But on the whole, the change was in the direction of greater freedom for women, a change facilitated by the existence of the pill. "We are now living in a contraceptive culture," claimed the famed sex research team of Masters and Johnson.[22]

Rock, as he well knew, bore some responsibility for this new culture even though he disapproved of women's liberation and could by no stretch of the imagination be called a feminist. But as we have seen, he did admire strong women—Margaret Sanger, Katharine McCormick, Mary Breckinridge, several of his female colleagues, his own wife, his daughters, two of whom combined parenthood with work. A. J. Levinson, his second daughter, had been a teacher and then became executive director of Concern for Dying, which promoted living wills and advocated social policies that allowed for death with dignity. Her quick wit, irreverence, and liberal political views could always be counted on to stir up family discussion. Rachel Achenbach, his oldest daughter, was a cytologist, although with six children she worked part time. (His other two daughters did not hold down paying positions, although both were dedicated volunteers to various causes.) But in spite of his admiration for some individual women, he believed that men and women were inherently different, and always argued that a good marriage and motherhood, if they were achievable, ought to be the most important aspects of a woman's life. Rock had never resolved his contradictory attitudes toward women, and it was too late for him to start now.

· · ·

Rock turned ninety on March 24, 1980. His daughter Rachel and her husband, Hart, threw him a surprise party, attended by his daughters, the husbands of the three who were still married, and all nineteen of his grandchildren. The milestone was also marked by articles on him in the *Boston Globe* and the medical press. But perhaps the highlight of his year was a tribute at the University of Pennsylvania School of Medicine in October, organized by two of his most distinguished protégés, Celso-Ramon Garcia and Luigi Mastroianni. The joy of the event was tinged by sadness, however. Just a month before, William Mulligan, who had assisted and then succeeded Rock at the Free Hospital, died at seventy-two after a long struggle with heart and lung disease.[23]

Rock had trained and mentored dozens of young MDs over the course of his career. Many of them continued to remember him with cards, letters, wedding photographs, and pictures of their children. But next to Bill Mulligan, perhaps none were as loyal as Celso-Ramon Garcia and Luigi Mastroianni. Garcia and Mastroianni had both served, at different times in the 1950s, as Sydney Graves Fellows in infertility and gynecology under Rock. The Graves Fellows, according to one account, later became responsible for the development of "contemporary reproductive medicine" in the 1980s and 1990s.[24]

Although there were certainly leaders in the field who did not trace their own or their teachers' training back to Rock, a number of his fellows did go on to have major careers in reproductive medicine. Rock had the final say in the selection of the fellows and took a personal interest in their later successes. Garcia and Mastroianni, after taking different paths—Garcia worked for Gregory Pincus, then became head of the infertility clinic at Massachusetts General Hospital, and Mastroianni went from Rock's clinic to Yale and then to UCLA—joined forces in the 1960s at the medical school at the University of Pennsylvania to create one of the leading academic centers in reproductive medicine—the Division of Reproductive Biology.

The two men held professorships named after famous Philadelphia obstetricians and gynecologists. Mastroianni was the William Goodell Professor and Garcia held the William Shippen, Jr., Professorship. Over the course of their careers, each man would serve as president of the American Society for Reproductive Medicine, and each of them earned a host of honors. Mastroianni would become the first to accomplish successful in vitro fertilization in the Philadelphia area in 1983, and Garcia would be nominated at least once for a Nobel Prize.[25]

Rock thought of the two younger men almost as surrogate sons. He had been the best man at Mastroianni's wedding, and one of Luigi's children is named John. Both Garcia and Mastroianni frequently came to visit him in Temple. They planned the Rock Commemorative Symposium to honor their mentor for his leadership in the field of fertility research. Since the event was underwritten by the Searle Company, it focused on the development of the oral contraceptive. Frank Colton, the chemist who invented the compound that became Enovid, gave a presentation. I. C. Winter, with whom Rock had worked so closely during the pill approval process, was among the attendees. All four of Rock's daughters attended, as did Mike DeLargey, the young man who today might be called Rock's caregiver but who had become his friend as well. At the dinner that followed the symposium, Rock received the first G. D. Searle Award for Research in the Benefit of Mankind, which included an impressive gold medal.[26]

By this time Rock had grown quite frail. He was less and less able to get around. Fortunately, Richard McDonough had found his writer for the Rock biography—Loretta McLaughlin, medical reporter for the Boston Globe. McLaughlin had been brought up a Catholic and was particularly interested in the relationship between Rock and the Catholic Church. She would later go on to become the editorial page editor of the Globe and in retirement to develop an expertise on the global HIV-AIDS health crisis. She interviewed Rock at length as part of her research, and he enjoyed his time with her despite complaining to his diary that she asked too many personal questions.[27] The Pill, John Rock, and the Church—in those years there was no need to say which church—appeared in 1982.

McLaughlin devoted more than half the book to the pill and particularly to the religious controversy it engendered. She interviewed Rock's colleagues and collaborators, giving the story the immediacy of living history. "John Rock belongs now and forever to that select company of mortals who profoundly changed the world," the biography begins. McLaughlin admired him most for serving "as champion of the pill and challenger to the Church," a role in which, she declared, his "greatness looms largest."[28]

Once the book appeared, Rock's former patients who read it or saw reviews wrote him long and chatty letters, altogether creating a remarkable record of the profound impact he had made on the lives he touched. Women whose babies he delivered as far back as the 1920s told him how fondly they remembered him. Others whose infertility he treated in the 1950s wrote that even after all these years, they kept him in their hearts. As one of them said, the "2 beautiful babies" she was able to bear as a result of her infertility treatment "made all the difference in my life, and I am eternally grateful." A woman whom he had seen as a "premarital" patient—her future mother-in-law had insisted on the visit—remembered thirty-four years later that as a result of his advice, she and her husband "had a resoundingly happy honeymoon." One man recalled his and his wife's "desperation" over their infertility, which Rock successfully treated, and wrote him proudly of the accomplishments of their three children. Old friends chimed in with their own reminiscences. Somers Sturgis, Rock's first Graves Research Fellow and by this time a distinguished Harvard physician, sent a letter recalling the hectic but satisfying days in the Fertility and Endocrine Clinic during the early years of the baby boom.[29]

Frederick Flynn, a Catholic theologian with whom Rock had been friendly during the 1960s, wrote his old friend with considerable satisfaction that some Catholics, like himself, still continued to support contraception. Flynn was fortunate, he said, to have spent his career at an institution that allowed him a "remarkable degree of academic freedom for a Catholic college in those years." Even the three archbishops who chaired the governing board never called him to account, Flynn informed Rock, and one of them continued to seek his advice on theological matters. The letter was a reminder—not that Rock needed one—that while the official stance of the Church remained opposed to contraception, many within it continued to agree with his own views.[30] It was gratifying for Rock to hear from so many in his past, although in characteristic fashion, he masked his pleasure with self-deprecation.

...

McLaughlin's book brought back warm memories among Rock's patients and received a number of favorable notices and reviews. Hilton Salhanick, writing in the *New England Journal of Medicine*, called it "the story of an indomitable man of conscience in conflict with authorities who make institutional decisions." It did not fare so well, however, among some feminist critics.[31] Barbara Ehrenreich lambasted the book in the *New York Times*, calling it "close to . . . a cover up" for what, in Ehrenreich's opinion was "the stuff of medical scandal." Accusing Rock of exploiting both "unwitting . . . charity patients" whom she believed he tricked into participating in the embryo studies and "impoverished Caribbean women [used] as guinea pigs" in the pill trials, Ehrenreich expressed outrage that McLaughlin not only did not acknowledge Rock's "ethical insouciance," but joined him in it. A year later, writer Gena Corea would make much the same argument. In both women's eyes, Rock was certainly not a hero but rather the epitome of all that was wrong with American medicine.[32]

For Corea and Ehrenreich, it required no leap of faith to jump from the documented fact that Rock performed hysterectomies on women who had recently conceived in order to track the progress of a fertilized egg from fallopian tube to implantation in the uterus, to assertions that the women were unwitting victims of overweening medical arrogance. They were wrong about Rock. He was scrupulous in explaining to the patients exactly what the research was and why he was asking them to participate.

Luigi Mastroianni, who had been involved in the progesterone studies that led to the pill, recalled in 2007 that working with Rock "gave me an opportunity to witness the concept of informed consent." The attacks on Rock by Ehrenreich and Corea make Mastroianni's remarks on this subject worth quoting in some detail. Rock wanted the young doctor to understand how important it was to make sure a patient was fully informed. He invited Mastroianni to join him while he interviewed one of them:

> He said, I'm going to interview a patient to see whether she would consider allowing us to do this [have her participate in a study], and I want you in the office with me. From then on, I had the entrée to come in anytime with infertility patients and any consults. But this informed consent was an eye opener. The way this man communicated with patients was something I'll never forget . . . I sat there. He made several points: "Look, you're here for infertility. What I propose to do will last for three months. There is no guarantee at all that this will help your infertility, but it may give us information that will eventually help a lot of women. As far as risks go, this medication has been extensively studied in animals and has been given to some patients, some volunteers, to test its safety. We don't know what the short-term or the long-term effects are because it hasn't been given in this way." And then he would say: "This will involve a series of visits where you will be seen by one of our physicians, most likely Dr. Mastroianni, who will make sure that the pills are taken properly, coordinate the collection of

your urine, do an endometrial biopsy in the presumed postovulatory phase of the menstrual cycle to check the effect of this hormone on your endometrium."[33]

Mastroianni said that medicine was indeed paternalistic during the period that Rock practiced. We would go further and call it patriarchal. Corea and Ehrenreich did not know anything about Rock, but they did not approve of the way medicine was often practiced. They simply decided that he must have been an emblem of medical patriarchy.

What they read in McLaughlin's book confirmed their conviction that reproductive science, and the people who practiced it, demeaned and exploited women. McLaughlin was writing about a single individual. She admired him greatly for his courage in facing down his own church, which was a powerful institution in Massachusetts and an increasingly powerful one in the nation. Rock risked his reputation—and some said even his soul—in fighting for the rights of couples to decide how many children they would have. For a Catholic reporter in Catholic Boston, who knew the depth of the power of the Church, Rock's support of contraception—not simply in developing and promoting the pill, but in thirty years of supporting legislative change—was indeed courageous. Rock neither condescended to his patients nor misled them. But to some, he was a symbol of all that was wrong with American medicine's attitudes toward women.

McLaughlin in some ways had written a book more attuned to the sensibilities of a slightly earlier age, when science and medicine were revered and when physicians could still be seen as heroes. By the time her book came out in 1982, both ideas were under attack. As historian Elizabeth Siegel Watkins has noted, there had been "a general loss of confidence in medicine in the 1970s." Among the critics were "feminists [who] protested a whole host of injustices perpetrated on women by the largely male medical establishment, including gender discrimination in medical school admissions, lack of informed consent in medical decision-making, and medicalization of too many aspects of women's lives, such as birth control, pregnancy, childbirth, and menopause."[34]

Paul Starr's Pulitzer Prize–winning book on the social transformation of American medicine in the twentieth century, which was published the same year as McLaughlin's biography of Rock, captured that disaffected mood. Charting the rise of several "health rights movements" that had taken hold in the United States by the early 1980s, he observed a "diminished faith in the efficacy of medicine and increased concern about its relation to other moral values." Feminists who "challenged the authority and power of the profession" were joined by others who had lost their faith in doctors. "For the first time in a century," Starr concluded, "American physicians faced a serious challenge simultaneously to their political influence, their economic power, and their cultural authority."[35] Public opinion research confirmed this decline in prestige. Almost three-quarters of Americans expressed considerable confidence in the medical profession in 1966; just ten years later, the number had dropped to only 42 percent.[36]

The fact that John Rock's behavior did not conform to their stereotype would have hardly mattered to those angry about the larger issues. Besides, there was good reason for women to mistrust medical expertise overall in the 1970s and 1980s that went well beyond the pill controversy. We might begin with the DES revelations. In the 1950s, a synthetic estrogen, diethylstilbestrol (DES), was widely used to prevent miscarriage. Beginning in the early 1970s, evidence emerged that the daughters of women who had taken the drug faced a higher risk of developing cervical cancer as well as what had until then been a rare type of vaginal cancer. Many others had abnormalities of the uterus and cervix. That the AMA attempted initially to dismiss the findings as insignificant did nothing to counter the growing public mistrust of doctors.[37]

Close on the heels of these reports came the Dalkon Shield scandal, which rocked the contraceptive world beginning in the mid-1970s. Hundreds of thousands of cases of infections, hysterectomies, miscarriages, uterine perforations, and other gynecological problems were attributed to this device. Women who had placed their faith in what turned out to be fraudulent medical research were left childless and worse.[38]

And then there was the first controversy (not to be confused with the current one) over the long-term use of estrogen by menopausal women. Estrogen replacement therapy, as it was called then, had been prescribed for the short-term treatment of menopausal symptoms, such as hot flashes, since the 1940s. Beginning in the 1960s, the hormone was advertised as a miracle drug that could virtually erase the effects of aging in women. But by the late 1970s, the picture had darkened as long-term estrogen use, now widespread, became clearly linked with a rise in endometrial cancer.[39]

The diminished faith in medicine and in those who practiced it touched the entire profession, and John Rock, as the nation's most visible symbol of the first great era of reproductive medicine, became a target. His patients had loved and respected him for his candor and kindness as well as his expertise, and Loretta McLaughlin nearly canonized him, but in the 1980s that was not enough to fend off the critics. Just a year after McLaughlin's book came out, *Esquire* magazine chose to include John Rock as one of "50 Who Made the Difference," for its special Golden Anniversary Collector's Issue. The magazine's president, Philip Moffitt, wrote Rock to congratulate him for his inclusion among the fifty men and women to be honored in "a special issue celebrating the power of the individual to make a major contribution to society." Moffitt went on to say that one of "America's greatest living writers" would be assigned to "honor" him as "one of these individuals."[40]

Unfortunately for its promise to "honor" Rock, the magazine chose writer Sara Davidson to profile him. Davidson was then best known for her fictionalized sixties memoir *Loose Change*, which chronicled her life and the lives of two other young women who met at Berkeley in the 1960s. *Loose Change* was a bestseller. The *New York Times* reviewed the book twice. John Leonard dismissed it as self-indulgent, and Erica Jong praised it as an authentic portrait of a generation—opinions that in retrospect may not have been as contradictory as they seemed at the time.[41]

Esquire's editors no doubt believed that a writer who lived through the sexual revolution would be the best person to interview one of the progenitors of that revolution. Davidson was not an oral contraceptive enthusiast and believed that by the 1980s, "the very concept of the pill seemed bizarre." Her source for such a surprising statement (after all, throughout the 1980s more women used the pill than they did any other reversible method of birth control) was her own social circle. Among her friends, "the pill was out of favor and . . . in any case [they] seemed more intent on trying to conceive babies." Although she mentioned that Rock was a noted fertility researcher, she seems not to have considered that his work on infertility might have had any relevance to young women in the 1980s.[42]

Davidson's essay was not so much about Rock as it was about her reactions to him. Seemingly unable to fathom that such an old man had been a key player in the transformation of the sexual and reproductive behavior of her own generation, she focused almost exclusively on his physical and mental frailties rather than his contributions to reproductive medicine, and she seemed angry that he would not overcome his physical limitations to pay more attention to her. His hearing aid squeaked, he had difficulty remembering, and he tired easily, she complained. Yes, he was well into his nineties, he did have memory lapses, and he was quite deaf. But she described his infirmities as if they were a personal insult to her and misread his modesty about his achievements as senility, expressing considerable frustration at having been given the job of interviewing "a person of extraordinary accomplishments at an age when he can no longer remember much about them."[43] And to add to the other insults, she was clearly annoyed with the conventional views he claimed to hold about the roles of women.

Whether she caught Rock on a particularly difficult day, whether now in the closing year of his life he had begun to recede from the world, or whether he simply did not like her, his famed courtesy seems to have deserted him when Davidson came to visit. Finally tiring of her questions, he moved to the sofa, lay down, and closed his eyes. When she tried to continue the interview, he simply tuned her out, falling asleep or feigning it.

It is hard to imagine more opposing images of John Rock than those of McLaughlin and Davidson. McLaughlin's Rock at ninety-two was "ramrod straight, his six-foot-three frame lean as a pole, his good sense and self-deprecating wit still intact." He radiated charm and grace, and she recalled his face "light[ing] up" when she reminded him that "he was once known as 'the saint of Radcliffe.'"[44]

Davidson's Rock was "dapper," but his eyes "wandered" and he "looked confused" when she asked questions. She wanted to engage him in conversation, and she took his refusal to be engaged as an insult. She thought he was choosing deliberately not to think about his achievements or to consider any possible problems with them. He fell asleep in the middle of a conversation. She said that she, too, would like to "curl up in a chair beside him, escape from my own responsibilities," but then "the impulse passes, and I let myself out and drive to the airport."[45]

Read a quarter-century later, when Americans frown on the public ridicule of old age simply because it is old age, Davidson's portrayal of Rock comes off as gratuitously cruel. Luckily for him, however, before the issue appeared he was able to enjoy being honored at Esquire's Lincoln Center gala for those who were being profiled. If the article itself hurt him terribly, he didn't leave a record of his feelings.

By that time, Rock was only a year away from death. Over the past four decades, he had lived with a number of ailments, but the worst was his heart disease, and it was heart disease that claimed him in the end. On Sunday, December 3, 1984, Rock telephoned his daughter Rachel and asked her to come to Temple to take him to the hospital. By now it had become almost a ritual; Rock had been in and out of the hospital several times in the last year. When she arrived, Rachel found him ready to go, dressed up in shirt and tie. Once they arrived at the emergency room at Peterborough Hospital, the doctors quickly moved him to the intensive care unit. After he was made comfortable, Rachel offered to stay the night. Her father demurred, so she told him that she would be back the next day. "I'll be here," Rock replied.[46]

In the early hours of the morning, on December 4, John Rock died. The nurse who had sat up with him during the night recalled that before he died, he told her he was seeing angels. The sight would have given him comfort. During the last year or so, he had been returning to his faith, a nearby priest often visiting him and bringing communion. Now the same priest would say his funeral Mass. In keeping with his wishes, the family had a private funeral, beginning with the Mass in Peterborough and concluding with his burial in Forest Hills Cemetery in Jamaica Plain. Celso-Ramon Garcia was there, and a few of Rock's other old friends joined his extended family. His biographer Loretta McLaughlin came. Tip Martin flew in for the burial.

Rock was buried beside Nan, Jack, and a stillborn son born to A. J. His daughter Ellen, who had died at the age of fifty of an aneurysm just two years before, was buried near her home. His three other daughters, nineteen grandchildren, and five great-grandchildren survived him. The obituaries in the *New York Times*, the *Boston Globe*, and elsewhere highlighted his work on the oral contraceptive, although the *Times* recalled that he had also been "the first scientist to fertilize a human egg in a test tube, and among the first to freeze sperm cells for a year without impairing their potency."[47] Celso-Ramon Garcia and Luigi Mastroianni called him a "true visionary" in their memorial essay, and columnist Ellen Goodman eulogized him as the most important of the pill's developers: "He was Number One, the man who became the pill's public defender, who became the popularizer and point man for the social medicine that initiated a sexual revolution." Goodman called the pill a form of "sexual security," by 1980 used by some 60 million women. Like Loretta McLaughlin, and like the editors of *Esquire* (if not by the writer the magazine chose to profile him), Ellen Goodman told her readers that Rock was one of the most important figures of the twentieth century, "a certified member of that small band of human beings who change the world."[48]

· · ·

In 2010 the pill will celebrate its fiftieth birthday, and Louise Brown will turn thirty-two. Rock would be pleased to know that today 93 percent of all Americans, and 90 percent of Catholics, approve of the use of contraceptives. As Elizabeth Siegel Watkins, the leading expert on the social history of the oral contraceptive, declared when the pill was just about to turn forty, it is "still going strong," remaining "the most popular reversible method among American women," and "unlikely to lose its first-place ranking to another method." But would Rock ever have imagined, in the early twenty-first century, a conservative backlash in the United States that has resulted, as the *New York Times Magazine* described it, in a new "War on Contraception"?[49] We doubt it, just as we doubt that this "war" will be lasting. For the overwhelming majority of American women—and men—the right to prevent pregnancy is considered an entitlement.

Viewed as almost as much of an entitlement is what is increasingly seen as the "right" to bear children. If hormonal contraception can guarantee that a woman won't become pregnant while she earns her PhD, makes partner in a law firm, completes her medical residency, or acquires her first million, then why can't modern reproductive technology make it possible for her to choose to conceive whenever she is ready? And even beyond that rarified group of women, what of many others—the young woman robbed of her ovaries by disease, another who marries at forty or who never marries at all, the gay men and lesbians forming their own nuclear families? Many of them feel entitled as well to experience pregnancy or to have biological offspring.

The separation of sex from reproduction—this is a major part of John Rock's legacy. Would he mind, we sometimes wonder, if he knew where the technologies that he had pioneered ended up? We don't know for sure. We do know that he would have felt great satisfaction in knowing that in vitro fertilization now provides a way for women to bear children who in past decades would never have been able to do so, women with irreversible damage to their fallopian tubes, for example. IVF has made it possible to bypass them.

Donor eggs, we believe, would also have met with his approval, particularly given his views on donor insemination. First used in the mid-1980s by a few women in their twenties and thirties who had undergone premature menopause or whose ovaries had been removed in surgery, donor eggs became more widely available in the 1990s. While hardly as commonplace as conventional IVF, this form of assisted reproduction now allows women to make, in writer Peggy Orenstein's words, an "end run" around their biological clocks. And although there have been a few cases of women in their sixties taking advantage of donor eggs, most of the recipients, in addition to the younger women, are those in their forties who for one reason or another did not have children in their earlier, more fertile years.[50]

What would he have said about donor embryos? We can only imagine the spirit of John Rock in the office of a twenty-first-century reproductive endocrinologist, looking over her shoulder as she sits at her desk, flipping through a pile of what looks like patient histories—detailed, thorough information about what appears to be couples seeking treatment for infertility. A closer look, however, reveals that these are not the files of couples currently in treatment. Instead they are the files of the lucky couples, those who have already successfully conceived through in vitro fertilization. Why haven't the charts been sent to storage?

The files are still on the desk because these couples had decided to donate their remaining frozen embryos to others who had not been successful.[51] Today, a couple, having been unsuccessful with the woman's own eggs or those of a donor, can have a child using another couple's embryo. Although embryo "adoption" is by no means a common practice, it does exist and has recently captured the imagination of antiabortion advocates and those opposed to embryonic stem cell research. There was even a television feature about a meeting between a couple who had donated embryos and the couple who "adopted" them through a program known as Snowflake, which is run by Nightlight Christian Adoptions. Nightlight claims that in the last decade, 134 children have been born as a result of its program.[52]

Donor eggs and particularly donor embryos have challenged conventional ideas of biological parenthood. And now, as a recent article in *Obstetrics and Gynecology* suggests, uterine transplantation could be next on the horizon.[53] Ethical controversies swirl around such techniques as they once dominated discussions of in vitro fertilization using a married couple's eggs and sperm, which is now commonplace and widely accepted. We don't know what Rock would have said about these specific techniques. We do know this about Rock, however. In his eyes, it was the family, and the desire of couples to be parents, that mattered most.

We asked Luigi Mastroianni, who knew Rock well, what he thought his mentor would have made of the issues surrounding reproductive technologies today. Now eighty, he told us that in considering all the current controversies, John Rock, if he were alive today, "would still be the voice of compromise and dialogue," navigating through the complexities and contradictions, urging his successors to listen to their patients and work for their benefit.[54] For Rock, the oral contraceptive was one of the best means to ensure that an unwanted child did not come into the world. But wanted children were equally important to him, and he devoted much of his professional life to making it possible for men and women to have their desired children. John Rock believed that both foolproof birth control and advances in reproductive technology were in themselves good, if used ethically and responsibly. He had a profound faith in the common sense of the ordinary individual, and in his or her ability to make the right choice.

Acknowledgments

Readers of our last book, *The Empty Cradle: Infertility in America from Colonial Times to the Present*, will know that the two of us are sisters—Margaret Marsh is a historian, and Wanda Ronner, a gynecologist. We have been collaborators since 1988. For two decades now, we've been thinking, talking, and writing about the history and cultural significance of reproductive medicine and its practice. We bring our specific fields of expertise, Margaret in the study of women and gender and Wanda in women's health, to bear on the work we do together. We've learned a lot from each other, including how to look at the issues from the point of view of a different discipline and how to make our patterns of analysis work in complementary ways instead of opposing ones. Even when we disagree occasionally, we have a wonderful time working together.

Margaret first encountered John Rock in the Rare Books and Manuscripts Division of the Countway Library of Medicine at Harvard University in the early 1990s, where she and two of her research assistants, Julie Berebitsky and Sally Dwyer-McNulty (then PhD students at Temple University and now professors themselves) were rummaging through some forty or so uncataloged boxes of his papers. We were there to do research on the dramatic growth of infertility treatment during the baby boom for *The Empty Cradle*. All we knew about John Rock at the time was that he had been the codeveloper of the oral contraceptive and that, before the pill, he had spent his professional life as a specialist in infertility. Our interest then was in the emergence of infertility clinics in the postwar era. As it turned out, Rock came close to taking over that chapter of the book, and as we read through his papers, we realized that in his life and work there was a much larger story to be told.

After *The Empty Cradle* was published, we sent a copy to Rachel Achenbach, John Rock's eldest daughter, who controls the literary rights to his papers. Once Margaret met her, she became captivated by the idea of writing a book based on his experiences. She had only to persuade Wanda, which did not take long. We owe our greatest debt of gratitude to Rachel Achenbach, both for her belief in the significance of our project and her generosity of spirit. Without her, this book *literally* could not have been written. As it turned out, the Rock papers in the Countway were only a fraction of the materials John Rock left behind. Mrs. Achenbach had the rest, amounting to around seventy boxes of diaries, personal and professional correspondence, research records of all kinds, drafts of papers and books, transcripts of meetings, the original photographs of the first human embryos fertilized outside the body, and much more. She allowed us privileged and unrestricted access to the papers, also granting us permission to quote from them even before she had any idea of what many of the boxes contained—or what we would say. About three years into our research, Margaret took ten or so boxes of papers to the Countway, which was about to close Rock's papers to catalogue them. Those ten boxes are now catalogued with the Countway's collection.

For a few years, Margaret regularly made the trip to Massachusetts to work on the papers in Rachel's dining room, which the Achenbachs had set up as a kind of office for that purpose. Margaret also met other members of the Rock family, who have graciously given their time and memories. We are grateful to Hart Achenbach, MD, Rachel's husband, who had once served as one of John Rock's research fellows, for his insights, and to their daughter Susan Achenbach, who helped us to understand Rock's last decade. We spent one day of formal interviews with the Achenbachs and Ann Jane (A. J.) Levinson, Rock's second daughter, who died in 2002. If Rachel reminded us of John Rock— her dry sense of humor and attitude to life echo his—A. J. was close to their mother and had a somewhat different perspective of her distinguished father than did Rachel. We are also grateful to Hank Levinson, A. J.'s husband, and their daughters Martha M. Levinson and Katharine Ewing, for talking with us and sharing their views. Rachel and Hart Achenbach also read an earlier draft of our manuscript and saved us from several factual errors. But they never asked us to change an interpretation or assessment. Rachel and Margaret often talked about the fact that the John Rock that would emerge from our book would be Margaret and Wanda's John Rock, not necessarily the family's. We intended, to the best of our ability, to write a book that would situate Rock in the medical and cultural history of twentieth-century America, that would be both scholarly and readable, and that would be as objective as a historian and gynecologist could make it.

In addition to Rock family members, we talked to three distinguished figures in the field of reproductive medicine. Dr. Edward Wallach discussed with

Wanda his insights into the practice of reproductive medicine in the 1960s and 1970s. Rock's protégés Dr. Celso-Ramon Garcia, who died in 2004, and Dr. Luigi Mastroianni, who spent much of their careers together at the University of Pennsylvania School of Medicine, were generous with their time and expertise. We owe a special debt of gratitude to both of them.

We also owe a similar debt to a person we have never met, journalist Loretta McLaughlin, author of *The Pill, John Rock, and the Church: The Biography of a Revolution*. Ms. McLaughlin interviewed Rock, his collaborator Arthur Hertig, Rock's long-serving research assistant Miriam Menkin, and many of those involved with the pill's development and the controversies over its use. Her book is essential reading in order to understand the pill controversy in the 1960s and 1970s. It has the immediacy of living history.

For almost the entire time we worked on this book, Margaret was serving as a dean, provost, or chancellor. Wanda is a full-time practicing physician as well as teacher of medical students and residents. If it were not for a major multiyear grant from the National Endowment for the Humanities (RZ-20431-99), we'd likely be halfway through our research right about now. We are grateful to the Endowment, and we are especially grateful to two of its senior program directors: Daniel Jones, now retired, and Elizabeth Arndt. We cannot praise either of them highly enough. This grant made it possible for Margaret to take six months of research leave and for Wanda to take two, and for the two of us to cover myriad research expenses. It also allowed us to hire several wonderful graduate and undergraduate research assistants.

Our two graduate researchers for this project were Katherine "Katie" Parkin and Diana Reinhard, both of them, while they worked for us, PhD candidates at Temple University. Katie is now a full-time faculty member and a prize-winning scholar. Diana, as of this writing, has just completed her dissertation. Both Katie and Diana not only conducted research, organized materials, and tracked down many elusive sources, but they also offered their own important insights and intellectual judgments. They supervised our outstanding undergraduate research assistants—Jessica Bluebond-Langner, Diana Postemsky, Vanessa Cantarella, and Mary Vesper.

The undergraduates were enormously helpful to the project, while also gaining experience in the complexities of historical research and writing, and learning about the joy of discovery. Vanessa, for example, was a biology major. While she was taking an embryology course, she saw in one of her textbooks a picture of Rock and Menkin's fertilized eggs—the first human eggs ever fertilized in vitro. She told us how incredibly excited she was to be able to tell the whole class that she had seen the original photograph of those eggs in the files of the researchers who had created them.

We also owe a considerable debt of gratitude to the people who made it possible for us to take advantage of the NEH grant. Margaret is grateful to Rutgers University for its support and to two administrations, that of former president Francis Lawrence and current president Richard L. McCormick. She also thanks Executive Vice President Philip Furmanski. Her provost for eight years, Roger Dennis, made it possible for her to be away for six months of research leave and to spend one month each summer working on this book. Associate Dean Daniel Hart took over as acting dean during her leave. He also held down the fort in the dean's office every July from 2000 through 2005, as did Associate Dean Michael Palis for July 2006. Associate Dean Nancy Rosoff, Business Manager Maria Garcia, and Senior Executive Assistant Iris Rodriguez did everything they could to lighten her load during busy times. Harold Winshel, director of Computer and Instructional Technology, got her over her technological difficulties. Harold and Roman Volkovich of his staff digitized our images, and Scott Kuhnel excelled at trouble-shooting. Margaret also wishes to thank Arts and Sciences Associate Deans Luis Garcia and Christopher Dougherty; former Associate Dean Marie Cornelia; and Nancy Hoover, Louise Waters, Andrea Ohrenich, and Julie Strasser of her office. In the chancellor's office she is especially grateful to Vice-Chancellor Larry Gaines, Associate Chancellor Mary Beth Daisey, Director of Campus Event Planning Kristin Walker, Director of Communications Mike Sepanic, Kathy Boyle, Mary Falls, and Celeste Fisher.

Wanda is especially grateful to her department chair at Pennsylvania Hospital, Dr. Jack Ludmir, for his unfailing support and interest in her historical pursuits. Dr. Beverly Vaughn covered her patients in 2000 so that she could spend some uninterrupted time on the project. Dr. Lee Huppert provided ongoing encouragement and insights into the practice of reproductive endocrinology today. Wanda also wants to thank Dr. Deborah Driscoll, chair of the Department of Obstetrics and Gynecology at the University of Pennsylvania School of Medicine, and Dr. Christos Coutifaris, director of the Division of Reproductive Endocrinology and Infertility, for providing the photograph of Gregory Pincus and Celso-Ramon Garcia reproduced in this book. Wanda is grateful to her office staff—Wanda Byrd, Elizabeth Peeler, Angela Pasquini, and Helen Queensbury for their support, and she also thanks Joan Faraone, Arlene Reichert, and Dee Milliner of the Department of Obstetrics and Gynecology at Pennsylvania Hospital for all that they do. In addition, she thanks the residents and Penn medical students at Pennsylvania Hospital for politely listening to her tales of the development of the pill and the emergence of the field of reproductive medicine.

The two of us have given formal and informal talks, papers, and lectures over the past decade to different groups, separately and together, on various facets of the history of reproductive medicine, including John Rock's role in its development—from grand rounds, to medical groups, to conferences in the United States and Australia. For the opportunity to participate in the University of Melbourne conference *Women's Bodies, Women's History*, Margaret is especially grateful to Rima Apple, who coordinated the conference and secured a grant from the National Science Foundation for the American scholars. She is also grateful to our cousin, Kathleen Sammartino, for attending with her and for unparalleled support throughout decades of friendship. We are grateful for all the comments and suggestions made by commentators and other participants at these various conferences and talks.

We and our research assistants would like to thank, for their generosity and patience, the staffs of all the universities, colleges, libraries, and archives in which we worked: the Rare Books Division of Harvard's Countway Library of Medicine, especially Jack Eckert and Jessica Murphy; the Library of Congress, especially the Manuscript Division; Smith College for the Margaret Sanger Papers; Simmons College; Bryn Mawr College; and the College of Physicians of Philadelphia. Although we did not use the Rockefeller Archives Center collections in writing this book, we cite several documents used in our previous book, *The Empty Cradle*, and we want to acknowledge the center once again. We cannot praise highly enough the librarians of Rutgers University, who responded to our requests for hundreds of articles with both grace and dispatch.

We owe several special debts. One is to fellow historian of medicine Alan Kraut, for his excellent advice at a critical stage of this project. Another is to the work of Peter Conn, whose extraordinary 1996 biography of Pearl Buck inspired our own approach to the life of John Rock. We also want to thank our spectacular editor at the Johns Hopkins University Press, Jacqueline Wehmueller, for taking us on for a second book and for working with us all the way through the finishing stages. We owe an enormous debt to the external reviewer for Hopkins, Elizabeth Siegel Watkins. As the author of books on the oral contraceptive and the history of hormone replacement therapy, her insightful reading of the manuscript strengthened some of our arguments and caused us to rethink and redefine others. We are very lucky that the press assigned editor Melanie Mallon to work on this book. Much more than a copy-editor, Melanie lent us her expertise in all editorial matters. We are grateful for her outstanding work.

Throughout the process of writing this book, we received a great deal of good advice, and a good deal of great advice. If, in spite of all this help, errors remain, they are our fault.

Finally, we could not have written this book without the love, support, and tolerance of our family—Margaret's husband, Howard Gillette, Wanda's husband, Peter Ronner, who also helped us with PowerPoint presentations and provided other technological assistance, and Lukas Ronner, Wanda's son and Margaret's godson. We dedicate this book to the three of them.

Notes

Abbreviations

BSH   Bureau of Social Hygiene Collection, Rockefeller Archives

GP-LC Gregory Pincus Papers, Library of Congress

JR-CLM John Rock Papers, Harvard Medical Library in the
       Francis A. Countway Library of Medicine

JR-RA John Rock Papers, Rachel Achenbach Collection

MS-SS Margaret Sanger Papers, Sophia Smith Collection

Introduction

1. The history of IVF was the subject of a recent PBS *American Experience* documentary, for which one of us, Margaret Marsh, was a consultant. To our surprise, the filmmakers appeared to give Miriam Menkin too much of the credit for the first IVF because they were unable to portray the difference between the researcher who designs the protocols and makes the major research decisions (Rock) and the technician who carries out the technical work (Menkin). The film did, however, generate considerable interest in the history of IVF and did an excellent job of illustrating the social and political controversies that are generated by new technologies. See www.pbs.org/wgbh/amex/babies/filmmore/fd.html.

2. Loretta McLaughlin's *The Pill, John Rock, and the Church: The Biography of a Revolution* (Boston: Little, Brown, 1982), written during Rock's lifetime, includes interviews with many of Rock's colleagues and family. Although its focus is different from ours, it conveys the immediacy of living history.

3. Rock's daughter Rachel Achenbach, who is the custodian of his papers, has given us unrestricted permission to quote and cite from them. Historian Harry Marks notes that because of the nature of the typical historical record, studies that incorporate patients' voices have been virtually impossible to undertake: "I have yet to encounter a source that would tell me much about patients, other than as researchers imagined them." Harry Marks, *The Progress of Experiment: Science and Therapeutic Reform in the United States, 1900–1990* (Cambridge: Cambridge University Press, 1997), 13.

Chapter 1. Family Matters

1. The genealogical information comes from records in possession of Rachel Achenbach, including census materials, birth records, and pages copied from Marlborough city directories.

2. See Frank Rock to John Rock, Oct. 18, 1909, JR-RA.

3. Maisie is spelled just like this in her early life; later, others spelled it Mazie or Maizie.

4. Ann Jane "Annie" Rock to Frank Rock, March 9, 1910, JR-RA.

5. See Joseph C. Ryan, "The Chapel and the Operating Room: The Struggle of Roman Catholic Clergy, Physicians, and Believers with the Dilemmas of Obstetric Surgery, 1800–1900," Bulletin of the History of Medicine 76, no. 3 (Fall 2002), esp. 470–74, for a discussion of cesarean sections. Hysterectomy was often performed at the same time to prevent what could be a life-threatening postoperative infection. Historians know less than we would like about the intimate lives of regular people like Frank and Annie, even if we have learned much about nineteenth-century fertility and sexuality in general. Family size had declined dramatically in the nineteenth century—from an average number of births in 1800 of 7.04 to 3.56 by 1900, although Catholic families, like the Rocks, tended to be larger. Margaret Marsh and Wanda Ronner, The Empty Cradle: Infertility in America from Colonial Times to the Present (Baltimore: Johns Hopkins University Press, 1996), 31, 77.

6. James Reed, From Private Vice to Public Virtue: The Birth Control Movement and American Society since 1830 (New York: Basic Books, 1978), chap. 3, and Janet Farrell Brodie, Contraception and Abortion in Nineteenth-Century America (Ithaca: Cornell University Press, 1994), esp. chap. 7, provide good summaries of the contraceptives available in the nineteenth century. Beginning at the end of the nineteenth century, California physician Clelia Duel Mosher asked forty-five married upper-middle-class women about their contraceptive habits, and most of them acknowledged using some form of contraception. Besides withdrawal and periodic abstinence, the women mentioned condoms and douching as other preferred contraceptive means. Clelia Mosher's survey has been edited and published, with a title supplied by the editors that she would never have chosen. Clelia Mosher, The Mosher Survey: Sexual Attitudes of 45 Victorian Women, ed. James MaHood and Kristine Wenburg (New York: Arno Press, 1980).

7. Robert Dallek, An Unfinished Life: John F. Kennedy, 1917–1963 (Boston: Little, Brown, 2003), 23.

8. Frank Rock to John Rock, Oct. 18, 1909, JR-RA.

9. See Elizabeth "Lizzie" McCarthy to John Rock, July 24, 1908, in which she mentions John's popularity; letter from Angela (Gately), July 31, 1908, in which she tells stories of Eddie Gately and others in Lakeside, JR-RA.

10. The Simmons information comes from the college's website: www.simmons .edu. Maisie's major from e-mail from Donna Webber, Simmons College archivist, to Diana Reinhard, research assistant to Margaret Marsh, Jan. 2, 2005.

11. Interview by Margaret Marsh with Rock family: Rachel (Rock) Achenbach, A. J. (Rock) Levinson, John Rock's daughters, and Hart Achenbach, Rock's son-in-law, June 3, 1998.

12. Ibid. Apparently Rock kept a diary or journal all his life. Only some of it survives. The diaries are in the possession of Rachel Achenbach.

13. John Rock diaries, Jan. 2, 1905, JR-RA.

14. John Rock diaries, March 2, 1904, and March 10, 1905, JR-RA.

15. See diary entry April 20, 1905, JR-RA. Holy Thursday is the day the Last Supper is observed during the week before Easter. Protestants call it Maundy Thursday.

16. When he was fourteen, he was upset for several days about an incident in which he and a group of friends "jollied" their friend Henry Brigham over the phone. Whatever prank they played, an angry Henry told John that he didn't think "'it' [whatever "it" was] was a nice thing to do." As for John, he was "very sorry. I was mean today." Henry stayed angry and hurt for several days, and John felt especially sad because Henry was his closest male friend—a walking companion with whom he felt comfortable discussing serious matters. John Rock diaries, Jan. 2, 1905, JR-RA.

17. See, for example, John Rock diaries, March 1, 1905; Eddie Gately to John Rock, Dec. 19, 1905, JR-RA.

18. Harry Rock to John Rock, Aug. 19, 1909, JR-RA. In the same letter, Harry also complains about anti-Irish discrimination at his workplace.

19. John Rock diaries, May 21, 1907, JR-RA.

20. Ella (Hogan) to John Rock, Oct. 4, 1905, JR-RA. She gleefully recounted to John how she had singled out one of her classmates, an "Indian girl," to see just how miserable she could make this poor young woman. She continued writing him until at least mid-November.

21. Interview with Rock family, June 3, 1998. Also see Frank Rock to John Rock, March 28, 1912, JR-RA.

22. Eddie Gately to John Rock, June 27, 1905, Dec. 19, 1905, and Jan. 16, 1906, JR-RA.

23. McLaughlin, *The Pill, John Rock, and the Church*, 10. Ernest A. Wreidt, William J. Bogan, and George Herbert Mead, *A Report on Vocational Training in Chicago and Other Cities* (Chicago: City Club of Chicago, 1912), 245–47.

24. Ann Jane Rock to John Rock, undated letter written in 1908, JR-RA.

25. John Rock diaries, March 6, 1907, JR-RA.

26. John Rock diaries, undated, but just before March 15, 1907, entry torn out. John Rock diaries, Nov. 25, 1972, JR-RA. Ben and Ray may have been the same person, with Ray just choosing, in true adolescent fashion, to change his name to a middle name or Ray itself being a school nickname later dropped. Alternatively, they could have been brothers.

27. John Rock diaries, March 15, 1907, JR-RA.

28. We have been unable to find out what happened to Ray. If he and Ben were brothers, then probably Ray became permanently disabled and therefore simply no longer talked about, or he died.

29. This is generic textbook history of the early twentieth century, but it has stood the test of time. One good textbook version is Gary Nash et al., *The American People: Creating a Nation and Society*, vol. 2, 5th ed. (New York: Longmans, 2001), 651–55. Its assessment conforms to what has become a truism of American history.

30. For example, John Rock to Charlie Rock, July 6, 1908; John Rock to "Papa," July 21, 1906; John Rock to Maisie Rock, July 30, 1908; John Rock to Harry Rock, Aug. 6, 1908; and John Rock to Charlie Rock, Aug. 14, 1908. Frank Rock as delegate to Democratic Convention mentioned in Lizzie (Rock) to John Rock, July 20, 1908, JR-RA.

31. John Rock to Charlie Rock, July 10, 1908, JR-RA.

32. The University of Vermont was the first college to elect a woman to Phi Beta Kappa, in 1875.

33. Howard Morse to John Rock, Aug. 1, 1908; Elizabeth Rock to John Rock, Sept. 17, 1909; quotation from Ella Conway to John Rock, Dec. 5, 1909, JR-RA.

34. John Rock diaries, Dec. 8, 1908, JR-RA.

35. Ibid.

36. On the early history of United Fruit, see, for example, Charles David Kepner, Jr., *Social Aspects of the Banana Industry* (New York: Columbia University Press, 1936). On Minor Keith, see John Keith Hatch, *Minor C. Keith: Pioneer of the American Tropics* (privately printed, no place of publication, 1963), and Charles David Kepner and Jay Henry Soothill, *The Banana Empire* (New York: Vanguard Press, 1935), esp. 53–55.

37. See Charles Morrow Wilson, *Empire in Green and Gold: The Story of the American Banana Trade* (New York: Henry Holt, 1947), esp. 123–27; Diane Stanley, *For the Record: The United Fruit Company's Sixty-Six Years in Guatemala* (Guatemala: Centro Impresor Pudra Santa, 1994), 2; Paul J. Dosal, *Doing Business with the Dictators: A Political History of United Fruit in Guatemala, 1899–1944* (Wilmington, Del.: Scholarly Resources, 1993), 47.

38. Dosal, *Doing Business with the Dictators*, 37, 46–47. The Guatemala Railway Company was incorporated in New Jersey and was owned by Keith and two of his former rivals, William Van Horne and Thomas Hubbard. See also Jason M. Colby, "'Banana Growing and Negro Management': Race, Labor, and Jim Crow Colonialism in Guatemala, 1884–1930," *Diplomatic History* 30, no. 4 (Sept. 2006), 605–6.

39. Victor Cutter, *Trade Relations with Latin America* (Boston: United Fruit Company, 1929), 27.

40. Wilson, *Empire in Green and Gold*, 204–9 and 124–27; quotation on 127. Dosal, *Doing Business with the Dictators*, 75.

41. Stanley, *For the Record*, 84–87; see clipping from *Daily Enterprise*, 1909, and additional unidentified clipping, both indicating that John Rock would be working for United Fruit. See F. V. Thompson to John Rock, Nov. 30, 1909, and typed draft (never mailed) of letter from John Rock to Victor Cutter, April 4, 1910. Also see letter from Neil MacPhail to "Tommy" [H. E. K. Thompson], Oct. 20, 1947, in which he discussed John Rock's experiences on the Dartmouth plantation, JR-RA.

42. See also Colby, "'Banana Growing and Negro Management,'" 608.

43. Stanley, *For the Record*, 101–3.

44. Ibid., 118.

45. Colby, "'Banana Growing and Negro Management,'" 596, quotes one of Cutter's friends on his temper and discusses the company's racial policies on 609–10.

46. John Rock diaries, Aug. 17, 1909, JR-RA.

47. Frank Rock to John Rock, undated, but definitely fall 1909; Frank Rock to John Rock, Dec. 22, 1909; Frank Rock to John Rock, Jan. 5, 1910; Frank Rock to John Rock, undated, but envelope postmarked Nov. 6, 1909, JR-RA.

48. Maisie Rock to John Rock, Oct. 26, 1909, JR-RA.

49. Stanley, For the Record, 125–27. Aldous Huxley, Beyond the Mexique Bay (New York: Harper Bros., 1934), 36.

50. Neil MacPhail to "Tommy" (Dr. H. E. K. Thompson) Oct. 20, 1947, JR-RA.

51. John Rock diaries, Dec. 21 and 22, 1909. Rock to Smith, transcript of telegraphic transmissions among the farms and offices of the Guatemala division, Dec. 16 and 17, JR-RA.

52. "MacPhail to Haxworth," transcript of telegraphic transmissions, Dec. 16, 1909, JR-RA.

53. Colby, "'Banana Growing and Negro Management,'" quotes Cutter on 611.

54. It's not clear whether the shooting took place on the 16th of Dec. or the 22nd or if there may have been two shootings. Draft of letter from John Rock to, we think, Ben Williams, because Ben was one of his closest friends and Ben's sister Mary figures in the same letter. Dec. 25, 1909, JR-RA. Colby, "'Banana Growing and Negro Management,'" 610–11, names another man as the shooter, but since more than one worker was killed, there may have been more than one shooter. Rock, who was there and knew everyone involved, surely knew who had committed this particular killing.

55. John Rock to [Ben Williams?], Dec. 25, 1909, JA-RA. Also letter from John Rock to Victor Cutter (typed but with a notation in JR's hand that it was never sent), April 4, 1910, JR-RA.

56. MacPhail to John Rock, April 21, 1910. John and MacPhail remained friends throughout MacPhail's life. MacPhail visited John in Boston while the latter was a medical student and whenever he could afterwards. His letters during these early years offer advice about the practice of medicine. Much later, in 1947, in a letter addressed to a friend (that somehow made it to Rock), MacPhail recalled these early years and that during the six days Rock had spent with MacPhail before leaving Guatemala, John had set his sights both on Harvard and on a medical career. MacPhail to Tommy, Oct. 20, 1947, JR-RA.

57. See, for example, Lizzie (Rock) to John Rock, Sept. 17, 1909, and Nov. 13, 1909; L. T. Wall to John Rock, March 12, 1912; and F. V. Thompson to John Rock, Nov. 30, 1909. Also Ben Williams to John Rock, Aug. 29, 1911, JR-RA.

58. See, for example, letters from Neil MacPhail to John Rock, Nov. 20, 1910, and Dec. 7, 1911, JR-RA. In the second letter, he says, "Go ahead John, and if you decide on medicine cram hard and then come down to be my right hand."

59. Henry B. Sawyer to John Rock, July 25, 1910, JR-RA. Also see McLaughlin, The Pill, John Rock, and the Church, 11.

Chapter 2. Choosing Medicine, Coming of Age

1. John T. Bethell, *Harvard Observed: An Illustrated History of the University in the Twentieth Century* (Cambridge, Mass.: Harvard University Press, 1998), 33–37. J. Pierpont Morgan gave a million dollars to finance three new buildings for the medical school in 1901. John D. Rockefeller not only donated a million dollars to the medical school but also supplied half the seed money needed to create the Harvard Business School.

2. Bethell, *Harvard Observed*, 13.

3. Marcia Graham Synnott, *The Half-Opened Door: Discrimination and Admissions at Harvard, Yale, and Princeton, 1900–1970* (Westport, Conn.: Greenwood Press, 1979). Lowell's letter to Alfred Stearns of Andover is quoted on 7.

4. Bethell, *Harvard Observed*, 22, indicates that Charles William Eliot, Lowell's predecessor and the president credited with building Harvard as a national institution, also sought "public school" boys, but it was Lowell who really focused on undergraduate education, who insisted on reining in the excesses of the elective system (which allowed students who so wished to coast to a degree), and introduced the New Plan.

5. John Brett Langstaff, ed., *Harvard of Today from the Undergraduate Point of View* (Cambridge, Mass.: Harvard Federation of Territorial Clubs, 1913).

6. Synnott, *Half-Opened Door*, 31. She describes Lowell as nativist and anti-Semitic, and her evidence on this is quite persuasive. See esp. 34–38.

7. Samuel Eliot Morison, *Three Centuries of Harvard, 1636–1936* (Cambridge, Mass.: Harvard University Press, 1936), especially chap. 16.

8. *Harvard Class Album for 1915* (Cambridge, Mass.: Harvard University, 1915). We estimated the numbers of Irish Catholics by considering their names and by looking to see if, in addition to an Irish name, they were members of St. Paul's Catholic Society; the Jewish students were similarly estimated by looking at their names, supplemented by membership in the Menorah Society and sometimes the Zionist Club. The African Americans we deduced by photograph (and a hometown in the United States rather than in Africa). Two students were obviously African American, and two more may have been. We could not get any closer than these rough estimates.

9. Bethell, *Harvard Observed*, 22–23; Morison, *Three Centuries*, 422.

10. Morison, *Three Centuries*, 442, 418; Langstaff, *Harvard of Today*, 60–61.

11. Term bill for John Rock, Jan. 20, 1912, JR-RA.

12. *Harvard Class Album*, entry for John Rock, 176. The students themselves provided the copy for these entries, JR-RA.

13. Morison, *Three Centuries*, 423–24; Langstaff, *Harvard of Today*, 64.

14. *Harvard Class Album*, 176; Morison, *Three Centuries*, 427. Invitation for Pi Eta in JR-RA.

15. As an alumnus, John may have found it easier simply to mention Hasty Pudding. He recounts his interview with McLaughlin in his diary. See John Rock diaries, March 18, 1979, JR-RA. Loretta McLaughlin, *The Pill, John Rock, and the Church: The Biography of a Revolution* (Boston: Little, Brown, 1982), 12. There was no Newman Club when John

Rock was an undergraduate, although the St. Paul's Catholic Society did meet at the new Newman House.

16. Frank Rock to John Rock, Oct. 17, 1911, JR-RA.

17. Frank Rock to John Rock, March 28, 1912, JR-RA.

18. Frank Rock to John Rock, Oct. 17, 1911, JR-RA.

19. Note from L. T. Wall to John Rock, March 12, 1912, wondering why John hadn't responded to an invitation to meet with his old friends (indeed, his closest friends from those years) from the High School of Commerce. Also, Neil MacPhail to John Rock, Dec. 7, 1911, and Feb. 15, 1915, JR-RA.

20. Kenneth M. Ludmerer, *Learning to Heal: The Development of American Medical Education* (New York: Basic Books, 1985), 50–54.

21. Ibid., 57–58.

22. In fact, President Eliot feared it was too ambitious, so the two professors who devised it, Henry Bowditch and J. Collins Warren, went over his head to Robert Bacon, a member of the university's board of overseers. Persuaded, Bacon then helped Bowditch and Warren secure gifts not only from John D. Rockefeller and J. P. Morgan, but also from others, including Arabella Huntington (the widow of railroad magnate Collis Huntington) and the Sears family. Morgan gave three buildings, and Huntington and the Sears family each gave one. Major Higginson, who had planned and endowed the Harvard Union, headed a group that gave one. The total cost of the land and buildings was $2.7 million, which would be more than half a billion dollars today. Bethell, *Harvard Observed*, 35; Ludmerer, *Learning to Heal*, 147–48.

23. On the Harvard teaching hospitals and clinical clerkships, see Ludmerer, *Learning to Heal*, 226–27.

24. The quotation about Folin comes from Ludmerer, *Learning to Heal*, 104. All these subjects were covered in the school's second general examinations of Feb. 1918, JR-RA.

25. Charlie Rock to John Rock, Jan. 22, 1917, JR-RA.

26. Annie Rock's role in the theater business is detailed in the court records of the litigation over Frank Rock's estate. *Kathryn G. Rock et alii., Executors of the Estate of Charles E. Rock et alii., Appellants, vs. Delia M. Rock individually and as Administratrix d.b.n. et al., Appellees.* Estate of Frank Rock, First and Final Account, Suffolk County, Commonwealth of Massachusetts Probate Court, no. 253457 (n.d., approx. 1940), 135, 137, 144–45, 149. On Charlie Rock paying for John's education, see 140.

27. Charlie Rock to John Rock, Jan. 22, 1917, JR-RA.

28. Charlie Rock to John Rock, Feb. 28, 1917, JR-RA.

29. Charlie Rock to John Rock, Jan. 22, 1917, JR-RA.

30. From "Pers. S" (probably Bill Sefton's brother) to John Rock, Sept. 22, 1917, JR-RA. Underline in original.

31. Rock told later interviewers that before beginning his internship, he had been an assistant to a general surgeon in Brockton, but he began an internship at MGH on July 1, 1918, according to his office records. If both are correct, he must have finished

his medical requirements by the beginning of March 1918. See "Check of Dr. Rock's Biographical Data," typewritten, Dec. 1954, p. 1, JR-RA. For the story of his failed attempt to serve in the military, see McLaughlin, *The Pill, John Rock, and the Church*, 12–13.

32. Rusty (Rustin) McIntosh (in Paris assigned to the Peace Commission) to John Rock, Feb. 21, 1919; Frank Berry (in Dijon, France) to John Rock, March 24, 1919, JR-RA.

33. McIntosh to Rock, Aug. 16, 1920, JR-RA.

34. Kenneth Ludmerer, *Time to Heal: American Medical Education from the Turn of the Century to the Era of Managed Care* (New York: Oxford University Press, 1999), 80–85.

35. In the United States today, laws limit the hours that interns and residents can work. Doing so cuts down on the errors these young doctors make; some also say that such regulation means that although the young doctors will be less fatigued, they will also see fewer cases and therefore not learn as much as they could during their residencies. In the early twentieth century, physicians and hospitals did not concern themselves with such issues.

36. Ludmerer, *Time to Heal*, 96.

37. Nell had often wondered about her future even before her mother's death. See Nell Rock to John Rock, undated but sometime in summer 1909, JR-RA, in which she says, "Of course I fully realize that I am the thickest one of the bunch, but nevertheless there ought to be something in this world for poor little fat me to do." In the court records detailing the dispute over Frank Rock's estate, it is evident that Frank worried about what would happen to Nell when he remarried. *Kathryn G. Rock et alii. vs. Delia M. Rock et alii.*, 188.

38. Neil MacPhail to John Rock, Feb. 15, 1915, and Dec. 21, 1915, JR-RA.

39. MacPhail to Rock, March 10, 1917, JR-RA.

40. "Dr. Rock's Career," typescript, Dec. 1954, JR-RA.

41. Charlie Rock to John Rock, June 18, 1919, JR-RA.

42. John Rock to Dr. H. E. K. Thompson, Oct. 10, 1956, JR-RA.

43. George V. Smith, *My Professional Life with Women* (privately printed, no date, but sometime in the early 1980s), 13, JR-RA. We discuss Sims's work, and the Woman's Hospital, in Margaret Marsh and Wanda Ronner, *The Empty Cradle: Infertility in America from Colonial Times to the Present* (Baltimore: Johns Hopkins University Press, 1996), 48–64 and 71–74.

44. The controversial Sims, founder of the Woman's Hospital, was the first surgeon to cure the condition of vesico-vaginal fistula, which is a tear that results in an opening between the vagina and the bladder. It can occur after a difficult delivery. For centuries before Sims, physicians had been trying unsuccessfully to cure the condition, which doomed a woman to experience constant leakage of urine from the bladder into the vagina. Medical historians now believe that rickets, a vitamin D deficiency, resulted in pelvic deformity, which made childbirth more difficult and vesico-vaginal fistulas more likely. While not life threatening, the condition caused women constant

discomfort and made it impossible for them to live normal lives. It was no respecter of social or economic status. This awful condition still ravages parts of the developing world, especially in Africa. Although Sims cured the condition, he learned how to do so by operating on enslaved women, repeatedly and without anesthesia. This earned him in his own day considerable antipathy among some quarters in the North and (at best) a morally compromised historical legacy. Thomas Addis Emmet, *Reminiscences of the Founders of the Woman's Hospital Association* (New York: Stuyvesant Press, 1893), 14, 17; Deborah Kuhn McGregor, *Sexual Surgery and the Origins of Gynecology: J. Marion Sims, His Hospital, and His Patients* (New York: Garland Publishers, 1989), 176–77; Ann Dally, *Women Under the Knife: A History of Surgery* (New York: Routledge, 1991), 22.

45. The Woman's Hospital in New York was itself moving into new and grander facilities in 1875, when William Baker became the founding director of the Free Hospital for Women. Baker would later become Harvard Medical School's first professor of gynecology. Holmes was hardly optimistic about the hospital's potential to cure disease, noting that in the case of women's diseases, a physician could hope "to cure, seldom, to alleviate, often, to comfort, always." Smith, *My Professional Life with Women*, 13. Holmes is quoted on 37.

46. George V. Smith, "The Life of a Physician," unpublished memoir, typescript, 1982, esp. 38, 72, 74, JR-RA. The "teaching material" quotation is on 46.

47. His knowledge of urology (at that time the only specialty that focused on the male reproductive organs) would hold him in good stead later as an infertility specialist.

48. Interview with Rock family: Rachel Achenbach, A. J. Levinson, and Hart Achenbach, June 3, 1998. Rachel and A. J. said their father told them this story sometime in the 1940s.

49. Ibid.; Frank Rock to Charlie Rock, undated but sometime in late 1920, reprinted in *Kathryn G. Rock et alii. vs. Delia M. Rock et alii.*, 191.

50. The documentation of this expectation is detailed in the court records of the litigation over Frank Rock's estate. *Kathryn G. Rock et alii. vs. Delia M. Rock et alii.*, esp. 187–88.

51. Ibid.

52. Frank Rock to Charlie Rock, Dec. 28, 1920, in ibid., 188. The letters in the court documents are in the order they were entered as exhibits, not the order in which they were written.

53. Frank Rock to Charlie Rock, Jan. 17, 1921, in ibid., 192. Nell's "so upset" quotation is from her testimony on 136.

Chapter 3. New Discoveries in Human Reproduction

1. In 1924 the two men published a book on the subject: Edward Reynolds and Donald Macomber, *Fertility and Sterility in Human Marriage* (Philadelphia: W.B. Saunders, 1924). The contents—a compendium of cliches—failed to live up to the ambitious title. From the idea that female orgasm promoted conception, a discredited notion

that had been around for at least two centuries, to a caution that postpubertal girls and young women should not exert themselves too strenuously either physically or mentally lest they doom themselves to a sterile marriage, which had been around for only half a century, this pair of distinguished gynecologists had little new to offer. They even brought out the Victorian-era warnings to avoid "over frequent" sex, advising couples to limit intercourse to five or six times between menstrual periods. "Modern life," they warned, could diminish sperm production, and the use of contraception could result in female sterility. One of the few new ideas they had was that dietary deficiency, especially of vitamins and minerals, could affect fertility, and they did recognize the concept of relative fertility. See esp. 45, 123, 166, 210–11, 229–31.

2. Margaret Marsh and Wanda Ronner, The Empty Cradle: Infertility in America from Colonial Times to the Present (Baltimore: Johns Hopkins University Press, 1996), is a medical and cultural history of infertility in the United States. Elaine Tyler May, Barren in the Promised Land: Childless Americans and the Pursuit of Happiness (New York: Basic Books, 1995), is an excellent study of the social, cultural, and political dimensions of childlessness, including voluntary childlessness as well as infertility. For the 16% figure, see Samuel Meaker, Human Sterility: Causation, Diagnosis, and Treatment. A Practical Manual of Clinical Procedure (Baltimore: Williams and Wilkins, 1934), 244–45.

3. Marsh and Ronner, The Empty Cradle, chaps. 3 and 4, 75–108 and 131–70.

4. Although in 1926 Rock gave up his surgical privileges at MGH, he reactivated them in 1929. Notes for "Dr. Rock's Biographical Data: Harvard University Class of 1915 Anniversary Reports," undated, handwritten, JR-RA.

5. George V. Smith, My Professional Life with Women (privately printed, no date, but sometime in the early 1980s), 13, JR-RA. Graves is quoted in George V. Smith, "Life of a Physician," unpublished memoir, typescript, 1982, 42, JR-RA.

6. See typescript with handwritten corrections for an article by Sam Berkow, dated March 7, 1960, JR-RA. The article appeared as Sam Gordon Berkow, "After Office Hours: A Visit with Dr. John Rock," Obstetrics and Gynecology 15 (May 1960), 665–72.

7. Rachel Thorndike to John Rock, June 27, 1919, JR-RA.

8. Letters from Anna Thorndike to her mother and her sister Martha. None of the letters are dated, but the ones to Martha have postmarked envelopes. They were from 1912 and 1913 and sent from Montreal to Paris, where Martha was probably at school. Letter to Martha, postmarked March 14, 1913, JR-RA.

9. Thomas was its second president. She succeeded James E. Rhoads.

10. This description, and the ones that follow, are summarized from Helen Lefkowitz Horowitz's excellent biography of Thomas, The Power and Passion of M. Carey Thomas (New York: Knopf, 1994), esp. 60–71, 147–53, 318–19. Horowitz's biography was recommended to our research assistant, Diana Reinhard, by the current library staff at Bryn Mawr for its brilliant portrayal of Thomas and its insight into the Bryn Mawr experience for students.

11. Thomas constantly chafed under her nominal Quakerism, a requirement for her position at Bryn Mawr. Her belief in the intellectual equality of women and men was

uncompromising, but she was contemptuous of Jews, African Americans, and most immigrants.

12. Horowitz, *The Power and Passion*, 192–93.

13. Anna Thorndike, Bryn Mawr College transcript, handwritten, 1919, Bryn Mawr College Archives.

14. *Bryn Mawr Yearbook, Class of 1919*, Bryn Mawr College Archives, 22, 36, 39, 54, 76.

15. Photograph album in possession of Rachel Achenbach. See also Loretta McLaughlin, *The Pill, John Rock, and the Church: The Biography of a Revolution* (Boston: Little, Brown, 1982), 16–17. McLaughlin has Nan in France in 1923, but the photograph album indicates 1921 or 1922.

16. One of the few others had been the 1914 wedding of Joseph Kennedy and Rose Fitzgerald, daughter of HoneyFitz, the city's colorful mayor. Rose and Joe Kennedy, of course, were the parents of that great twentieth-century political dynasty, which included a president, two senators, and more than a fair share of family tragedy.

17. McLaughlin, *The Pill, John Rock, and the Church*, esp. 16–22.

18. See for example, Margaret Marsh, *Suburban Lives* (New Brunswick, N.J.: Rutgers University Press, 1990), 98, 106.

19. Nan talked about the family's domestic arrangements in 1929 in a letter—Nan Rock to John Rock, undated, but internal evidence shows to be April 1929, JR-RA.

20. John Rock diaries, Oct. 8, 1929, JR-RA. For conversion of the $800 into today's dollars, see the Federal Reserve Bank of Minneapolis Consumer Price Index Calculator, http://minneapolisfed.org/Research/data/us/calc/index.cfm. We have used this calculator for all conversions in the text.

21. John Rock diaries, Oct. 8, 1929, JR-RA.

22. John Rock, "Progress in Obstetrics," *Boston Medical and Surgical Journal* 197, no. 19 (1927), 858–65. (This journal became the *New England Journal of Medicine* in 1928.)

23. Preeclampsia is characterized by swelling, increase in blood pressure, protein-urea, and fetal compromise. An introduction to this condition for a general audience is Jane E. Brody, "For Mother and Child, a Lurking Danger," *New York Times*, Nov. 23, 2004, D9.

24. Rock, "Progress in Obstetrics" (1927), 858; Rock, "Progress in Obstetrics," *New England Journal of Medicine* 200, no. 18 (May 2, 1929), 919–27, and 206, no. 2 (Jan. 14, 1932), 77–87.

25. Rock, "Progress in Obstetrics" (1927), 858; Rock, "Progress in Obstetrics" (1929), 919.

26. Rock, "Progress in Obstetrics" (1927), 859–60.

27. Joseph C. Ryan, "The Chapel and the Operating Room: The Struggle of Roman Catholic Clergy, Physicians, and Believers with the Dilemmas of Obstetric Surgery, 1800–1900," *Bulletin of the History of Medicine* 76, no. 3 (Fall 2002), 492.

28. On progressive obstetrical opinion, see Leslie Reagan, *When Abortion Was a Crime: Women, Medicine, and Law in the United States, 1867–1973* (Berkeley: University of California Press, 1997), 143.

29. Rock, "Progress in Obstetrics" (1932), 78.

30. See Judith Walzer Leavitt, *Brought to Bed: Childbearing in America, 1750–1950* (New York: Oxford University Press, 1986).

31. John Rock, "Prenatal and Maternal Care," paper presented to the White House Conference Institute, Springfield, Mass., Oct. 9, 1931 (partly typewritten, partly handwritten), p. 4, JR-RA.

32. First quotation, ibid., p. 3-c. He had written the words "and ability" after "qualifications" but struck those words out of his spoken version. Second quotation is on the next to the last page, page not numbered.

33. "Final Draft: Medical Progress: Obstetrics: Labor and Delivery," for the *New England Journal of Medicine* 221, no. 18 (Nov. 2, 1939), 694–98, JR-RA.

34. Rock, "The Problem of Sterility," *New England Journal of Medicine* 199, no. 2 (July 12, 1928), 79–85. He also wrote the "Progress in Obstetrics" pieces for the *New England Journal* in 1929 and 1932.

35. John Rock to Nan Rock, Aug. 28, 1928, and "Friday A.M." [also Aug. 1928], JR-RA.

36. John Rock to Nan Rock, April 22, 1929, JR-RA.

37. Nan Rock to John Rock, "Friday" [April 26, 1929], JR-RA.

38. John Rock to Nan Rock, April 27, 1929. Nan to John Rock, undated, but written during John Rock's stay at Hopkins, JR-RA.

39. Walter E. Duka and Alan H. DeCherney, *From the Beginning: A History of the American Fertility Society, 1944–1994* (Birmingham, Ala.: The American Fertility Society, 1994), 19, noted that the society's founder, Walter W. Williams, confined his medical practice to infertility. But he was also a former veterinarian who continued to do research on cattle, which may have provided him with additional income. It became easier to specialize in this field after World War II, exemplified by Rock's career and that of others described in this history.

40. Interview by Margaret Marsh with Rock family: Rachel (Rock) Achenbach, A. J. (Rock) Levinson, and Hart Achenbach, June 3, 1998; John Rock budget ledger, 1921–29 (very incomplete), JR-RA.

41. Charles Rock, "Is Advertising an Exact Science?" speech given to an unnamed advertising group in Philadelphia on March 28, 1935, typescript, 8 pages, quotation on 4, JR-RA.

42. *Kathryn G. Rock et alii. vs. Delia M. Rock et alii.*, 190. Charlie funneled his support for Delia through John. We have no idea why; perhaps he was simply too angry with Delia to deal with her directly.

43. Ibid., table facing 190 but unpaginated.

44. Adele E. Clarke, *Disciplining Reproduction: Modernity, American Life Sciences, and the Problems of Sex* (Berkeley: University of California Press, 1998), is a history of the life sciences in the United States, including the study of sex and reproduction in animals as well as humans. It is not about reproductive medicine.

45. Robert Latou Dickinson's Committee for Maternal Health funded Moench's research. Marsh and Ronner, *The Empty Cradle*, 150–51.

46. For discussion of the Rubin test, see the comments following N. Sproat Heaney, "A Simple Method of Testing the Patency of the Fallopian Tubes," *Gynecological Transactions* 48 (1923), 218. Some physicians attributed as much as 70% of tubal inflammation and blockage to gonorrhea, and as much as 25% to 50% of all cases of sterility to this disease.

47. This discussion is drawn from the more extended one in Marsh and Ronner, *The Empty Cradle*, 135–42.

48. There is more than one estrogen, but that discovery came later.

49. Marsh and Ronner, *The Empty Cradle*, 134.

50. See Victor Cornelius Medvei, *The History of Clinical Endocrinology: A Comprehensive Account of Endocrinology from Earliest Times to the Present* (Pearl River, N.Y.: Parthenon Publishing, 1993), and John G. Gruhn and Ralph R. Kazer, *Hormonal Regulation of the Menstrual Cycle: The Evolution of Concepts* (New York: Plenum, 1989).

51. See Medvei, *The History of Clinical Endocrinology.*

52. Henry R. Harrower, *Practical Endocrinology* (Glendale, Calif.: Pioneer Printing, 1932).

53. Theodoor van de Velde et al., *Fertility and Sterility in Marriage: Their Voluntary Promotion and Limitation* (New York: Medical Books, 1931).

54. For example, Marsh and Ronner, *The Empty Cradle*, 142–47.

55. Ibid., 142.

56. Ibid., 141. Smith, "The Life of a Physician," esp. 79–82. Elizabeth Siegel Watkins, *The Estrogen Elixir: A History of Hormone Replacement Therapy in America* (Baltimore: Johns Hopkins University Press, 2007), 10–11, 18–24.

57. George Corner, *Anatomist at Large: An Autobiography and Selected Essays* (Freeport, N.Y.: Books for Libraries Press, 1969), 48–50.

58. Marsh and Ronner, *The Empty Cradle*, 141.

59. There were indirect indications, such as the rise and fall of a woman's basal body temperature, but temperature readings did not predict ovulation, nor could they determine its exact timing. Stephen Fleck, Elizabeth F. Snedeker, and John Rock, "The Contraceptive Safe Period: A Clinical Study," *New England Journal of Medicine* 223 (1940), 1005–9, in summarizing the findings of K. Ogino, H. Knaus (the separate theorists of the rhythm method of contraception), and Carl Hartman, author of *The Timing of Ovulation in Women* and an expert on primate reproduction, say as follows: "The theory may be expressed thus: The fertile period extends from and including the nineteenth day before the *earliest* likely menstruation up to and including the ninth day before the *latest* likely menstruation" (1005). In other words, precision about this matter was not possible with the current state of knowledge.

60. McLaughlin, *The Pill, John Rock, and the Church*, 41.

61. Susan Lederer, *Subjected to Science: Human Experimentation in America before the Second World War* (Baltimore: Johns Hopkins University Press, 1995), xv. She does not deny that there were many abuses in the system. We discuss this subject further in the context of Rock's clinical studies in the next chapter.

62. Smith, "The Life of a Physician," 46. Smith did care about his patients, but it is

hard to read the paragraph in which this term appears without sensing a demeaning attitude.

63. John Rock and Marshall Bartlett, "Biopsy Studies of Human Endometrium: Criteria of Dating and Information about Amenorrhea, Menorrhagia and Time of Ovulation," *Journal of the American Medical Association* 108 (June 12, 1937), 2022-28; quotation on 2026.

64. Ibid.

65. L. B. #29645 under OVA, JR-RA.

66. James M. Snodgrass, John Rock, and Miriam Menkin, "The Validity of 'Ovulation Potentials,'" *American Journal of Physiology* 140, no. 3 (Dec. 1943), 394-97.

67. Ibid., 398. Miriam Menkin discussed this study in an informal talk to scientists at Cold Spring Harbor on July 18 or 28 (the first numeral not legible), 1949. Untitled typescript of twenty pages, with note in Menkin's hand at the bottom, "Final Draft, Talk at CSH, July [18 or 28], 1949," p. 6. JR-CLM.

68. Snodgrass, Rock, and Menkin, "The Validity of 'Ovulation Potentials,'" 415.

69. Smith, "The Life of a Physician," 84.

70. Regina Markell Morantz-Sanchez, *Sympathy and Science: Women Physicians in American Medicine* (New York: Oxford University Press, 1985), 328-31.

71. See McLaughlin, *The Pill, John Rock, and the Church*, 72-75.

72. For Menkin's work history, letter of application, and resume, Miriam Menkin to John Rock, March 2, 1938, JR-RA.

73. J. D. Ratcliff, "No Father to Guide Them," *Collier's* (March 20, 1937), 19, 73.

74. Menkin resume, 1938, JR-RA.

Chapter 4. Firing the First Shot in the Reproductive Revolution

1. This is the first of two chapters about this critical period in Rock's career. Here, we concentrate on the two research studies that made his reputation in the field that would eventually be called reproductive medicine. The next chapter brings us into the world of Rock the practitioner, where we will meet women he treated and who participated as research subjects in his studies. Rock would sternly disapprove of our dividing his life this way. He never made a distinction between research and practice. From his earliest days as a resident, he made clear his commitment to his patients. The patients returned his regard. See Mrs. W. to John Rock, Dec. 1919, and Mrs. W.'s daughter to Rock, Oct. 20, 1919, JR-RA. Indeed, the confidence his patients had in him no doubt made it easier for him to recruit research participants. We separate his research and practice here only for the convenience of describing each more fully.

2. The car story was recalled by Rock's son-in-law Hart Achenbach. Interview by Margaret Marsh with Rock family: Rachel (Rock) Achenbach, A. J. (Rock) Levinson, and Hart Achenbach, June 3, 1998. Whenever Rock attended meetings or gave lectures abroad, he always tried to get Nan to go with him, which she often did. He wasn't alone in this. Few of his male colleagues, it seemed, could stand to go on long trips without their wives.

3. Loretta McLaughlin, *The Pill, John Rock, and the Church: The Biography of a Revolution* (Boston: Little, Brown, 1982), 23. John Rock to Nan Rock, undated, but internal evidence suggests early 1930s, JR-RA.

4. John Rock to Nan Rock, undated, but internal evidence suggests early 1930s, JR-RA.

5. It would take several more decades for such a method to be developed.

6. Until this book the most complete source of published information has been Loretta McLaughlin, *The Pill, John Rock, and the Church*. See also John Rock, *The Time Has Come: A Catholic Doctor's Proposals to End the Battle over Birth Control* (New York: Knopf, 1963); Margaret Marsh and Wanda Ronner, *The Empty Cradle: Infertility in America from Colonial Times to the Present* (Baltimore: Johns Hopkins University Press, 1996), 171–202; John Rock's obituary in *New York Times*, Dec. 5, 1984; "John Rock," in Margot Levy, ed., *The Annual Obituary, 1984* (London: St. James Press, 1985), 656–58; Walter E. Duka and Alan H. DeCherney, *From the Beginning: A History of the American Fertility Society, 1944–1994* (Birmingham, Ala.: The American Fertility Society, 1994), 77–83. The society, begun as the American Society for the Study of Sterility, changed its name in the mid-1990s to the American Society for Reproductive Medicine.

7. Duka and DeCherney, *From the Beginning*, 79.

8. Hertig called them the Rock-Hertig study, and Rock the Hertig-Rock study.

9. The term conceptus is rarely, if ever, used today, but since Rock and Hertig did so, we are retaining the term. On the disuse of conceptus in popular literature: Robin Marantz Henig, *Pandora's Baby: How the First Test Tube Babies Sparked the Reproductive Revolution* (New York: Houghton Mifflin, 2004), never once uses this term, though she talks of blastocysts, embryos, and ova.

10. John Rock, transcript of a talk given to the Pacific Coast Obstetrical and Gynecological Society, San Francisco, Nov. 1946, pp. 13–14, JR-RA. (Actually the third page of this document. The other pages, which are not included, were transcripts of other material from that meeting.)

11. See Marsh and Ronner, *The Empty Cradle*, 149–50, 175–76.

12. Ibid., 148–51.

13. A "graded" series means one organized by age of the embryo. Each stage would be numbered. For a series called Our Scientific Heritage, Hertig, with some input from Rock, described the embryo study in A. T. Hertig and J. Rock, "Searching for Early Fertilized Human Ova," *Gynecologic Investigation* 4 (1973), 112–39. Description of Hertig's work at the Carnegie, 122–23. See also Hertig obituary, *New York Times*, July 22, 1990; McLaughlin, *The Pill, John Rock, and the Church*, 61–62.

14. Arthur T. Hertig, "A Fifteen Year Search for First Stage Human Ova," *Journal of the American Medical Association* 261, no. 3 (Jan. 20, 1989), 434–35.

15. Hertig obituary, *New York Times*, July 22, 1990; McLaughlin, *The Pill, John Rock, and the Church*, 61–62.

16. The study formally concluded in 1954, but there are patient files marked "Rock-Hertig" that date to as late as 1955 (but no later), Series II, Reproductive Research

Files, 1925–1972, undated, boxes 7, 8, and 9, JR-CLM. Others in JR-RA. Our guess is that what is usually called a formal "series" concluded in 1954, but that the informal search for embryos kept going for a year or so later. The study achieved its research objective by 1954, and Hertig's appointment as chair of the Pathology Department at the Harvard Medical School had brought on other obligations. See also McLaughlin, *The Pill, John Rock, and the Church*, 61–62.

17. The Department of Embryology of the Carnegie Institution of Washington held the collection of embryos (including those we would call fetuses), and it was to this institution that the embryos collected in the Rock-Hertig study were sent. The Carnegie Institution sectioned and photographed the embryos Hertig discovered.

18. Rock performed many of the surgeries on these patients, but inevitably clinic patients were also operated on by other physicians, including residents. This project was built on the cooperation of an entire group of colleagues, staff, and patients. On Rock's generosity in crediting others, see John Rock, transcript of a talk given to the Pacific Coast Obstetrical and Gynecological Society, 13. On their joint public recollection of the origins of the study, see Arthur T. Hertig, John Rock, and Eleanor Adams, "A Description of 34 Human Ova Within the First 17 Days of Development," *American Journal of Anatomy* 98, no. 3 (May 1956), 4356.

19. George V. Smith, "The Life of a Physician," unpublished memoir, typescript, 1982, 84, JR-RA. It is hard to know what provoked such an outburst against a longtime friend and colleague, his wife's doctor, and the person who delivered his children. Perhaps he simply believed that Rock, who had become an international celebrity in the 1960s, did not deserve such fame. Perhaps his bitterness came from the opprobrium he and his wife, Olive Watkins Smith, faced in the early 1970s over their championing of the use of DES to prevent miscarriage. He may have felt that he and Olive were maligned unfairly, while Rock was lionized. We have no way of knowing. If Rock, to whom Smith sent a copy of his memoir, had any reaction, we have not found it.

20. In later years, Hertig often uses the number 210. Perhaps later information caused them to eliminate one of the cases, but originally it was 211.

21. We discuss the rhythm clinic in more detail in chapter 5. Almost all the published reports of this study suggest that the patients were not originally Rock's and that they were all clinic patients, but unless the patient records are in error, some of the women were Rock's private patients and a number of the clinic patients had been seen by Rock before they were selected for the study. Ronner reviewed records of fifty patients in this study. Series II A 2b, Reproductive Research Patient Files, undated, boxes 7–10, JR-CLM, and Patient Records, 1938–1955, JR-RA. Rock had examined at least twenty of these patients prior to surgery, and had operated on sixteen. While records are not complete on each patient, Rock seems to have done more of the examinations and surgery in the early years. Later, other physicians (Mulligan, Smith, Younge, Tucker, Johnson, and Easterday) performed the surgeries, with Mulligan performing at least eighteen procedures. Ronner also analyzed the extant records for the parallel ova study, and learned that 10% of the participants were private patients.

22. Miriam Menkin, untitled talk at Cold Spring Harbor, 1949, p. 3, Series III B, Lectures, Speeches, and Speaking Engagement Records, 1946–1972, undated, box 19, folder 23, JR-CLM, talks about the logistics of the clinics.

23. Hertig, "A Fifteen Year Search for First Stage Human Ova," 434.

24. This was a constant in the study. See, for example, John Rock and Arthur T. Hertig, "Some Aspects of Early Human Development," paper presented at the 67th Annual Meeting of the American Gynecological Society, Sky Top, Pa., June 15, 1942, JR-RA; and Hertig and Rock, "Searching for Early Fertilized Human Ova," 124.

25. The case records are principally from JR-RA.

26. Ronner closely analyzed fifty records from the embryo study. The oldest patient was forty-six, and the youngest was twenty-five. The majority were in their thirties. Twenty-four percent were over forty, and 8 percent were in their twenties. Patient Records, 1938–1955, JR-RA.

27. Hertig, "A Fifteen Year Search for First Stage Human Ova," 434.

28. Sometimes the hysterectomy was not the surgery first recommended but was resorted to only after the failure of less drastic measures. For example, in 1938 a thirty-four-year-old patient with pelvic pain and uterine prolapse had surgery to repair the prolapse. Several months later, still complaining of significant pain, she was recommended for a hysterectomy and agreed to participate in the study. Arthur T. Hertig and John Rock, "Two Complete Normal Human Ova of the Pre-Villous Stage, Estimated at 11 and 12 Days of Age," typescript, pp. 2–3, JR-CLM.

29. Patient Records, 1938–1955, JR-RA.

30. Ibid.

31. Because they are more accessible to the reader, and since so much of this research is from a private collection, we have chosen these quotations from published sources. They conform to the patient records. See Arthur T. Hertig and John Rock, "Two Human Ova of the Pre-Villous Stage, Having a Developmental Age of about Eight and Nine Days Respectively," Contributions to Embryology 33 (1949), 169, 177, and "Two Human Ova of the Pre-Villous Stage, Having a Developmental Age of about Seven and Nine Days Respectively," Contributions to Embryology 31 (1945), 67, 74. Also, Chester Heuser, John Rock, and Arthur T. Hertig, "Two Human Embryos Showing Early Stages of the Definitive Yolk Sac," Contributions to Embryology 31 (1945), 87, 91.

32. Hertig, "A Fifteen Year Search for First Stage Human Ova," 435. Regarding the patient who might have missed the preperiod deadline, his exact words were, "Only once, I think, did we operate after the patient might have had a period, and that's too bad." He did not express any worry over having terminated a potential pregnancy, but he was concerned enough about public opinion to edit this remark out of the transcript of his talk before it was published. John Rock, transcript of a talk given to the Pacific Coast Obstetrical and Gynecological Society, 12, JR-RA.

33. Jean Nauss to Mrs. [name redacted], Dec. 19, 1950, Series II A b1, Patient Research Files, 1925–72, undated, box 7, folder 29, JR-CLM.

34. Hertig, "A Fifteen Year Search for First Stage Human Ova," 435. Bouin's fluid was picric acid and formalin (p. 434).

35. Rock and Hertig, "Some Aspects of Early Human Development," 1, Series III A, Reproductive Research Writings, 1937–72, undated, box 15, folder 104, JR-CLM.

36. Hertig, "A Fifteen Year Search for First Stage Human Ova," 435; A. T. Hertig and J. Rock, "Searching for Early Fertilized Human Ova," 136; also see acknowledgment of grant funding on the cover of "The Human Conceptus During the First Two Weeks of Gestation," paper presented at the Annual Meeting of the American Gynecological Society, Montebello, Canada, June 17, 1947, JR-RA.

37. Rock and Hertig, "Some Aspects of Early Human Development," 1–5.

38. Ibid.

39. Arthur T. Hertig and John Rock, "Two Human Ova of the Previllous Stage, Having an Ovulation Age of About Eleven and Twelve Days Respectively, *Contributions to Embryology* 29, no. 184 (1941), 129–56.

40. Unidentified clipping, May 16, 1950, JR-RA.

41. Hertig, "A Fifteen Year Search for First Stage Human Ova," 435.

42. Susan Lederer, *Subjected to Science: Human Experimentation in America before the Second World War* (Baltimore: Johns Hopkins University Press, 1995), is an excellent study of nontherapeutic clinical research. Lederer does not mention the Rock-Hertig study, but the study fits the parameters she describes.

43. Hertig, "A Fifteen Year Search for First Stage Human Ova," 434.

44. We found only the one possible instance, described above, of a patient who may not have had her surgery exactly when it was scheduled.

45. L. Lee to [name redacted], June 19, 1943, box 10, folder 68, JR-CLM.

46. Luigi Mastroianni, interview by Wanda Ronner, July 7, 2007.

47. See Patient Records 1947 and 1948, JR-RA.

48. The cumulative effect of reading dozens of boxes of Rock's papers, at the Countway Library and in the Achenbach Collection, persuades us that Rock deserved the affection bestowed on him by his patients and his staff.

49. Leslie Reagan, *When Abortion Was a Crime: Women, Medicine, and Law in the United States, 1867–1973* (Berkeley: University of California Press, 1997), 109–10.

50. Lederer, *Subjected to Science*, 120–21. Also see James H. Jones, *Bad Blood: The Tuskegee Syphilis Experiment* (New York: Free Press, 1981), and Susan Reverby, ed., *Tuskegee's Truths: Rethinking the Tuskegee Syphilis Study* (Chapel Hill: University of North Carolina Press, 2000).

51. Lederer, *Subjected to Science*, 120.

52. Ibid., 97–98. Lederer notes that the physician who proposed the AMA resolution—which never happened—in 1916 was a defender of human experimentation responding to public criticism of it. He wanted to influence public opinion in favor of such research. The idea never got off the ground because many physicians believed that even "those procedures that, although unrelated to an individual's treatment, contributed to clinical research" would be interfered with by such a resolution.

53. As journalist Gena Corea put it, Rock and Hertig took advantage of poor charity patients, making them wait months until their surgery was scheduled so that Rock

and Hertig could monitor the women's ovulation patterns. Then, and without their consent, the researchers experimented on their unfertilized ova and their fertilized embryos. "Rather than performing the operation at just the time physicians diagnosed a need for it," she insisted, "Rock had the women spend several months taking their temperatures daily and charting their ovulatory cycles so the researchers could predict a date for the operation when they were most likely to find an embryo. Week after week, the charity patients brought their charts to the hospital until a surgical date optimal for the research could be determined." The patient records clearly and decisively contradict such an assessment; but of course, at the time no one had access to the records, which included the women's voices. We have not been able to obtain a copy of the antiabortion activists' representation of this study, of which we have oral information from one of the activists. For the antitechnology feminists' representation, see Gena Corea, *The Mother Machine: Reproductive Technology from Artificial Insemination to Artificial Wombs* (New York: Harper and Row, 1985), 101–3. Quotation on 102.

54. Herbert Ratner, "The Rock Book—I: A Catholic Viewpoint," *Commonweal* 78 (July 5, 1963), 393.

55. Janice Raymond, *Women as Wombs: Reproductive Technology and the Battle over Women's Freedom* (San Francisco: HarperSanFrancisco, 1993), viii; Corea, *Mother Machine*, 102–3. For more writings by this group of feminists, see Renate D. Klein, ed., *Infertility: Women Speak Out about Their Experiences of Reproductive Medicine* (London: Pandora, 1989).

56. Loretta McLaughlin relied on interviews with Rock, Hertig, and Menkin for her assessment of the Rock-Hertig study, and their memories were apparently affected by the contemporary political climate.

57. Contemporary opponents of abortion may find the study morally indefensible because women were asked to try to conceive prior to a scheduled hysterectomy. It is important to consider both the historical and medical context, however.

58. Editorial, "Conception in a Watch Glass," *New England Journal of Medicine* 217 (Oct. 21, 1937), 678. See also Miriam Menkin, "Notes for Lecture, American Association of Anatomists," 1948, typescript, p. 3, Series VII, Miriam Menkin Personal Records, 1918–1979, undated, box 22, folder 62, JR-CLM. See also oversized box 25, folder 34.

59. Henig, *Pandora's Baby*, 42–44; George L. Streeter to John Rock, July 12, 1944, JR-CLM.

60. J. D. Ratcliff, "No Father to Guide Them," *Collier's* (March 20, 1937), 19, 73.

61. Miriam Menkin, untitled talk on IVF at Cold Spring Harbor on July 18 or 28 (first number not legible), 1949. Untitled typescript of twenty pages, with note in Menkin's hand at the bottom, "Final Draft, Talk at CSH, July [18 or 28], 1949," Series III B, box 19, folder 33, JR-CLM. Quotation on 5.

62. Because it is not directly related to IVF, although it was related to Hertig's expertise, we have not discussed the ways in which the macaques (then called rhesus monkeys) were handled at the Carnegie Institution, but we were utterly appalled by their

treatment at the hands of the researchers and others. Equally appalling, in our view, is that even now, in the early twenty-first century, the attitude toward the animals seems so callous. The scientists at the Carnegie did not perform IVF on them but studied their reproductive habits. Elizabeth Hanson, "How Rhesus Monkeys Became Laboratory Animals," in Jane Maienschein, Marie Glitz, and Garland E. Allen, *Centennial History of the Carnegie Institution of Washington*, vol. 5, *Department of Embryology* (Cambridge: Cambridge University Press, 2004), 63–81.

63. Rabbit Experiment files, 1940–42, JR-RA. On Olive Smith and the Fearing Laboratory, see George V. Smith, "The Life of a Physician."

64. Miriam Menkin, untitled talk beginning "This seems to be too long," 1944, p. 1, and untitled talk at Cold Spring Harbor, 1949, pp. 5–6, JR-CLM.

65. Menkin talk, 1944, 3.

66. Menkin, "Figures on Number of Patients Studied (ova research July 1, 1938–June 30, 1944)," JR-RA. Her overall number is 1,032, but she includes the 85 women to date who were part of the embryo study in that figure.

67. McLaughlin, *The Pill, John Rock, and the Church*, 79–80, describes these years from Menkin's vantage point.

68. Menkin talk at Cold Spring Harbor, 1949, p. 14.

69. Ibid.

70. Ibid.

71. John Rock and Miriam Menkin, "In Vitro Fertilization and Cleavage of Human Ovarian Eggs," *Science* 100, no. 2588 (Aug. 4, 1944), 105–7; Miriam Menkin and John Rock, "In Vitro Fertilization and Cleavage of Human Ovarian Eggs," *Am. J. Obst. & Gynec.* 55, no. 3 (March 1948), 440–51. Letters between Menkin and members of Rock's staff, as well as between Rock and Menkin, document her dogged search for references. Rock kept asking for the paper to be sent back so it could go to the journal. She kept demurring, saying that she just needed to check a few more things. See, for example, Sue Hedge to Menkin, March 1, 1946; Menkin to Rock, Feb. 8, 1946; Menkin to Rock, Oct. 8, 1946; Menkin to Hedge, March 8, 1946; Menkin to Rock, April 9, 1946, JR-RA.

72. Clipping, Robert S. Bird, "A Human Ovum Is Fertilized in Test Tube for the First Time," undated but appears to be a Boston newspaper from Aug. 1944, Series II A1, Research Records, 1936–1983, undated, In Vitro Fertilization, Misc. Notes, Reports, 1944–1968, box 3, folder 54, JR-CLM. See also, "Momentous Conception: A New Human Life Formed under the Microscope," *Science Illustrated*, Sept. 1944, 49. McLaughlin, *The Pill, John Rock, and the Church*, 85–86, discusses how the news spread across the country via the Associated Press.

73. *Time* (Aug. 14, 1944), 75. Another article, Joan Younger, "Life Begins in a Test Tube," *Collier's* 115, no. 10 (March 10, 1945), 27ff., described the IVF study and noted, "If and when these experiments are developed, other eggs such as this one may be implanted in the mother's womb where they may grow into normal offspring," 49.

74. Mrs. E. C. to "President, Harvard University, New Haven Connecticut," Sept.

22, 1944, Series II A1, Research Records, 1936–1983, undated, Correspondence, Media Clippings, Pamphlets, 1944–1971, box 2, folder 63, JR-CLM. The letter got to the right place anyway, and ultimately made its way to Rock.

75. Carl Hartman to John Rock, June 8, 1954, Series II A1, Hartman, C.G., In Vitro Fertilization, Ortho Research File, 1954, box 3, folder 55, JR-CLM. By then, Hartman was the associate director of the Ortho Pharmaceutical Company's research foundation. Some skepticism remains even today about Rock and Menkin's IVF experiments. But most of their contemporaries then, and the Society for Reproductive Medicine today, credit them with this accomplishment.

76. George L. Streeter to John Rock, July 12, 1944, box 15, folder 103, JR-CLM.

77. Paul White to John Rock, Nov. 25, 1935, with copy of letter attached from Paul White to Dr. Norton S. Brown, Nov. 25, 1935, JR-RA.

78. Charles Rock to John Rock, Dec. 7, 1935, JR-RA.

79. See Charles Rock to John Rock, Feb. 17, 1939, JR-RA.

80. Although we are sure that Gillette stock is involved, there was another story about the stock, that Charlie had told Frank *not* to sell, but Frank thought the stock was about to fall so he sold it prematurely. In any case, there was definitely a flap about the stock.

81. John Rock to Kathryn Rock, undated but 1940, within weeks after Charlie's death, JR-RA.

82. *Kathryn G. Rock et alii. vs. Delia M. Rock et alii.*

83. Nell Rock Malloy to John Rock (with draft of letter from Nell to Maisie), Dec. 13, 1944, JR-RA.

84. Rachel Achenbach remembers that late in her aunt Maisie's life, John and she did see each other again, but Rachel did not recall any details.

85. John Rock to Jack Rock, July 14, 1945, and John Rock to Jack Rock, Oct. 10, 1945, JR-RA.

86. See McLaughlin, *The Pill, John Rock, and the Church,* 30–31. McLaughlin interviewed Rock about his son when he was nearly ninety, and her description poignantly shows how long he mourned.

87. Sue Hedge to Miriam Menkin, Sept. 4, 1946, JR-RA.

Chapter 5. The World of the Patients

1. John Rock to Deborah C. Leary, MD (of the staff of the National Research Council), Nov. 24, 1948, JR-RA.

2. Adele E. Clarke, *Disciplining Reproduction: Modernity, American Life Sciences, and the Problems of Sex* (Berkeley: University of California Press, 1998), offers a detailed history of the development of scientific ideas about reproduction in the first half of the twentieth century.

3. For example, although he had Miriam Menkin, before she embarked on laboratory work for the human IVF studies, conduct a series of experiments at the Free Hospital on rabbits, the principal goal, as near as one can figure out from the surviving

data, was to perfect her technique for the work on the human ova. Rabbits in Fearing folders, JR-RA.

4. George V. Smith, "The Life of a Physician," unpublished memoir, typescript, 1982, p. 84, JR-RA.

5. There could be some disagreement about our assertion here that the reproductive disorders described here were "real," since it could be argued that medical scientists and practitioners in the twentieth century turned natural processes into medical conditions. We do know that conditions such as infertility were medicalized, as we argue in The Empty Cradle: Infertility in America from Colonial Times to the Present (Baltimore: Johns Hopkins University Press, 1996), but we also know that painful menstruation, prolapse of the uterus, pelvic inflammatory disease, and infertility, for example, were as "real" to the women who experienced them in 1840 as in 1930. Even with pregnancy and menopause, the lines are not entirely clear. The hot flashes, night sweats, mood swings, and memory disorders that many women experience may have been tolerated because there was no alternative, but that doesn't mean they didn't trouble and upset those who had them. The same might be said for eclampsia and preeclampsia, or ectopic pregnancies. They weren't typical, but they did occur. What was beginning to change was the possibility of treating some of these problems, and that certainly did mean that previously accepted conditions had become, or were in the process of becoming, medicalized, which brought them into the realm of the expert and beyond the complete control of women themselves. Clarke, Disciplining Reproduction, especially chaps. 8 and 9, provides an excellent summary of the dominant feminist scholarship in these matters. See also Nelly Oudshoorn, Beyond the Natural Body: An Archeology of Sex Hormones (New York: Routledge, 1994), esp. 13, for a nuanced interpretation of the "social reality" of illness.

6. See, for example, Marsh and Ronner, The Empty Cradle, introduction and chaps. 3 and 4, for examples.

7. The problem with knowing the extent to which Rock differed from his colleagues is that we have so many records for him and so few for other physicians. Luigi Mastroianni, interview by Wanda Ronner, July 5, 2007.

8. Rock destroyed his regular patient records. He did not destroy the patient information in his research files, which often include correspondence in addition to patient information. After 1944, when media reports of his work in IVF made national and international news, Rock's newfound fame brought him a flood of letters from women and men who were struggling with infertility. Such rich records are a rare resource; they help make it possible to follow Rock in his everyday interactions with patients and other ordinary men and women.

9. Elmer Osgood Cappers, History of the Free Hospital for Women, 1875–1975 (Boston: Boston Hospital for Women, 1975), 62–64.

10. Interview by Margaret Marsh with Rock family: Rachel Achenbach, A. J. Levinson, and Hart Achenbach, June 3, 1998. As young women, both Rachel and A. J. worked for their father. Rachel became a cytologist.

11. Nearly all the patients we know a great deal about were potential surgical cases (although not all of them, in the end, actually underwent surgery).

12. See Marsh and Ronner, The Empty Cradle, 150, which cites the following: Memo from Lawrence Dunham to Raymond Fosdick, Dec. 14, 1927, and Fosdick's Dec. 22 reply, folder 173, box 7, series 3, BSH. Also R. L. Dickinson to K. B. Davis, Jan. 14, 1925, folder 172, box 7, series 3, BSH; and a memo that says only "Topping" in upper right, undated, folder 175, box 7, series 3, BSH. The Committee for Maternal Health funded Gerald Moench's research on sperm.

13. Marsh and Ronner, The Empty Cradle, 150, citing Louise Bryant, "Appeal to the Bureau of Social Hygiene from the Committee on Maternal Health," Dec. 8, 1928, folder 173, box 7, series 3, BSH.

14. Meaker had an excellent reputation, a thriving infertility practice, and no scruples against birth control. The last was central to one of the purposes of the study as Dickinson envisioned it—to lay to rest a time-honored view that contraceptive practices brought on sterility. See Samuel R. Meaker, Human Sterility: Causation, Diagnosis, and Treatment: A Practical Manual of Clinical Procedure (Baltimore: Williams and Wilkins, 1934).

15. Meaker, vii, 9. Meaker's reasoned argument cut no ice with some of his colleagues. Samuel Berkow, writing for a general audience in Childless: A Study of Sterility, Its Causes and Treatment (New York: Lee Furman, 1937), used those very genealogical studies to say that sterility had increased six hundred–fold since the late eighteenth century (28–29). Contemporary readers who remember the alarmist rhetoric from the late twentieth century about an infertility crisis among educated women, which was equally inflated, may experience a sense of deja vu. See Marsh and Ronner, The Empty Cradle, 245.

16. Marsh and Ronner, The Empty Cradle, esp. 150–52 and 160–61; quotation on 161.

17. Meaker, Human Sterility; Samuel R. Meaker, "Two Million American Homes Childless," Hygeia 5, no. 11 (Nov. 1927), 346–48; Margaret C. Sturgis, "Fertility," Transactions of the 52nd Annual Meeting of the Alumnae Association of the Women's Medical College of Pennsylvania (1927), 65.

18. Marsh and Ronner, The Empty Cradle, 173.

19. The hysterosalpingogram is still part of a basic infertility evaluation. New York gynecologist Frances Seymour reported obtaining an astonishing 77% pregnancy rate with insufflation. However, she performed the insufflations over a period of up to nine months on women whose tubes already had some degree of patency; since both the hysterosalpingogram and insufflation could remove bits of debris and minor obstructions from the tubes, her report is at least somewhat plausible. However, for women with a blockage or occlusion, only surgery worked, and tubal surgery had a low rate of success, only about 7% even at clinics, such as Rock's, with highly skilled surgeons. See Marsh and Ronner, The Empty Cradle, 175.

20. Current statistics are from the website of the American Society for Reproductive Medicine: www.asrm.org. See "For Patients—Fact Sheets." Also see Marsh and Ronner, The Empty Cradle, 156–60.

21. The rhythm method was also known as periodic continence. It is still the only method of contraception approved by the Catholic Church.

22. Stephen Fleck, MD, Elizabeth F. Snedeker, BA, and John Rock, MD, "The Contraceptive 'Safe Period': A Clinical Study," 1940, typescript, Series III A1, Reproductive Research Writings, 1937–1972, undated, box 15, folder 101, JR-CLM. The study was published as Stephen Fleck, Elizabeth F. Snedeker, and John Rock, "The Contraceptive Safe Period: A Clinical Study," *New England Journal of Medicine* 223 (1940), 1005–9.

23. Stephen Fleck, "Incomplete Survey of Sterility Patients," handwritten, Series II B1, Patient Research Files, 1925–1972, undated, box 9, folder 2, JR-CLM.

24. Boston's Irish Americans and Italian Americans were overwhelmingly Catholic. The Italian surnames were sometime acquired by marriage, of course, but first names at that time were often a giveaway. We would have liked more information about race, but such information appeared only rarely.

25. The patients in this group are mostly from the 1940s. Embryo Study, 1948, JR-RA.

26. In this context, "careful" seems to indicate withdrawal.

27. Record of Mrs. [name redacted], 1954–55, Series II A2 b1, Patient Research Files, 1925–1972, undated, box 7, folder 141, JR-CLM.

28. Embryo Study, 1946, JR-RA.

29. Ibid.

30. Eleven were still living; two had died.

31. Record of Mrs. [name redacted], 1955, Series II A2 b1, Patient Research Files, 1925–1972, undated, box 7, folder 142, JR-CLM.

32. Ibid.

33. Embryo Study, 1954, JR-RA.

34. Personal communication, Rachel Achenbach and A. J. Levinson. See also, Loretta McLaughlin, *The Pill, John Rock, and the Church: The Biography of a Revolution* (Boston: Little, Brown, 1982), 27, for a discussion of the petition.

35. Dickinson wished to capitalize on practitioners' interest in learning about infertility treatment as an opportunity to build support for birth control. Rock, an up-and-coming infertility expert in Boston, was among the prominent practitioners Dickinson hoped to attract. For information on Dickinson and the NCMH, see James Reed, *From Private Vice to Public Virtue: The Birth Control Movement and American Society since 1830* (New York: Basic Books, 1978), 168–91.

36. John Rock diaries, Dec. 5, 1936, JR-RA.

37. Not everyone answered the question, and only a few of these forms survive, but those that do provide interesting reading, and the following conclusions are derived from this information. Patient Records, 1947, 1949, 1951, and 1952, JR-RA.

38. There are twenty-five questionnaires that contain birth-control information, and scattered additional patient charts mention contraception. Only fifteen women answered the question about their frequency of sexual relations on the charts, but this information also appears in scattered patient records. This is certainly not much of a

sample, but it does offer a glimpse of the sexual lives of some of Rock's patients, and his asking the questions shows his interest.

39. "Old Embryo Cases Seen in Clinic" and "Embryo Cases: Follow Up," JR-RA.

40. Ibid.

41. Remember that at least 20% of Rock's patients failed to conceive because of this problem, and some other physicians reported an even higher incidence of tubal disease than Rock did. Rock's incidence may have been lower than others because he had begun to use antibiotics for some of the pelvic infections that often led to tubal damage. Marsh and Ronner, The Empty Cradle, 160, 175. I. C. Rubin, the developer of tubal insufflation in the 1920s, had placed the figure as high as 47%.

42. Marsh and Ronner, The Empty Cradle, 178–81; quotation on 178.

43. There is only one biography of Merle Oberon. The family history seems to have been based at least in part on documentation kept by Charlotte's older daughter, Constance, and found by Constance's son after his mother's death. Charles Higham and Roy Moseley, Princess Merle: The Romantic Life of Merle Oberon (New York: Coward-McCann, 1983), 17–21.

44. Ibid., 31–33.

45. Merle Oberon's biographers either never knew what Charlotte had done or considered it too shocking to admit. Instead, they said that when Merle was twenty-one, she had cancer of the fallopian tubes, causing both of them (but none of her other reproductive organs) to be removed, and that she was never told that she would be sterile. But Rock remembered it differently. According to him, her surgery had occurred at her mother's initiative when Merle was only sixteen or seventeen. Merle did not know that its purpose was sterilization. But when she married and attempted to conceive, a laparotomy revealed that her fallopian tubes had been severed and portions removed. Higham and Moseley, Princess Merle, 51–52; McLaughlin, The Pill, John Rock, and the Church, 52–53.

46. Elaine Tyler May, Barren in the Promised Land: Childless Americans and the Pursuit of Happiness (New York: Basic Books, 1995), 96–107.

47. Clipping, undated in file but likely Boston, Aug. 4, 1944, JR-CLM.

48. Marsh and Ronner, The Empty Cradle, 179.

49. Ibid., 180–81.

50. Ovariotomy was the term used in the late nineteenth and early twentieth centuries for bilateral oophorectomy, or removal of the ovaries. The discussion that follows is taken from Margaret Marsh and Wanda Ronner, "Ovarian Transplantation: An Early Form of Reproductive Technology," ACOG Clinical Review 4 (Sept./Oct. 1999), 5.

51. McLaughlin, The Pill, John Rock, and the Church, 52.

52. William L. Estes, "A Method of Implanting Ovarian Tissue in Order to Maintain Ovarian Function," Pennsylvania Medical Journal (May 1910), 610–13; William L. Estes, Jr., "Further Results with Ovarian Implantation," Journal of the American Medical Association 83 (Aug. 30, 1924), 674–77; typewritten abstract of findings of A. Westman, Acta. Obst. et Gynec. Scandivav. 30: 186–202, reported in Yearbook of Obstetrics and Gynecology

(1951), 313–14. These abstract notes are in the John Rock Papers, Countway Library. They were doubtless taken by Menkin and were part of a series of abstracts she culled that year on the surgical treatment of infertility.

53. Marsh and Ronner, *The Empty Cradle*, 161.

54. Rock to Mr. M. H., Feb. 8, 1946, JR-RA.

55. See, for example, Rock to Elizabeth Quirk (his cousin), June 23, 1949, JR-RA.

Chapter 6. The Fertility Doctor Meets the Pill

1. Most accounts of the development of the pill tell one or another version of this story. Quotation from Bernard Asbell, *The Pill: A Biography of the Drug that Changed the World* (New York: Random House, 1995), 125. Discovery/Health Channel, "Sex and Serendipity," Spring 2002. Videotape in possession of the authors. One of us, Marsh, an academic "expert" who appeared on this program, tried unsuccessfully to disabuse the filmmakers of the idea of a spontaneous, accidental meeting. See also Loretta McLaughlin, *The Pill, John Rock, and the Church: The Biography of a Revolution* (Boston: Little, Brown, 1982), 108–9; Elizabeth Siegel Watkins, *On the Pill: A Social History of Oral Contraceptives, 1950–1970* (Baltimore: Johns Hopkins University Press, 1998), 29.

2. George Smith to Gregory Pincus, Oct. 1, 1937, GP-LC.

3. Woodbine was a fascinating turn-of-the-century farming community financed by philanthropy and founded for Jews displaced by pogroms and discrimination in their home villages. The town's synagogue is now a museum. There is a beautiful old cemetery, and many of the original houses are still standing. We grew up in nearby Vineland, New Jersey, and one of us revisited Woodbine in 2005.

4. Quoted in Asbell, *The Pill*, 121.

5. James Reed, *From Private Vice to Public Virtue: The Birth Control Movement in American Society since 1830* (New York: Basic Books, 1978), 322–23, 325.

6. R. Christian Johnson provides a brief history of the creation of the Worcester Foundation in "Feminism, Philanthropy, and Science in the Development of the Oral Contraceptive Pill," *Pharmacy in History* 19, no. 2 (1977), 68–70.

7. On Pincus and Hoagland, Reed's analysis is excellent, *From Private Vice to Public Virtue*, 327–31. Asbell, *The Pill*, 122–24, draws on Reed's work.

8. Letter (unsent) from Gregory Pincus to Al Raymond, undated, but probably the winter of 1951–1952, when Upjohn's success was about to be made public, written from the Stevens Hotel in Chicago (where Searle was located), GP-LC. For Upjohn, see John A. Hogg, "Steroids, the Steroid Community, and Upjohn in Perspective: A Profile of Innovation," *Steroids* 57, no. 12 (Dec. 1992), 617–23.

9. Letter (unsent) from Pincus to Raymond, undated, but probably the winter of 1951–1952, GP-LC.

10. I. C. Winter to John Rock, Dec. 20, 1950, JR-RA.

11. Winter to Rock, July 9, 1951, JR-RA, asks for confirmation of some data directly from Rock that he had heard about from Pincus regarding one of Searle's estrogen compounds.

12. NRC, Division of Medical Sciences, Minutes of the Committee on Human Reproduction, First Meeting, Sept. 22, 1947, esp. appendix A, JR-RA.

13. A review of Miriam Menkin's available bibliographic notes, the completeness of which we cannot ascertain, did not show any reference to Haberlandt or Fellner.

14. Nelly Oudshoorn, *Beyond the Natural Body: An Archeology of Sex Hormones* (New York: Routledge, 1994), 113–14; Joseph Goldheizer and Harry W. Rudel, "How the Oral Contraceptives Came to Be Developed," *Journal of the American Medical Association* 230, no. 3 (Oct. 21, 1974), 421–22.

15. Goldheizer and Rudel, "How the Oral Contraceptives Came to Be Developed."

16. Leo Loeb and William B. Kountz, "The Effect of Injection of Follicular Extract on the Sex Organs in the Guinea Pig," *Am J Physiol.* 84 (1928), 283–306; 422. Goldheizer and Rudel, "How the Oral Contraceptives Came to Be Developed," 422; also Oudshoorn, *Beyond the Natural Body,* 114, and Johnson, "Feminism, Philanthropy, and Science," 70–71.

17. Oudshoorn, *Beyond the Natural Body,* 114. In this early proto-research on oral contraceptives, the active hormone was presumed to be estrogen, which probably also militated against its widespread acceptance. Some physicians considered estrogen to be carcinogenic if used for a long period. Rock never accepted this idea, although he did believe that estrogen promoted the growth of existing cancers.

18. An excellent nontechnical explanation of antibiotics can be found at "What the Heck is an Antibiotic," by John C. Brown, http://people.ku.edu/ffijbrown/antibiotic.html.

19. Peter Temin, *Taking Your Medicine: Drug Regulation in the United States* (Cambridge, Mass.: Harvard University Press, 1980), 65–66.

20. Oudshoorn, *Beyond the Natural Body,* 114.

21. Although the baby boom cut across class and racial lines, fertility behavior changed most dramatically among educated white Protestant and Jewish women. Working-class white women and Catholics of all social classes had a higher overall birth rate than Protestants and Jews during the 1950s, but their fertility patterns remained consistent with the past. Fertility patterns of African Americans were more complicated. Although black women had a higher rate of childlessness than whites did in the 1950s, as they'd had for decades, at the baby boom's peak in 1957, the overall birth rate among black Americans was 100 percent higher than it had been in 1940.

Young married couples moved quickly into parenthood. In the mid-1950s, the average white woman was just under twenty-two when she gave birth to her first child; among African Americans, the average age was just over twenty. The average age for their mothers would have been about twenty-four and twenty-one respectively. Couples planned large families; Americans considered four children to be the most desirable number to have, and they wanted to have them soon after marriage. Birth control, except among Catholics, some orthodox Jews, Mormons, and a few nonmainstream Protestant denominations, had become a widely accepted means to space births, rather than a way of providing women with sexual freedom. See, for example, Margaret

Marsh and Wanda Ronner, *The Empty Cradle: Infertility in America from Colonial Times to the Present* (Baltimore: Johns Hopkins University Press, 1996), 183–89.

22. Elizabeth Siegel Watkins, *On the Pill*, 29, calls Rock "a relatively recent convert" to contraception. She did not have access to the bulk of Rock's papers, which were held by his family. In the 1930s through the mid-1940s, Rock was indeed circumspect outside of medical circles.

23. John Rock and David Loth, *Voluntary Parenthood* (New York: Random House, 1949), esp. 19–22. Quotation from 19.

24. Rock's brief time as chair was during the waning years of the NCMH, in the early 1950s. The NRC committee was chaired by Howard C. Taylor and had twelve members, including the pioneering hormone researcher Willard Allen. George Corner represented the Committee for Research in Problems of Sex, the NRC committee that had fueled twentieth-century research in reproductive endocrinology. NRC, Division of Medical Sciences, Minutes, Sept. 22, 1947, esp. Appendix A, JR-RA.

25. John Rock, "Physiology of Conception and Early Pregnancy," typescript [1948], p. 3, JR-RA.

26. Ibid., 2, 5, 6.

27. Ibid., 1–2.

28. Ellen Chesler, *Woman of Valor: Margaret Sanger and the Birth Control Movement in America* (New York: Simon and Schuster, 1992), 393.

29. The best and most complete biography of Sanger at this writing is Chesler's *Woman of Valor*. My characterization of Sanger's views is drawn from this work.

30. In reality, it does seem to be the other way around—greater prosperity and especially increased education for women appear to lead to fewer children.

31. Andrea Tone, *Devices and Desires: A History of Contraceptives in America* (New York: Hill and Wang, 2001), is an excellent recent history of contraceptives. Tone demonstrates convincingly how widely available birth-control devices were in the marketplace long before there was medical sanction for contraception.

32. Watkins, *On the Pill*, 12.

33. Tone, *Devices and Desires*, 205. Armond Fields, *Katharine Dexter McCormick: Pioneer for Women's Rights* (Westport, Conn.: Praeger, 2003), is the only full-scale biography of McCormick. Fields argues that McCormick's husband was impotent, 155.

34. Rock and Loth, *Voluntary Parenthood*.

35. For some reason, either the birth-control pill, or perhaps Rock's role in it, seems to lend itself to dramatic imagery. After we wrote the following paragraph, we saw that Loretta McLaughlin also used the drama metaphor, although her description is different from ours. See McLaughlin, *The Pill, John Rock, and the Church*, 106–7.

36. Reed, *From Private Vice to Public Virtue*, 340. Also, "Planned Parenthood Federation of America: *Research Projects in Progress*: Gregory Pincus, Sc. D.—Studies in Hormonal Contraception," typescript attached to letter from Margaret Sanger to David Rosenthal, March 10, 1952, reel 119, vol. 184, Sanger Papers, Library of Congress. Pincus's project began in April 1951 and the date on the typescript is 10/51.

37. Pincus and his chief biologist, Min-Chueh Chang, clearly had the expertise. For example, see Asbell, *The Pill*, 58–60; Fields, *Katharine Dexter McCormick*, 255–64.

38. Margaret Sanger to Katharine Dexter McCormick, March 10, 1952, MS-SS; McCormick to Sanger, May 31, 1952, SS. On Hoskins's research, see Reed, *From Private Vice to Public Virtue*, 338.

39. Telegram from McCormick to Sanger, May 20, 1953, MS-SS. Mrs. Hoskins (first name not recorded), the professor's wife, was also at the visit, perhaps to facilitate the introduction. Reed, *From Private Vice to Public Virtue*, 340.

40. Renee Michelle Courey, "Participants in the Development, Marketing, and Safety Evaluation of the Oral Contraceptive, 1950–1965: Mythic Dimensions of a Scientific Solution," PhD diss., University of California, Berkeley, 1994, 18, contends that funding for the pill was much greater among foundations and the government than previously supposed; however, not only was funding for reproductive science in general low compared with other areas of investigation, but what Pincus and later Rock would need was funding targeted toward the particular goal of contraception, not general funding. Only McCormick was willing. Even Planned Parenthood saw this project as far too expensive and risky. According to Walter E. Duka and Alan H. DeCherney, *From the Beginning: A History of the American Fertility Society, 1944–1994* (Birmingham, Ala.: The American Fertility Society, 1994), 59, Rock gave a speech in 1954 in which he claimed that while $2 billion was being spent on nuclear research, only $500,000 was devoted to the study of reproduction and fertility.

41. Gregory Pincus to Paul Henshaw, Feb. 19, 1953, box 14, GP-LC.

42. Marsh and Ronner, *The Empty Cradle*, 140.

43. The first study used progesterone continuously rather than cyclically. Women began by taking 5 mg of stilbestrol and 50 mg of progesterone, increasing the dose of stilbestrol by 5 mg and of progesterone by 50 mg every two weeks. By the end of twelve weeks, women were taking 30 mg of stilbestrol and 300 mg of progesterone. If they had vaginal bleeding at any time, the doses were increased. "Pseudopregnancy," typescript, July 15, 1954, GP-LC. Rock also summarizes his early studies in John Rock, Celso-Ramon Garcia, and Gregory Pincus, "Synthetic Progestins in the Normal Human Menstrual Cycle," *Recent Progress in Hormone Research*, vol. 13 (New York: Academic Press, 1957), 323–24.

44. John Rock to Paul R. Rollins, MD, Oct. 28, 1957, JR-RA.

45. Rock to Winter, Sept. 26, 1955, JR-RA.

46. Gladwell concluded from this practical decision that the pill was "a drug shaped by the dictates of the Catholic Church—by John Rock's desire to make this new method of birth control seem as natural as possible." Rock took advantage of the cyclical administration of the pill in the 1960s but never thought about it in the 1950s. Malcolm Gladwell, "John Rock's Error," *New Yorker*, March 13, 2000, 55.

47. Ibid.

48. McCormick to Sanger, July 21, 1954, MS-SS.

49. See Abraham Stone to Sanger, March 30, 1954, MS-SS, describing the earliest progesterone-only experiments.

50. As Rock was finding that the progesterone-only regimen—even at a dose of 300 mg a day—was not clearly suppressing ovulation, Pincus told Sanger that he and Rock now had "excellent evidence that in a good proportion of the patients in our series ovulation has been inhibited" and that if it could "be inhibited in a good proportion it should be possible to evolve a method for inhibition in 100%." Pincus to Sanger, March 31, 1954, MS-SS.

51. McCormick to Sanger, July 19, 1954, MS-SS

52. Ibid.

53. Ibid.; McCormick to Sanger, July 21, 1954; McCormick to Sanger, July 23, 1954, MS-SS.

54. McCormick's famous phrase is in McCormick to Sanger, May 31, 1955, MS-SS. Transcript from tape of Meeting of the Board of Trustees of the Rock Reproductive Study Center on Wednesday, Oct. 23, 1957, typescript, p. 17, JR-RA. The transcripts of these meetings are invaluable sources for Rock's unedited, and unscripted, views.

55. McCormick to Sanger, July 23, 1954, MS-SS.

56. Neither Pincus nor Rock expressed qualms about this study, although later, when female prison inmates in Puerto Rico refused to participate in a similar study, everyone, including Pincus, accepted their right to refuse.

57. McCormick to Sanger, July 21, 1954, MS-SS.

58. Sanger to Abraham Stone, March 2, 1954, MS-SS.

59. It became the American Fertility Society in 1965 and is now the American Society for Reproductive Medicine. A useful history is Duka and DeCherney, *From the Beginning*. The information on members in this paragraph can be found on 22, 26–27, 32, 45.

60. R. W. Noyes, A. T. Hertig, and J. Rock, "Dating the Endometrial Biopsy," *Fertility and Sterility* 1 (1950), 3–25. Duka and DeCherney, *From the Beginning*, 39, 237. Noyes, who performed most of the painstaking correlations, was first author. Rock, who no longer "needed" publications, tended to promote his junior colleagues by having them be first authors on papers, as he had done with Menkin on the longer and more detailed article about the first IVF. It didn't appreciably advance her career, but it did make her very, very happy.

61. Rock was a member of several medical societies, including the exclusive American Gynecological Society, and was not as active in the American Society for the Study of Sterility as were some of his colleagues, including Somers Sturgis and Fred Simmons. But as a member of the society, he was fully in agreement with its occasionally controversial positions on reproductive issues. Duka and DeCherney, *From the Beginning*, 67.

62. John Rock, "Physiology of Conception and Early Pregnancy," 3, notes that there were about six such facilities in the nation, JR-RA.

63. Marsh and Ronner, *The Empty Cradle*, 183.

64. Paul Starr, *The Social Transformation of American Medicine: The Rise of a Sovereign Profession and the Making of a Vast Industry* (New York: Basic Books, 1982), 352–53.

65. See for example, Brooks Ranney, MD, to Rock, Sept. 24, 1951, and Rock's reply,

Oct. 18, 1951, on polyethylene in tuboplasty, a subject on which Rock was speaking but had not yet published. On the same subject, H. O. Padgett, MD, to Rock, July 31, 1952, and Rock's reply, Aug. 5, 1952, and follow-up letter from Rock's secretary, Katharine Moore, Nov. 13, 1952, JR-RA. Rock was unfailingly helpful to his colleagues in these matters.

66. For example: Linton Smith, MD, to Rock, July 11, 1952, and Rock's reply, Aug. 11, 1952—a British gynecologist requesting information on the subject of success rates in the treatment of infertility; Joslyn W. Rogers, MD, to Rock, April 8, 1952, and Rock's reply, April 12, 1952, regarding a physician at the University of Toronto wishing to meet Rock; Newell W. Philpott, MD, to Rock, Nov. 28, 1952, and Rock's reply, Dec. 6, 1952, regarding a young physician at the Royal Victoria Hospital in Montreal; Robert N. Rutherford, MD, to Rock, Sept. 25, 1953, and Rock's reply, Oct. 3, 1953, in regard to some issues related to the opening of an infertility clinic in Seattle; L. M. Randall, MD, to John Rock, March 3, 1949, and Rock's reply, March 8, 1949, and again Oct. 5, 1953, and Rock's reply, Oct. 12, 1953, regarding a visit to Rock's clinic from different colleagues at Mayo Clinic. W. T. Pommerenke, MD, to Rock, March 11, 1955, and Rock's reply of March 17, 1955, in regard to a Japanese physician from the University of Tokyo who wished to visit. Physicians wrote Rock to introduce their colleagues to him and ask if these colleagues were welcome to observe at Rock's clinic. These and dozens of similar letters are in the JR-RA.

67. Some of the physicians from abroad kept up with Rock for years, including Aloys Naville from Zurich. See Aloys H. Naville to Rock, Dec. 31, 1964, JR-RA.

68. The Rock Papers at Harvard are full of notes to, from, and about the students, fellows, and practitioners who worked or observed at the clinic, and Rock's daughter Rachel Achenbach has many more. Letters in the JR-CLM include Anthony Cominos to Rock, Oct. 29, 1957; "the Mastroianni family" to Rock, May 4, 1957; Celso-Ramon Garcia to Luigi Mastroianni, June 25, 1958; Angeliki Tsacona to Rock, Sept. 30, 1956; and Rock to Tsacona, Dec. 11, 1965. Series I B, Rock Reproductive Study Center, Correspondence and Personnel Records, 1948–1972, box 2.

69. Hart Achenbach interview, June 3, 1998.

70. By the early 1950s, as demand for infertility services soared, some patients began openly protesting; others left. More than half of the new patients, Rock noted in 1953, did not stay around long enough for their evaluation to be completed. They were, he told his hospital board, dissatisfied "with clinic routine." By 1954 the clinic was better funded. With more staff and better facilities, Rock determined to provide clinic patients with as close to the same environment as his private patients received. He banned teaching from examining and consultation rooms, relying instead on full patient records that were presented in seminar fashion after the clinic closed. Apparently, the changes worked. Visits were up the next year, and patients were less likely to drift away. Annual Report: Free Hospital for Women (Boston, 1945), 19; Annual Report: Free Hospital for Women (Boston, 1955), 16; Annual Report: Free Hospital for Women (Boston, 1956), 18, Series I A2, Annual Reports, 1940–1968, folders 46 (1945), 56 (1955), and 57 (1956), JR-CLM.

71. Hart Achenbach interview, June 3, 1998; "Research Fellows in Fertility and Endocrinology," typescript [1962], JR-RA.

72. Noyes, Hertig, and Rock, "Dating the Endometrial Biopsy." See Edward E. Wallach and Serena H. Chen, "Five Decades of Progress in Management of the Infertile Couple," *Fertility and Sterility* 62 (Oct. 1994), 665–85; Records of Ovarian Resections, Series II A1, Reproductive Research Records, 1936–1983, undated, JR-CLM. Fred Simmons discussed the use of such treatments in "Medical Progress in Human Infertility," *New England Journal of Medicine* 255 (Dec. 13, 1956), 1190–91. A fellow Harvard faculty member who treated infertility at Massachusetts General Hospital, Simmons argued that too many physicians misdiagnosed endometriosis and performed unnecessary surgery on young women. "I have seen young women deprived of their gonads," he noted, "by well meaning surgeons who did not recognize that this disease could be resected from the ovary, with functioning ovarian tissue left behind" (1191).

73. Although one surgeon claimed to have achieved a pregnancy rate of 53% among women he operated on to repair damaged tubes, his numbers evoked considerable skepticism. The published literature by the early 1950s more commonly cited pregnancy rates ranging from about 4% to 13%. Some doctors, however, included cases in which only one tube was occluded, claiming success even though the other tube had never posed an obstacle to impregnation. Others included ectopic pregnancies in their success rates. And even more did not indicate the extent or location of the tubal obstruction in reporting their cases. "Tuboplasty," typescript abstract of studies to 1951, twenty pages, Series III A2, box 18, folder 48, JR-CLM; Simmons, "Medical Progress in Human Infertility," 1142–43.

74. Simmons, Medical Progress in Human Infertility," 1142–43.

75. John Rock, "Surgery for Infertility," page proof of an essay based on a paper read in Washington, D.C., in March 1956, p. 2, JR-RA. A review of the articles that appeared in the first decade of the publication of *Fertility and Sterility* (1950–1959), which was the U.S.'s most important infertility journal, demonstrates the surgical conservatism of the infertility elite.

76. Mulligan came up with the idea of using polyethylene. Tubal patency did seem improved, Rock and his colleagues believed, but the early report did not find that pregnancy rates were much improved. John Rock, William Mulligan, and Charles Easterday, "Polyethylene in Tuboplasty," *Obstetrics and Gynecology* 3, no. 1 (Jan. 1954), 21–28.

77. Rock, Mulligan, and Easterday presented the results of this series of cases at the First Annual Clinical Meeting of the American Academy of Obstetrics and Gynecology in 1952, and published them in *Obstetrics and Gynecology* 3, no. 1 (Jan. 1954): 21–29. Rock had also reported on several cases at the Central Association of Obstetrics and Gynecology in Sept. 1951. Letters to Rock from Brooks Ranney, MD, Sept. 24, 1951, and H. O. Padgett, MD, July 31, 1952. The quotations are from Rock's reply to Padgett, Aug. 5, 1952, JR-RA.

78. Casebook Records, 1950s, JR-RA. Simmons, "Medical Progress in Human Infertility," 1143.

79. For a more extended discussion of male infertility, see Marsh and Ronner, *The Empty Cradle*, 198–203.

80. Fred A. Simmons, "The Treatment of Male Sterility," *Fertility and Sterility* 1, no. 3 (1950), 193–98.

81. One of the few studies of physicians' willingness to perform the procedure was conducted in the 1930s. John Henry Caldwell, "Babies by Scientific Selection," *Scientific American* 150 (March 1934), 124–25, interviewed two hundred doctors from six major urban areas. Most who received requests for donor insemination were receptive. Fifty-six physicians had fielded a total of three hundred requests from wives of sterile husbands. Thirty-four of the doctors agreed to perform the procedure; the others decided against it. Of those who refused, some cited a fear of legal complications. Others worried that the husband, even if he agreed, might later reject the child. Still others did not want to be a party to concealment when confronted with wives who did not want their husbands to know about the donor insemination. This discussion of donor insemination is drawn from our previous work on the history of infertility. A more extended discussion can be found in Marsh and Ronner, *The Empty Cradle*, esp. 164, 203–4.

82. Duka and DeCherney, *From the Beginning*, 63–65; Milton Golan, "Paternity by Proxy," *Medico-Legal Digest* (May 1960), 17–20.

83. Marsh and Ronner, *The Empty Cradle*, 201.

84. L. Mastroianni, J. L. Laberge, and J. Rock, "Appraisal of the Efficacy of Artificial Insemination with Husband's Sperm and Evaluation of Insemination Technics," *Fertility and Sterility* 8, no. 3 (May–June 1957), 260–66. Quotation on 266.

85. See, for example, Luis Fernandez-Cano, Miriam Menkin, Celso-Ramon Garcia, and John Rock, "Refrigerant Preservation of Human Spermatozoa I: Factors Influencing Recovery in Euspermic Semen: Clinical Applications," *Fertility and Sterility* 15, no. 4 (July–Aug. 1964), 390–406. Edward Tyler, a pioneer in sperm freezing, told a reporter for the *Boston Globe* that in most of his recent cases, this was the way he had utilized the frozen sperm. Tyler, *Boston Globe*, June 24, 1971, clipping in Series II B, Male Misc., Infertility Notes, 1968–1971, box 12, folder 19, JR-CLM. See also, "Insemination Success Rate is 70% with Frozen Semen," *Ob/Gyn News* (Aug. 15, 1971), 1.

86. Mastroianni, Laberge, Rock, "Appraisal," 261, indicates that in this series of 506 inseminations, the overall success rate was 6.2%.

87. Horne and Rock, "Oral Terramycin Therapy of Chronic Endocervicitis in Infertile Women," *Fertility and Sterility* 3, no. 4 (July–Aug. 1952), 321–27.

88. John Rock, "Diagnosis and Treatment of Infertility" [1956], 2, 6–7, Series III A1, Reproductive Research Writings, 1937–1972, undated, box 17, folder 11, JR-CLM.

89. This was the Syntex progesterone preparation given in megadoses, not the progestin that would be used in the first pill. The progesterone in these studies only worked in very large doses. It also was not the micronized version used by physicians today.

90. McCormick to Sanger, July 19, 1954, MS-SS.

91. See John Rock, Celso-Ramon Garcia, and Gregory Pincus, "Synthetic Progestins in the Normal Human Menstrual Cycle," *Recent Progress in Hormone Research* 13 (1957), 323–46; John Rock, Celso-Ramon Garcia, and Gregory Pincus, "Clinical Studies with Potential Oral Contraceptives," *Report of the Proceedings of the Sixth Annual Conference on Planned Parenthood* (Feb. 14–21, 1959, New Delhi, India), 212–14; Gregory Pincus, Celso R. Garcia, John Rock, et al., "Effectiveness of an Oral Contraceptive," *Science* 130, no. 3367 (July 10, 1959), 81–83; and John Rock, Celso-Ramon Garcia, and Gregory Pincus, "Use of Some Progestational 19-Nor Steroids in Gynecology," *American Journal of Obstetrics and Gynecology* 79, no. 4 (April 1960), 758–69.

92. "Conversation with Dr. Pincus, June 30, 1955," typescript sent to Margaret Sanger from Katharine Dexter McCormick, MS-SS; John Rock to I. C. Winter, Sept. 26, 1955, JR-RA.

93. Rock to Winter, Oct. 17, 1955, JR-RA.

94. Winter to Rock, Nov. 25, 1955, and Rock to Winter, Nov. 30, 1955, JR-RA.

95. Rock to Winter, Nov. 10, 1955, JR-RA. Some accounts say ten women, but if that is so, then he must have been using Djerassi's Syntex formula on the other six. He clearly tells Winter that the number was four.

96. For example, McLaughlin, *The Pill, John Rock, and the Church*, 121, says that Rock was "greatly irritated" with Pincus for doing this.

97. McCormick to Sanger, June 29, 1955, MS-SS.

98. This is not to dispute the significant work of the Worcester Foundation. We are not the only scholars to observe this contrast between Rock and Pincus. Elizabeth Siegel Watkins also remarked on it, in *On the Pill*, 28–29. She makes a special point both of Rock's Harvard connections and his Catholicism.

99. For example, see Father Gregory Stevens to Rock, April 26, 1960, and Oct. 30, 1960; Rock to Stevens, April 20, 1960, July 8, 1960, Oct. 19, 1960, Oct. 21, 1960, Nov. 7, 1960, June 20, 1961, July 10, 1961, and Aug. 2, 1961; Rock to Rt. Rev. Francis J. Lally, March 17, 1960, Nov. 4, 1960, and Nov. 9, 1960; Lally to Rock, Nov. 7, 1960. Also see Monsignor Robert J. White to Rock, March 15, 1957, and Rock's reply, April 11, 1957; Father William Porras to Rock, Sept. 28, 1961, and Rock's reply, Oct. 10, 1961; Rock to Reverend Ernest Sullivan, July 22, 1964; Rock to Father Pete Murphy, June 11, 1973. All in JR-RA. McCormick to Sanger, July 21, 1954, MS-SS.

100. See Chesler, *Woman of Valor*, esp. chaps. 10 and 11 and p. 441.

101. Paul Vaughan, *The Pill on Trial* (New York: Coward-McCann, 1970), 32.

102. Understanding the endometrium remains important, and it is still measured for its "thickness," that is, its readiness for implantation. But today the follicles can be easily measured to predict ovulation, and procedures today, such as inseminations, are timed based on blood work (measuring levels of estrogen and progesterone) and follicle maturity.

103. Annette B. Ramirez de Arellano and Conrad Seipp, *Colonialism, Catholicism, and Contraception: A History of Birth Control in Puerto Rico* (Chapel Hill: University of North Carolina Press, 1983), 49, 55.

104. McCormick to Sanger, Oct. 21, 1954, MS-SS.

105. In the end, the medical school at the University of Puerto Rico pulled out. As the director of the cytology center told Pincus, "We reviewed the entire situation and decided that due to the inability to get subjects for the study, we will have to drop the project. We feel that we should not use any more of your money without being able to get some results." See E. Harold Hinman to Pincus, Jan. 23, 1956; Jose Diaz Carazo to Pincus, Jan. 31, 1956, box 22, GP-LC. They were using the older progesterone, and not the new progestins.

106. McCormick to Sanger, Jan. 28, 1956, MS-SS.

Chapter 7. The Era of the Pill Begins

1. For McCormick's favorite term for the space, "the hovel," see, for example, Katharine Dexter McCormick to Margaret Sanger, May 8, 1956, and May 25, 1956, MS-SS.

2. Elizabeth Quirk to John Rock, April 19, 1955, JR-RA.

3. See, for example, Rock to Quirk, July 7, 1958, and Oct. 20, 1959, JR-RA.

4. Rock to Quirk, July 31, 1958, JR-RA.

5. Rock to Rachel Achenbach, Sept. 3, 1963; Rock to Mr. and Mrs. Alex Thackara, Feb. 8, 1967, JR-RA.

6. "Sometimes she's peaceful and very helpful, and other times she's stormy and disturbing," he wrote, another time remarking that "Ellie . . . is gradually regaining to her troublesome self again." Rock to Barbara (Mrs. Wentworth) Brown, Aug. 29, 1955; Rock to Quirk, July 7, 1958, and Oct. 20, 1959, JR-RA.

7. Rock referred not only his regular patients to Southam, but also his friends. See Rock to Southam, June 22, 1960, JR-RA. Until the 1980s, gynecology was a male-dominated field, in part because it is a surgical subspecialty, and surgical fields were particularly unfriendly to women. Few women became fellows in elite professional societies, for example. On Rock and Howard Taylor's sponsorship of Southam to be a fellow in the AAOG, see Secretary to John Rock to Dr. Clayton T. Beecham, Feb. 20, 1963, JR-RA.

8. "Research Fellows in Fertility and Endocrinology," typescript, undated but attached card indicates Sept. 30, 1993. This list goes back to 1945, the first year Rock had official fellows. Another list, "Research Associates of Dr. Rock: 1937–," JR-RA, of the same date lists as a research associate Christine Sears, MD, for 1940, but does not list what she was doing at the clinic.

9. "Contemporary reproductive medicine was developed by its incumbents," according to an article on Garcia in 2005. It was at the Free Hospital that Garcia first met Luigi Mastroianni, another Graves Fellow (though not at the same time) and future leader of the field. Jerome F. Strauss III and Luigi Mastroianni, Jr., "Celso-Ramon Garcia, M.D. (1922–2004), Reproductive Medicine Visionary," *Journal of Experimental and Clinical Assisted Reproduction* 2, no. 2 (2005). Text at www.jexpclinassistreprod.com/content/2/1/2.

10. Edris Rice-Wray, "Study Project of SC-4642," typescript, Jan. 1957, p. 2. We used

the copy in the JR-RA, with underlining and marginal notes by Rock, but there is another copy in the GP-LC. Numerous historians have written about these trials. In addition to the primary sources individually cited in these notes, we are strongly indebted to James Reed, *From Private Vice to Public Virtue: The Birth Control Movement and American Society since 1830* (New York: Basic Books, 1978); Loretta McLaughlin, *The Pill, John Rock, and the Church: The Biography of a Revolution* (Boston: Little, Brown, 1982); and Lara V. Marks, *Sexual Chemistry: A History of the Contraceptive Pill* (New Haven, Conn.: Yale University Press, 2001), all of which provide excellent accounts. Reed had the advantage of speaking to many of the participants in the 1970s, when he was working on his study; McLaughlin talked at length with Rock in the late 1970s and perhaps the early 1980s, and Marks conducted interviews in the 1990s with additional members of the research team. Reed and Marks also conducted prodigious archival research.

11. Katharine Dexter McCormick to Margaret Sanger, May 8, 1956, and May 25, 1956, MS-SS.

12. He discussed his work on a male oral contraceptive informally at a board meeting of his new clinic. Transcript of Board of Trustees meeting, Rock Reproductive Study Center, April 10, 1958, p. 7, JR-RA.

13. The most important of the books attacking the pill is Barbara Seaman, *The Doctors' Case Against the Pill: 25th Anniversary Updated Edition* (Alameda, Calif.: Hunter House, 1995). The book was originally published in 1969.

14. "Translation: from El Imparcial, 4/21/1956. PILLS ARE DISTRIBUTED AGAINST THE BIRTH RATE," box 22, Puerto Rico, GP-LC.

15. Seaman, *The Doctors' Case Against the Pill*, 239. This statement by Seaman sent one of us (Marsh) back to the Pincus Papers, which I had already consulted in detail, for another complete review. I was convinced we had missed something, since Seaman seemed so sure of her facts. In a second review of all 137 boxes of papers, I found that controls were mentioned only once (with the exception of the study on side effects involving the antacids, in which the "controls" were taking placebos and using other birth-control methods). Aside from the side effects study, the sole other mention was of former pill users who were used as "matched" controls during the first year of the study, under Rice-Wray's direction. If there was any mention of what Seaman says she saw in the papers (she does not specify where in the papers), I could not find it, even when I was making a special effort to look for it.

16. In 1957 Rock told a group of his friends and supporters that the pill was not a panacea, but that it was successful in a place like Puerto Rico because the women taking the pill had, in his words, "a moderately high degree of culture." See transcript of Board of Trustees meeting, Rock Reproductive Study Center, typescript, Oct. 23, 1957, JR-RA. Annette B. Ramirez de Arellano and Conrad Seipp, *Colonialism, Catholicism, and Contraception: A History of Birth Control in Puerto Rico* (Chapel Hill: University of North Carolina Press, 1983), 83–85.

17. Edris Rice-Wray to Gregory Pincus, May 10, 1956, box 22, Puerto Rico, GP-LC.

18. Transcript of television program sponsored by the Family Planning Association

of Puerto Rico, of which first Rice-Wray and then Paniagua were the medical directors. The pointed questions were staged, of course, but the accusations that the researchers were treating the island's women as if they were laboratory animals were real. The transcript was translated from the Spanish. Box 40, GP-LC.

19. "Leila" to "Uncle Goodie" (G. P.), May 1, [1957?], GP-LC. Pincus had just come back from his first trip to India, and we think that was in 1957, but it could even have been 1956.

20. Rock and Garcia were responsible for the clinical trials at Rio Piedras; Clarence Gamble and Adeline Satterthwaite conducted the other Puerto Rican trials, in Humacao, under the overall direction of Pincus.

21. McLaughlin, The Pill, John Rock, and the Church, 130.

22. Marks, Sexual Chemistry, 110.

23. The clinical studies of the new progestins began in December 1954 and were reported in John Rock, Celso-Ramon Garcia, and Gregory Pincus, "Synthetic Progestins in the Normal Human Menstrual Cycle," Recent Progress in Hormone Research 8 (1957), 323–46.

24. Edris Rice-Wray, "Study Project of SC-4642," typescript, Jan. 1957, pp. 7–8. The English translation here is very inelegant.

25. "Steroid Op Cases," handwritten, Aug. 24, 1956, JR-RA. The operations took place from March through June 1956.

26. For a brief biography of Greenblatt, see "Robert B. Greenblatt (1906–1987)," www.georgiaencyclopedia.org. Rock, Garcia, and Pincus, "Synthetic Progestins in the Normal Human Menstrual Cycle," 344–45. The discussion printed here occurred in 1956.

27. Rice-Wray to Pincus, Dec. 20, 1956, box 22, Puerto Rico, GP-LC.

28. Ibid.

29. Rice-Wray, "Study Project," p. 6 and summary, JR-RA; Rice-Wray to Pincus, Dec. 20, 1956, box 22, Puerto Rico, GP-LC.

30. Rice-Wray to Pincus, Dec. 20, 1956, box 22, Puerto Rico, GP-LC; I. C. Winter to Garcia, Oct. 24, 1956, JR-RA.

31. Rice-Wray to Pincus, undated, but probably sometime in summer 1957, based on a letter from Pincus to Rice-Wray, Sept. 17, 1957, GP-LC.

32. Rock to Winter, Jan. 26, 1960, and Winter's reply, Feb. 4, 1960, JR-RA.

33. Ibid.

34. Rock, Garcia, and Pincus, "Synthetic Progestins in the Normal Human Menstrual Cycle," 345–46.

35. For the discussion of the four women, see Rock to Winter, Nov. 10, 1955, JR-RA.

36. Loretta McLaughlin has a nice report on the presentation at the Laurentian conference, including a later reminiscence of Rock, in The Pill, John Rock, and the Church, 122–23. In another part of the book, she describes his high spirits at the conference, 45; John Rock, Gregory Pincus, and Celso-Ramon Garcia, "Effects of Certain 19-Nor

Steroids on the Normal Human Menstrual Cycle," *Science* 124, no. 3227 (Nov. 2, 1956), 891–93.

37. Cable from Rock to Pincus, June 25, 1957; Clipping from the Quincy *Patriot Ledger* (with notation that it "also appeared in the Herald"). It was in the *Boston Globe* as well, according to Rock's colleague Somers Sturgis. Cable and clippings in box 29, GP-LC.

38. Rock to Pincus, June 26, 1957, box 29, GP-LC. Rock had direct quotations from Guttmacher's letter, which we have not found the original of, in this letter to Pincus.

39. Rock to Winter, Aug. 10, 1957, attached to Rock to Pincus, Aug. 11, 1957, box 29, GP-LC. See also Winter to Rock, Aug. 6, 1957, and Rock to Winter, Aug. 10, 1957, JR-RA.

40. Rock to Crosson, Nov. 18, 1957, JR-RA.

41. Rock, Garcia, and Pincus, "Synthetic Progestins in the Normal Human Menstrual Cycle," 344.

42. Rock's candid comments about the pill, and contraception more generally, were voiced in 1957, the second year of the pill's Puerto Rican trials, and are part of a transcript of tape-recorded minutes of trustees' meetings for the new Rock Reproductive Study Center. The quotation here is from Board of Trustees meeting, Oct. 23, 1957, p. 29, JR-RA.

43. Ibid., 30.

44. Ibid., 32.

45. Ibid., 9.

46. Hart Achenbach interview by Margaret Marsh, June 3, 1998. Rock had plenty of patients, but he still needed to figure out how to do what he wanted to do professionally and still pay his bills.

47. Transcript of Board of Incorporators meeting of the Rock Reproductive Study Center, May 1, 1957, p. 23, JR-RA.

48. Ibid., Mr. (Charles) Storey speaking, 23.

49. See list of participants for Board of Incorporators meeting, May 1, 1957, and Board of Trustees meeting, Oct. 23, 1957, Rock Reproductive Study Center.

50. Board of Trustees meeting, Oct. 23, 1957, Rock Reproductive Study Center, p. 4.

51. Ibid., 15.

52. There is extensive correspondence regarding what seemed to Rock and McCormick to be obstructionism over the renovations to Rock's new quarters, as well as on financial relations between the new center and the hospital. Throughout, Rock declares publicly that these are simple misunderstandings, without any malicious intent on the part of the hospital. For example, Richard C. Paine (a trustee at the Free Hospital and member of the hospital's executive committee charged with working on the separation of Rock's new center from the Free Hospital) to John Rock, June 7, 1956, and Rock's reply, June 12, 1956; Rock to Paine, Sept. 6, 1956; Benjamin Grant (the management consultant) to Paine, July 2, 1956; Grant to Rock, July 2, 1956, JR-RA. Nan seems to have believed, not unreasonably, that Rock was being taken advantage of.

53. Rock to Winter, March 26, 1957. But Rock never stinted his patients and remained chronically short of operating funds. He was back to Winter again in 1958, asking for both an early payment of the final quarter's grant for 1958 and an advance for 1959. Rock to Winter, Oct. 18, 1958, JR-RA.

54. "The Rock Reproductive Clinic," no date, but probably 1963, JR-RA. There is another copy in JR-CLM.

55. There are pages and pages of notes and minutes of staff meetings from this period, some gathered in the Office Policies files, beginning in 1957, JR-RA. "Co-operative Institutions" for Brookline (Mrs. Stanley McCormick grants, Jan. 1 to Dec. 31, 1958), box 34, McCormick, GP-LC.

56. John Rock to J. William Crosson, Aug. 14, 1962, and Nov. 15, 1962, JR-RA, contain early indicators of an increasingly difficult situation. Rock was already putting much of his own income into the clinic, and taking a smaller and smaller share for himself.

57. Or then again, maybe not. Nelly Oudshoorn, *The Male Pill: A Biography of a Technology in the Making* (Durham, N.C.: Duke University Press, 2003), seems to think that a male pill will be developed soon, but it is not here yet.

58. Rock to Winter, Nov. 13, 1958, JR-RA.

59. Board of Trustees meeting, Oct. 23, 1957, the Rock Reproductive Study Center, p. 16.

60. Lynwood Heiges, MD, to John Rock, May 8, 1958; Rock to Heiges, June 3, 1958; and Rock to G. D. Searle & Company, June 3, 1958, JR-RA. Although Rock found it impossible to answer every letter personally, this was a typical exchange.

61. Rock to Winter, Dec. 11, 1958, and Winter to Rock, Dec. 18, 1958, JR-RA.

62. McCormick to Sanger, Feb. 29, 1956, MS-SS.

63. James Ferguson, *Papa Doc, Baby Doc: Haiti and the Duvaliers* (Oxford, UK: Basil Blackwell), 34–41; quotation page 41.

64. Bernard Asbell, *The Pill: A Biography of the Drug that Changed the World* (New York: Random House, 1995), discusses Pincus's attitude toward Haiti, which did not keep him from his usual optimism, on 149–53.

65. For American Committee for Devastated France, see Mary Breckinridge, *Wide Neighborhoods* (Lexington: University Press of Kentucky, 1981), 60–109. This book is her autobiography, written in 1952 but not published until 1981. The pages cited include a chapter on her son and on the committee. She says very little about either of her marriages. On Nan Rock's involvement with the FNS, see the *Alumnae Association of Bryn Mawr College, Alumnae Survey, 1953*, Bryn Mawr College Archives. Rock's daughter Rachel told Margaret Marsh (interview, July 6, 2007) that Breckinridge was a frequent houseguest of her parents.

66. Breckinridge, *Wide Neighborhoods*, 49, 59–66, 73–74. Her first husband was Henry Ruffner Morrison, and her second, Richard Ryan Thompson. Nancy Dammann, *A Social History of the Frontier Nursing Service* (Sun City, Ariz.: Social Change Press, 1982), 5.

67. Dammann, *A Social History of the Frontier Nursing Service*, passim, but for a brief history with photographs, also see the FNS website, www.frontiernursing.org.

68. *Frontier Nursing Service Quarterly Bulletin* 33, no. 4 (Spring 1958), 43.

69. It is impossible to tell what Breckinridge truly believed about contraception since the FNS interviews are in direct conflict on this point. Our own sense is that her earlier disapproval had more to do with respect for the attitudes of the people she served, and that her real opposition was to tubal ligations, but that is only our impression.

70. Interview with Marianne Harper; interview with Helen Browne, March 27, 1979. Elsie Maier disagreed and did not think Breckinridge actually opposed contraception, but did oppose sterilization. Interview with Elsie Maier, Dec. 5, 1978. All in Frontier Nursing Service (FNS) Oral History Project, Special Collections, University of Kentucky.

71. Interview with Rachel and Ott Bowling, May 31, 1979, FNS Oral History Project.

72. Interview with Molly Lee, Feb. 6, 1979, FNS Oral History Project.

73. Interview with Helen Browne.

74. Ibid.

75. Quotation taken from interview with Betty Lester; interview with Elsie Maier. FNS Oral History Project.

76. Interview with Elsie Maier.

77. Minutes of Medical Committee Meeting, PPFA, Oct. 1, 1958, typescript, p. 3, box 34, GP-LC.

78. Memo to Winter from Venning, Sept. 19, 1958; Winter to Rock, Oct. 30, 1958; Rock to Winter, Nov. 7, 1958; enclosure for Swyer, "ENOVID-10 mg/day," Nov. 5, 1958, JR-RA. On Swyer's continued belief that the progestins did not have the same action as "natural" progesterone, see G. I. M. Swyer et al., "Determination of the Relative Potency of Some Progestogens in the Human," typescript [1960], JR-RA. Rock clearly disagreed, writing "Bunk!" in the margin on the first page.

79. Albert Raymond to Pincus, Aug. 24, 1955, box 14, GP-LC.

80. Rock's daughter Rachel recalled that after the pill was approved, Rock bought a few shares of Searle stock but immediately gave them away to his daughters because he did not want to leave himself open to criticism. For just one example of Rock's public praise of Pincus, see "Clinical Studies with Potential Oral Contraceptives," paper coauthored by Rock, Garcia, and Pincus, but presented by Rock in Feb. 1959 and published in *Report of the Proceedings of the Sixth International Conference on Planned Parenthood* (Feb. 14–21, 1959, New Delhi, India).

81. van Antwerp to Rock, Nov. 6, 1958, JR-RA.

82. Rock to van Antwerp, Nov. 18, 1958, JR-RA.

83. "ENOVID: Substitute expression for 'contraception' as obtained with *Enovid* . . ." Typescript, Nov. 18, 1958, JR-RA.

84. "ENOVID: FOR THE DOCTOR" #2, typescript, three pages, Nov. 18, 1958, JR-RA.

85. "ENOVID: FOR THE PATIENT" #2, typescript, two pages, Nov. 18, 1958, JR-RA.

86. Winter to Rock, Oct. 22, 1958, and Nov. 6, 1958, JR-RA.

87. For a very brief biography of Tyler, see Walter E. Duka and Alan H. DeCherney, *From the Beginning: A History of the American Fertility Society, 1944–1994* (Birmingham, Ala.: The American Fertility Society, 1994), 138.

88. Crosson to Rock, Nov. 25, 1959, JR-RA.

89. Rock to Crosson, Dec. 4, 1959, JR-RA.

90. Suzanne White Junod and Lara Marks, "Women's Trials: The Approval of the First Oral Contraceptive Pill in the United States and Great Britain," *Journal of the History of Medicine and Allied Sciences* 57, no. 2 (2002), 117–60, quotation on 132.

91. The following account of the pill approval is based largely on the Rock correspondence as a primary source, but it is also indebted to the work of Loretta McLaughlin, who interviewed many of the participants in the pill approval process, including Searle's I. C. Winter and the FDA's Pasquale DeFelice, into whose young lap the pill approval fell. McLaughlin, *The Pill, John Rock, and the Church*, 138–42. Our interpretation of the process is deeply indebted to the excellent article by Junod and Marks, "Women's Trials."

92. To give a sense of how understaffed the FDA must have been, with seven physicians, only three of them full time and the part-timers inexperienced and junior, consider that between 1952 and 1962, the FDA received 4,000 NDAs, and *averaged* 3,000 supplemental NDAs per year since 1957. Junod and Marks, "Women's Trials," 129–31.

93. Ibid., 140. The following demonstrates the concept of a "woman year": one woman is observed for one year, or two women are each observed for half a year.

94. The numbers of women who had taken the pills for twenty-four to fifty-two consecutive cycles is in Crosson to Rock, April 27, 1960, JR-RA.

95. Junod and Marks, "Women's Trials," 146–48.

96. DeFelice to Crosson, Sept. 25, 1959, JR-RA.

97. Crosson to DeFelice, Oct. 9, 1959, pp. 1–2, JR-RA.

98. Ibid., 1.

99. Winter and Rock quoted in McLaughlin, *The Pill, John Rock, and the Church*, 142–43. Rock recounted McLaughlin's interview in his diary, March 18, 1979, JR-RA. He wrote that he thought her name was Loretta McDonald. "Well, she came whatever her name is and stayed for fully four hours, asking all sorts of questions, many quite personal ones." He seems to have answered whatever she asked and wrote that he did not know what she intended to do with the interview.

100. Interview with John Rock, June 15, 1979, FNS Oral History Project, Special Collections, University of Kentucky. He also remembered it this way in his diary. On Dec. 4, 1979, he recalled how he and the two Searle scientists "went to Washington, and brow-beat the young squirt in the Food and Drug Administration to give their O.K. to Enovid." JR-RA.

101. McLaughlin, *The Pill, John Rock, and the Church*, 141, 143.

102. Crosson to Rock, Oct. 29, 1959; Winter to Rock, Nov. 3, 1959; Rock to Winter, Nov. 8, 1959. Rock to DeFelice, Feb. 24, 1960, mentions the date of their meeting as Oct. 23, 1959, JR-RA. Junod and Marks's revelation of the importance of Edward

Tyler's opinion in the FDA approval leads us to believe he may have been the outside referee.

103. Crosson to Rock, Feb. 12, 1960, JR-RA.

104. Junod and Marks, "Women's Trials," 131.

105. DeFelice to Rock, Feb. 12, 1960, JR-RA. This apparently was the standard letter sent out to all seventy-five physicians, since it gives no hint of direct knowledge of Rock's involvement in the pill's creation.

106. Rock to DeFelice, Feb. 24, 1960, JR-RA.

107. Crosson to Rock, April 12, 1960; Rock to Crosson, April 18, 1960; and Crosson to John Rock, April 27, 1960. Suzanne Junod, historian of the FDA, personal communication, Sept. 10, 2001, on Granger meeting with Tyler.

108. *Newsweek* 55 (May 23, 1960), 107B; *New York Times*, May 10, 1960, 75.

Chapter 8. The Face and Voice of the Pill

1. See, for example, Elizabeth Siegel Watkins, *On the Pill: A Social History of Oral Contraceptives, 1950–1970* (Baltimore: Johns Hopkins University Press, 1998), 29.

2. In 1940, Rock and his fellow researchers concluded that in women who ovulated regularly and who rigidly followed the directions (which included ten days of the month in which intercourse was prohibited), the method worked 97% of the time. However, of the 225 women who applied for treatment, 26 were simply too irregular in their cycles to make rhythm ever work, and another 76 found the method entirely too troublesome, which means that what they called the "true" failure rate of 2.9% only applied to "a self-selected group" with "no alternative in the way of birth control" and a need to avoid pregnancy. (The actual pregnancy rate was 10%.) Stephen Fleck, Elizabeth F. Snedeker, and John Rock, "The Contraceptive 'Safe Period': A Clinical Study," 1940, typescript, JR-CLM; published as Stephen Fleck, Elizabeth F. Snedeker, and John Rock, "The Contraceptive Safe Period: A Clinical Study," *New England Journal of Medicine* 223 (1940), 1005–9.

3. Loretta McLaughlin, *The Pill, John Rock, and the Church: The Biography of a Revolution* (Boston: Little, Brown, 1982), 154–55.

4. Rock to Quirk, March 23, 1959, and Rock to James W. Toumey, March 23, 1959, JR-RA. In these letters, Rock describes the month-long trip in which the couple traveled to India, Italy, and France.

5. Rock to Carlos E. Pinto, Oct. 7, 1960; Rock to Wilson Popenoe, MD, Oct. 28, 1960, JR-RA.

6. Dom Gregory Stevens to Rock, June 27, 1961; Rock to Lewis Scheffey, MD, July 20, 1961, JR-RA. The detail about Monsignor Lally comes from McLaughlin, *The Pill, John Rock, and the Church*, 158. McLaughlin interviewed Lally, who was not only Rock's friend and fellow Tavern Club member, but also the editor of the *Boston Pilot*, the newspaper of the archdiocese, and a close associate of its head, Richard Cardinal Cushing.

7. One of the best books about the sexual revolution in all its complexity is Beth Bailey, *Sex in the Heartland* (Cambridge, Mass.: Harvard University Press, 1999).

8. See, for example, Elaine Tyler May, *Homeward Bound* (New York: Basic Books, 1988), 139. Susan Householder Van Horn, *Women, Work, and Fertility* (New York: New York University Press, 1988), 95–96; National Center for Health Statistics, *Vital Statistics of the United States, 1989*, vol. 1, Natality. DHHS Pub. No. (PHS) 93-1100 (Washington, D.C.: U.S. Government Printing Office, 1993), 35–37.

9. The story of this cultural transformation has been told, often brilliantly, by a number of talented historians, including James Reed, *From Private Vice to Public Virtue: The Birth Control Movement in American Society since 1830* (New York: Basic Books, 1978), and Linda Gordon, *Woman's Body, Woman's Right: A Social History of Birth Control in America* (New York: Grossman, 1976). The life of the movement's founder, Margaret Sanger, is no better recounted than in Ellen Chesler's now classic biography, *Woman of Valor: Margaret Sanger and the Birth Control Movement in America* (New York: Simon and Schuster, 1992).

10. The historical assessment appears in John Von Rohr, "Christianity and Birth Control II: Protestant Views," *Christian Century* 77 (Oct. 19, 1960), 1209–12; the final quotation is from *Christian Century* 76 (Oct. 28, 1959), 1237.

11. Ronald F. Freedman, Pascal K. Whelpton, and Arthur A. Campbell, "Family Planning in the U.S.," *Scientific American* 200 (April 1959), 50–55; quotation from 51.

12. Margaret Marsh and Wanda Ronner, *The Empty Cradle: Infertility in America from Colonial Times to the Present* (Baltimore: Johns Hopkins University Press, 1996), chap. 6, esp. 183–91.

13. Freedman, Whelpton, and Campbell, "Family Planning in the U.S.," 51.

14. Ibid., 54.

15. John R. Connery, S. J. [Society of Jesus, i.e., the Jesuits], "Religious Pluralism and Public Morality," *America* 100 (Feb. 21, 1959), 597–99. Quotations from 598.

16. John Von Rohr, "Christianity and Birth Control I: The Roman Catholic View," *Christian Century* 77 (Sept. 28, 1960), 115–18, quotations on 115–16. See also Louis McKernan, C.S.P., "Population in a Changing World," *Catholic World* 190 (Feb. 1960), 286–93.

17. Two seminary textbooks quoted in Loretta McLaughlin, *The Pill, John Rock, and the Church,* 151.

18. "Planned Fertility," *Time* 51 (Feb. 9, 1948), 71. The occasion was the announcement that Rock had received the Lasker Award from Planned Parenthood for his research "into the causes and cures of sterility."

19. *Commonweal* authors, unlike those of *America,* tended to speak with multiple voices. See James O'Gara, "Catholics and Population," *Commonweal* 71 (Dec. 18, 1959), 339–42, and in the same issue, John Cogley, "The Bishops' Challenge," 350. (The quotation is from Cogley.)

20. James O'Gara, "Birth Control Laws Again," *Commonweal* 75 (Jan. 26, 1962), 450.

21. "Birth Control Pill Found Effective," *New York Herald Tribune*, May 28, 1958, 13. Clipping in JR-RA.

22. Monsignor Robert J. White to John Rock, March 15, 1957. (It isn't clear from this

letter exactly what issue prompted Rock to seek spiritual advice, but the letter appears in a file he kept on birth-control issues.) Rock to Alvah W. Sulloway, Oct. 16, 1959, JR-RA.

23. John Rock to Dom Gregory Stevens, April 20, 1960; Stevens to Rock, April 26, 1960; Rock to Stevens, May 19, 1960; Rock to Stevens, July 8, 1960; Rock to Stevens, Oct. 19, 1960 (quotation from JR from this letter), JR-RA.

24. John Rock, "We Can End the Battle Over Birth Control," *Good Housekeeping* 153 (July 1961), 44–45ff. Quotations from 107–8. John Rock, "Population Growth," *Journal of the American Medical Association* 177 (July 8, 1961), 58–60.

25. Rock, "We Can End the Battle Over Birth Control," 108.

26. Mrs. J. D. to Rock, July 22, 1960, and his reply July 28, 1960, JR-RA.

27. Mrs. E. C. to Rock, June 2, 1960, and his reply, June 7, 1960. Mrs. J. D. to Rock, July 22, 1960, and his reply, July 28, 1960. Rock to Donald B. McKean, MD, Sept. 13, 1961, JR-RA. (This letter is part of an exchange of views carried over six months between the two doctors.)

28. Rock to Mrs. M. H., March 5, 1962, to Mrs. F. B., March 16, 1962, and to Mrs. A. S., March 16, 1962, all in response to letters from them, JR-RA.

29. Rock went public with his views on contraception in a way that he was never willing to do for abortion, even though he did not entirely agree with the Church on abortion, either.

30. An excellent book on both the development of a consensus on the population problem and the later involvement of the U.S. government in international family planning assistance is Donald T. Chritchlow, *Intended Consequences: Birth Control, Abortion, and the Federal Government in Modern America* (New York: Oxford University Press, 1999). The above discussion is drawn from this book, esp. 16–33.

31. Rock to Sax, March 26, 1956, JR-RA.

32. Christian Herter to Rock, Jan. 13, 1959. See, for example, on the personal side, Rock to Lewis C. Scheffey, MD, Jan. 19, 1959. He also lobbied his senator, Leverett Saltonstall, whom he knew personally. Rock to Saltonstall, May 5, 1965; Saltonstall to Rock, May 13, 1965, JR-RA.

33. Rock to Crosson, Aug. 14, 1962, JR-RA. This interchange was specifically about two Chicago priests with whom Rock had met in January.

34. At the time, both men insisted that their involvement never be revealed, but later in his life, Best claimed coauthorship of the book. See *University of North Carolina Gazette Online*, January 26, 2005, http://gazette.unc.edu/archives/05jan26/facstaff/html.

35. Rock insisted that the two men share equally any royalties he might receive as well. John Rock diaries, Oct. 1, 1979; Frederick Jaffe to Rock, July 9, 1962, and July 19, 1962; Jaffe to Henry Robbins (of Knopf), Sept. 28, 1961. This letter copies Winfield Best, the other writer. The drafts of the manuscript and the rest of the material are all in JR-RA.

36. The emphasis is in the original work. John Rock, *The Time Has Come: A Catholic Doctor's Proposals to End the Battle over Birth Control* (New York: Knopf, 1963).

37. Ibid. Father Finnick appears on xi.

38. Kennedy's remarks cited in editorial, "Catholic Physician Favors Birth Control," *Christian Century* 80 (May 29, 1963), 699. Michael Novak, letter to the editor, *Commonweal* 78 (July 5, 1963), 399–400. On Jewish attitudes, see Milton Himmelfarb, "The Spirit Giveth Life?" *Commentary* 36 (Sept. 1963), 250–51.

39. Himmelfarb thought that Jewish commentators should be a little more sympathetic to Catholic legalisms, even if he agreed that Rock was trying "to untie a Gordian knot" when what was needed was to cut it. Himmelfarb, "The Spirit Giveth Life?"

40. *America* was an important official mouthpiece for the clergy. Fr. Joseph S. Duhamel, S.J., review of *The Time Has Come*, *America* 108 (April 23, 1963), 608–11. These quotations are representative of conservative Church opinion.

41. Not a single other Catholic reviewer expressed any concern about Rock's embryo studies, which were described in the book. The fact that no one else criticized Rock for the embryo research remains something of a mystery to us as well. But this was in the pre–Roe vs. Wade age, and most readers did not find Rock's description of his research to be morally problematic.

42. Herbert Ratner, "The Rock Book—I: A Catholic Viewpoint," *Commonweal* 78 (July 5, 1963), 393.

43. In the late 1920s Rock either assisted one of his patients, a young married woman with one child, to find a physician to perform an abortion, or perhaps performed it himself. The woman did not say why it was so "necessary" for her to have an abortion, but Rock not only made sure she obtained one but also helped her conceal the fact from everyone except her husband. Rock later delivered at least one of her two sons. Here are the relevant quotations, from letters written to Rock in 1983: "My daughter . . . was born in 1926—E[name redacted] and I were married in 1925. In 1929, much to my sorrow, it was considered necessary for me to have an abortion. As it was considered illegal it was kept secret even from my mother. She never did know about it." From Mrs. M. B. T. to Rock, Feb. 1, 1983. A note from her son was enclosed, which said in part, "I thought I would tuck my own note into my mother's letter . . . I have always known that the physician who delivered me into the world was a leader in obstetrics, and both of my parents used to refer to your courageous position with respect to certain matters which, since they were speaking to a little boy, they did not explain." To Rock, Feb. 2, 1983, JR-RA.

44. Interview with John Rock, June 15, 1979, FNS Oral History Project, Special Collections, University of Kentucky.

45. Ratner, "The Rock Book—I," 394–95.

46. "Dr. Rock's Book," *Commonweal* 78 (May 17, 1963), 213–14.

47. Richard Cardinal Cushing quoted, respectively, in *Newsweek* 61 (April 29, 1963), 62, and *Science Digest* 54 (July 1963), 9. The *Science Digest* article was condensed from the *National Observer*. Cushing's spokesperson was Monsignor Francis Lally, editor of the *Boston Pilot* and one of Rock's close friends, according to Loretta McLaughlin. See *John Rock, the Pill, and the Church*, 158. Cushing considered Rock a conscientious Catholic.

48. "Roman Catholics: A New View on Birth Control," *Time* 83 (April 10, 1964), 59. Portions of Janssens' essay were translated as "Morality of the Pill," *Commonweal* 80 (May 5, 1964), 332–35. Quotation on 334. Richard A. McCormick, S.J., "Whither the Pill," *Catholic World* 199 (July 1964), 209, also takes note of Janssens' reliance on Rock's view of the way the pill worked.

49. The author of this widely syndicated article was Father Edward Duff. For *Time's* assessment, see "Roman Catholics: A New View on Birth Control," *Time* 83 (April 10, 1964).

50. Editorial, "*Time's* Bomb," *America* 110 (April 25, 1964), 563.

51. *America* published this letter from *Time* reporter Robert B. Kaiser in vol. 110 (May 30, 1964), 751.

52. Letter to the editor, "The Pill," *Commonweal* 80 (April 24, 1964), 149.

53. *Commonweal* 80 (June 5, 1964), 312; Richard A. McCormick, S. J., "Toward a Dialogue," ibid., 315; George W. Casey, "The Pastoral Crisis," ibid., 317, 319; Bernard Haring, "Responsible Parenthood," ibid., 327. This issue contains several articles by priests and lay Catholics, all urging change on the Church in the matter of birth control.

54. Rock to Searle, Sept. 30, 1963, JR-RA; McLaughlin, *The Pill, John Rock, and the Church*, 183–84.

Chapter 9. The Pill Falls from Grace

1. See John D'Emilio and Estelle B. Freedman, *Intimate Matters: A History of Sexuality in America* (New York: Harper and Row, 1988), esp. chap. 10; Peter Gay, *The Education of the Senses* (New York: Oxford University Press, 1984), 71–95.

2. Beth Bailey, *Sex in the Heartland* (Cambridge, Mass.: Harvard University Press, 1999), 217.

3. Standing at 23.7 per thousand in 1960, the U.S. birth rate slipped to the Depression-era rate of 18.4 in 1970, and to 15.9 in 1980. See Susan Householder Van Horn, *Women, Work, and Fertility* (New York: New York University Press, 1988), 151–54; Stephanie Coontz, *The Way We Never Were: American Families and the Nostalgia Trap* (New York: Basic Books, 1992), 24; Victor Fuchs, *How We Live: An Economic Perspective on Americans from Birth to Death* (Cambridge, Mass.: Harvard University Press, 1983), 259.

4. As Victor Fuchs argued as long ago as 1956, "the direction and change of income," rather than "the absolute level of income," serve as the best predictors of a nation's fertility rate. By the 1970s, Fuchs concluded, the failure of the economy "to meet the rising tide of expectations undoubtedly contributed to the increase in the age of marriage and the low fertility rate of that decade." This notion of a change in income relative to expectations, rather than an absolute decline in prosperity, helps to explain why, although fertility rates declined across the entire spectrum of young Americans, the sharpest downward trend emerged among the most highly educated. Victor Fuchs, *How We Live*, 22. See also, Claudia Goldin, *Understanding the Gender Gap: An Economic History of American Women* (New York: Oxford University Press, 1990), 140–41. Van Horn, *Women, Work, and Fertility*, 157.

5. Barron H. Lerner, *Breast Cancer Wars: Hope, Fear, and the Pursuit of a Cure in Twentieth-Century America* (New York: Oxford University Press, 2001), demonstrates that this reliance on clinical experience was a common practice. For example, Lerner's research showed that American physicians continued to endorse mastectomies even after European data showed that lumpectomies seemed to be just as effective. They based their endorsement on their own experiences.

6. John Rock, "Let's Be Honest about the Pill!" *Journal of the American Medical Association* 192 (May 3, 1965), 401–2. See for example, on medical supervision, John Rock, "Contraceptive Methods for Global Control of Population, *Lowell Lecture, Dr. 3*" (the one presented), typewritten, 1967, p. 24, JR-RA.

7. Rock's views on abortion were complicated. At a speech to the Connecticut Medical Society in 1968, he grappled with the question of when the fetus became a human being, citing conflicting early Catholic thinkers such as Ambrose, who said, in effect, that the soul entered the fetus at conception, and Thomas Aquinas, who, in Rock's words, "proposed ensoulment only after several more weeks, even months, of pregnancy, i.e., when the fetus became recognizable as human." While not endorsing abortion (Rock refers to the "deep repugnance to doing an abortion which practically all of us physicians have"), he does say that "one may ask whether the time has come to . . . prevent species-harmful parentage, if contraception fails." And so, "the doctor's dilemma regarding induced abortion consists, on the one hand, of his responsibility to furnish his patient, rich or poor, with all the care that medical science affords; and on the other, to keep such care within the bounds of his own conscience, as well as those set by society, and presumably expressed in law." "Abortion: For Connecticut Medical Society, Hartford, 4/30/68," typewritten, JR-RA. Quotations on 2, 4, and 5.

8. For an excellent analysis of this and other works of Catholic intellectuals on the subject of sexuality, birth control, and abortion, see Patrick Allitt, *Catholic Intellectuals and Conservative Politics in America, 1950–1985* (Ithaca, N.Y.: Cornell University Press, 1993), 163–203. The discussion of Noonan is on 168–69. *Time* 86 (July 16, 1965), 74.

9. See, for example, "Birth Control Fight Spreads," *U.S. News and World Report* 65 (Oct. 7, 1968), 56.

10. See "Talks and Discussions of Dr. John Rock, M.D.," typescript, Oct. 9, 1963; Secretary (to Rock) to G. R. Venning, Feb. 11, 1965; John Rock diaries, April 19, 1966, and May 13, 1966, JR-RA. The diary, unfortunately, is sporadic. It seems he wrote in it only when he was in Temple, New Hampshire.

11. William F. Buckley, Jr., "The Birth Rate," *National Review* 17 (March 23, 1965), 231.

12. "Birth Control: A New Catholic Policy Soon?" *U.S. News and World Report* 58 (April 12, 1965), 16; "Division on Birth Control," *Time* 85 (April 2, 1965), 80.

13. "Papal Statement on Birth Control," *America* 113 (Nov. 13, 1965), 558–59; "Birth Control Decision," *Commonweal* 83 (Dec. 10, 1965), 296–97; Gregory Baum, "Birth Control—What Happened?" *Commonweal* 83 (Dec. 24, 1965), 371.

14. "Breakthrough in Birth Control," *Reader's Digest* 88 (Jan. 1966), 64; "Contra-

ception among Catholics," *Scientific American* 219 (Dec. 1968), 50; "Birth Control and American Catholic Women," *Trans-Action* 6 (Dec. 1968), 4; "The Report Revealed," *Newsweek* 67 (May 1, 1966), 94; Norman B. Ryder and Charles F. Westoff, "Use of Oral Contraception in the United States, 1965," *Science* 153 (Sept. 9, 1966), 1203.

15. The articles, letters to the editor, and editorials themselves in such Catholic magazines as *America* and *Commonweal* are nearly endless. For example, see Richard A. McCormick, S.J. (an assistant editor at *America*), "The Council on Contraception," *America* 114 (Jan. 8, 1966), 47–48, and a heated rejoinder from conservative John C. Ford, S.J., in Letters to the Editor, *America* 114 (Jan. 22, 1966), 103–7; a letter to the editors of *Commonweal* complaining about Gregory Baum from (Rev.) Cronan Regan, C.P., and a rejoinder from Baum himself in *Commonweal* 83 (Feb. 4, 1966), 542–43. *Catholic World* interviewed John Noonan (author of the aforementioned *Contraception*) in 203 (June 1966), 153–56. Both *Time* and *Newsweek* had ongoing coverage of the turmoil within the Catholic Church over birth control. "Roman Catholics: Lex Dubia Non Obligat," *Time* 87 (April 22, 1966), 60; *Newsweek* 67 (Feb. 14, 1966), 62.

16. "A Change on Birth Control?" *Time* 88 (July 1, 1966), 45; "Deadlock on Birth Control," *Newsweek* 67 (June 20, 1966), 74; Paul VI quoted in "The Pope and Birth Control," *Commonweal* 85 (Nov. 11, 1966), 157.

17. "The Pope Delays his Decision," *America* 115 (Nov. 12, 1966), 576–77; "The Pope and the Pill," *Newsweek* 68 (Nov. 14, 1966), 64; "Pope Postpones Decision on Birth Control," *Christian Century* 83 (Nov. 16, 1966), 1401; "Time for a Change," *Time* 89 (April 28, 1967), 62; "The Report Revealed," *Newsweek* 69 (May 1, 1967), 61; "The Symbol of Birth Control," *Commonweal* 86 (April 28, 1967), 163–64; Allitt, *Catholic Intellectuals and Conservative Politics*, 172.

18. "Birth Control: Pronouncement Withdrawn," *Time* 91 (June 21, 1968), 63–64.

19. Allitt, *Catholic Intellectuals and Conservative Politics*, 174; "The Pope and Birth Control," *Time* 92 (Aug. 9, 1968), 40–42; "Letter from Vatican City," *New Yorker* 44 (Nov. 2, 1968), 131–34ff., quotation on 136–37 (A series of "Letters from Vatican City" were published under the name Xavier Rynne. This was the pseudonym of Fr. Francis X. Murphy, a member of the Second Vatican Council, see Arthur Jones, "Another Luminary Lost," *National Catholic Reporter* [May 3, 2002]); "The Birth Control Encyclical," *Commonweal* 88 (Aug. 9, 1968), 515–16.

20. Kathleen Teltsch, "Encyclical Stuns Dr. Rock," *New York Times*, Aug. 8, 1968, 1, 18.

21. "The Birth Control Encyclical," 516; "An Editorial Statement on 'Human Life,'" *America* 119 (Aug. 17, 1968), 94–95.

22. "The Theologians Retort," *Commonweal* 88 (Aug. 23, 1968), 562; "Catholic Priests: Growing Split Over Birth Control," *U.S. News and World Report* 65 (Sept. 16, 1968), 16; "Roman Catholics: Soft Line on Contraception," *Time* 92 (Oct. 4, 1968), 57; "Bishops' Ruling on Birth Control," *U.S. News and World Report* 65 (Nov. 25, 1968), 10. Allitt, *Catholic Intellectuals and Conservative Politics*, 175, notes that "U.S. Catholics after 1968, . . . acted almost as though the Pope had said what they had hoped he would say rather than what he had said in fact."

23. Rock to H. Curtis Wood, Jr., MD, July 26, 1961, JR-RA.

24. Rock to Crosson, June 25, 1962; Rock to Pincus, July 24, 1962, JR-RA.

25. Phlebitis is an inflammation of a vein; thrombosis is the formation, development, or presence of a thrombos (a standing blood clot along the wall of a vessel). Definition from *Dorland's Illustrated Medical Dictionary* (Elsevier: Philadelphia, 2003).

26. Winter to William Kessenich, MD, Medical Director of the FDA, Dec. 20, 1961; Winter to E. R. Kassous, MD, Dec. 20, 1961, JR-RA. The early articles and commentaries on the pill focused on concerns about the mechanism of action on the ovary, the risk of permanently suppressing fertility or postponing menopause, its carcinogenic potential, and immediate side effects such as nausea, bloating, headaches, breast tenderness, and skin changes. Concern was expressed that the mode of action was incompletely understood. See R. L. Holmes, "Oral Contraceptives. An Assessment of Their Mode of Action," *Lancet* 1 (June 1962), 1167–68. At the same time, other articles were cataloging the noncontraceptive benefits, such as a decrease in menstrual flow, menstrual regulation, improvement in cramping and premenstrual tension, and as treatment for endometriosis and sterility. See *International Journal of Fertility* 8 (July–Sept. 1963), 600–755. Edward T. Tyler published in 1961 his four-year experience with another product, norethindrone. No serious side effects were noted, and no mention was made of thromboembolic disease. Tyler commented on the FDA ruling limiting contraceptive use to a two-year period, agreeing that it was justified, and noting that more data on longer usage was being acquired. E. T. Tyler et al., "An Oral Contraceptive—A 4-Year Study of Norethindrone," *Obstetrics and Gynecology* 18 (Sept. 1961), 363–67.

27. Mary Steichen Calderone, MD, "Survey of Enovid Use in Planned Parenthood Centers," typewritten, Aug. 20, 1962, pp. 1–3, JR-RA.

28. Rock to Winter, Oct. 1, 1962, JR-RA.

29. The activated partial thromboplastin time is used to assess the intrinsic and common pathways of coagulation. A prolonged time can indicate a deficiency in a number of clotting factors. (Definition from *Dorland's Illustrated Medical Dictionary*.) Typewritten instructions to all doctors at the Rock Reproductive Clinic, Jan. 10, 1963, written on the clinical laboratory's announcement of Jan. 3, 1963, that the test would be available, JR-RA.

30. Lara V. Marks, *Sexual Chemistry: A History of the Contraceptive Pill* (New Haven, Conn.: Yale University Press, 2001), 77–79.

31. Marks, *Sexual Chemistry*, chap. 6, 138–57, provides an excellent summary and analysis of the thromboembolic disease question in the United States and Great Britain.

32. In *The Use of Progestins in Obstetrics and Gynecology* (Chicago: Year Book Medical Publisher, 1969), Kistner lists pill side effects from numbers 1 to 35, noting that 29 to 35 are rarely reported, and he finishes his lists with the three side effects under the category of "Cause and Effect Not Definitely Established."

33. An early mention of thrombophlebitis, some with fatal embolism, appeared in

E. J. DeCosta, "Those Deceptive Contraceptives," *Journal of the American Medical Association* 181 (July 14, 1962), 122–25. The study on Provest (ethinyl estradiol, .05 mg and medroxyprogesterone acetate 10 mg), funded by Upjohn, found no cases of thromboembolic disease in 843 accumulated cycles. The author commented that the women stopped the trial after reading a newspaper article about Enovid and blood clots. J. T. Dingle, "Preliminary Report on Provest Study," *International Journal of Fertility* 8 (July–Sept. 1963), 711–19. In this same journal, there was a report by another researcher who looked for changes in the coagulation system in three volunteers before and after the use of Provest. They found no change in the lab values and concluded that no hypercoaguability existed. E. F. Mammen et al., "Provest and Blood Coagulation Tests," *International Journal of Fertility* 8 (July–Sept. 1963), 653–63. Echoing Rock's belief, the authors conclude that the pill had the same risk of thromboembolic disease as pregnancy, and that a woman who has had a thromboembolic disease event in pregnancy should not use the pill.

34. "Dear Doctor" letter from Searle, Dec. 26, 1962, JR-RA.

35. The committee found that among African American women, there were no reported deaths, so they looked at mortality in white women on the pill (12.1/1 million versus the general population, 8.4/1 million). They reported their findings in Ad Hoc Advisory Committee for the Evaluation of a Possible Etiologic Relation with Thromboembolic Conditions, "FDA Report on Enovid," *Journal of the American Medical Association* 185 (Sept. 7, 1963), 776. See also David A. Grimes, MD, and Melinda Wallach Grimes, MD, eds., *Modern Contraception: Updates from the Contraception Report* (Totowa, N.J.: Emron, 1997). In 1964, Edward Tyler noted that the FDA felt further statistical information was necessary to compare the incidence of naturally occurring pulmonary embolisms to those occurring in women on the pill. E. T. Tyler, "Current Status of Oral Contraception," *Journal of the American Medical Association* 187 (Feb. 22, 1964), 562–65.

36. "Birth Control Pill Found Safe for 11,711 Women," *Science News Letter* 87 (April 17, 1965), 242.

37. Reported in "Popular, Effective, Safe: Birth-Control Pills," *Newsweek* 68 (Aug. 22, 1966), 92.

38. "The Better Way: Birth Control Pills: An Up-to-Date Report," *Good Housekeeping* 161 (Sept. 1965), 159–61. The article includes quotations from Rock.

39. "Popular, Effective, Safe: Birth-Control Pills," 92.

40. Lawrence Lader, "Three Men Who Made a Revolution," *New York Times Magazine*, April 10, 1966, 8–9ff; Elizabeth Siegel Watkins, *On the Pill: A Social History of Oral Contraceptives, 1950–1970* (Baltimore: Johns Hopkins University Press, 1998), 34; Andrea Tone, *Devices and Desires: A History of Contraceptives in America* (New York: Hill and Wang, 2001), 239.

41. See, for example, Bill Surface, "Controversy over the Pill," *Good Housekeeping* 170 (Jan. 1970), 65–66ff.

42. Ibid., 125.

43. Reports of deaths in Great Britain among women taking oral contraceptives

continued to cause concern. The Committee on Safety of Drugs reviewed the prior year's data, noting that sixteen deaths from thromboembolic disease had been reported when thirteen would be expected. In response to growing concerns, in April 1965, the College of General Practitioners began a pilot survey to see if the effects of oral contraceptives could be ascertained by looking at patient records. The results showed that the risk of thromboembolic disease (venous thrombosis or pulmonary embolism) was increased sixfold in women who were pregnant or had recently delivered, and threefold in women taking oral contraceptives. Both studies cited in "Preliminary Communications. Risk of Thromboembolic Disease in Women Taking Oral Contraceptives—a Preliminary Communication to the Medical Research Council by a Subcommittee," British Medical Journal 2 (May 6, 1967), 355–59. A second British study evaluated women who had been hospitalized for thromboembolic disease at nineteen general hospitals. The authors concluded that the risk of requiring hospital admission for thromboembolic disease was about nine times greater in women who use oral contraceptives. M. P. Vessey and R. Doll, "Investigation of Relation Between Use of Oral Contraceptives and Thromboembolic Disease," British Medical Journal 2 (April 27, 1968), 199–205. In yet another study that investigated deaths from thrombosis or embolism in England, Wales, and Northern Ireland in 1966, a relationship was found with oral contraceptive use and death from pulmonary embolism or cerebral thrombosis, but no relationship was found with death from coronary thrombosis and pill use. W. H. W. Inman and M. P. Vessey, "Investigation of Deaths from Pulmonary, Coronary, and Cerebral Thrombosis and Embolism in Women of Child-bearing Age," British Medical Journal 2 (April 27, 1968), 193–99.

44. In the United States, Edward Tyler described continuing attempts to determine whether a relationship existed between the use of oral contraceptives and thromboembolic disease, citing several studies of blood-clotting factors. The women were on various pill formulations, and length of use varied. Some changes in clotting factors were noted, but their significance was unknown. E. T. Tyler, "Antifertility Agents," Annual Review of Pharmacology (Palo Alto, Calif.: Annual Reviews, 1967), 381–98.

45. American researchers were putting some of their efforts into understanding changes in the coagulation profiles of oral contraceptive users and comparing them to the changes that occurred in pregnancy. The Medical Letter on Drugs and Therapeutics in Aug. 1968 reported that five new oral contraceptives had become available, also noting that two reports provided statistically significant evidence linking embolic disease with the use of oral contraceptives. In this issue the Inman and Vessey hospital study of fatalities was cited, as was the Vessey and Doll examination of hospital admission for thromboembolic disease. See Medical Letter on Drugs and Therapeutics (New Rochelle, N.Y.: Medical Letter), Aug. 23, 1968. Debate continued in 1968 in the U.S. medical literature about the risks of clots and pill use. V. A. Drill and D. Calhoun, "Oral Contraceptives and Thromboembolic Disease," Journal of the American Medical Association 206 (Sept. 30, 1968), 78–84, concluded that data in the U.S. did not demonstrate an increase in death rate from pulmonary embolism. They also noted that the

vital statistics for England did not show an increase in the ratio of women to men dying from thromboembolic disease since the introduction of oral contraceptives, thus challenging some of the British data. As these discussions continued, drug manufacturers were warning physicians about possible risks. A 1968 brochure describing Ovral (0.5 mg ethinyl estradiol, 0.5 mg Norgestrel—Wyeth Labs, Philadelphia) lists thrombophlebitis, thromboembolic disorder, and cerebral apoplexy—or a history of these conditions—as contraindications to pill use. Under "Adverse Reactions," it is written that a statistically significant association has been demonstrated between use of oral contraceptives and thrombophlebitis and pulmonary embolism (Wyeth publication, Philadelphia, June 15, 1968). So while clearly the pharmaceutical companies had accepted this possible risk based on the preliminary data of the three major British studies, American researchers continued to look at the British data as well as their own, but not always reaching the same conclusions. Phillip E. Sartwell and colleagues at the Johns Hopkins School of Hygiene and Public Health published a retrospective study of thromboembolism using data from five American cities. This study was begun in the fall of 1965 and was of the same case-control design as the British studies cited. In addition to evaluating actual events, the researchers sought to identify which oral contraceptive products women had used. The women were shown lists of brand names and oral contraceptive sample packs to identify what they had used. The researchers found that of the fifteen patients using sequential oral contraceptives (estrogen taken alone for fourteen to sixteen days of the cycle), seven had a pulmonary embolism. Thus they concluded that those pills with high estrogenic activity were the most strongly associated with thromboembolism; P. E. Sartwell et al., "Thromboembolism and Oral Contraceptives: An Epidemiologic Case-Control Study," *American Journal of Epidemiology* 90, no. 5 (Nov. 1969), 365–80. In reviewing the studies previously reported, Sartwell commented on Vessey and Doll's follow-up paper in 1969—M. P. Vessey and R. Doll, "Investigation of Relation between Use of Oral Contraceptives and Thromboembolic Disease, A Further Report," *British Medical Journal* 2 (June 14, 1969), 651–57—in which the previously noted relationship between oral contraceptive use, smoking, and pulmonary embolism was no longer apparent. (They were not correct in this finding.)

46. See David A. Grimes, one of the country's most well-known experts on contraception, Grimes and Melinda Wallach, eds., *Modern Contraception: Updates from the Contraception Report* (Totowa, N.J.: Emron, 1997), preface. Grimes noted that contraception and related fields of women's health are rapidly evolving. That being said, some of the same issues discussed at the time of the pill's first appearance continue to be debated and research is ongoing. Books such as this, aimed at residents in training and clinicians in practice, offer lists of benefits and risks with headings such as "Well-documented, Noncontroversial, Growing Evidence, Still Controversial." This format was used in the 1970s and remains commonly used today. There has been a recent controversy regarding the Ortho Evra patch with possible higher rates of thromboembolic disease and higher circulating blood levels of estrogen.

47. Russell E. Schlitter, MD, to Rock, Feb. 17, 1966; Rock to Schlitter, March 1, 1966; Schlitter to Polly Porter (Rock's secretary), May 29, 1966, JR-RA. Rock's film, *The Role of the Endometrium in Conception and Menstruation*, was reviewed in *Journal of the American Medical Association* 204 (April 8, 1968), 181.

48. Rock first appealed to Searle for a major donation in 1962. Instead of a major gift to Rock's clinic, Jack Searle funded the Rock Chair at Harvard and the Searle Foundation began in that year to provide an annual grant of $5,000 to the clinic for operating purposes as long as Rock remained in practice. In some years, the grant was higher, but the records are not entirely clear when the higher amount—$10,000–$12,000—became regularized. See for example, Rock to Searle, Dec. 4, 1962; Searle to Rock, Dec. 14, 1962; Rock to Searle, Dec. 18, 1962; Searle to Rock, Aug. 3, 1966; Rock to Searle, Jan. 6, 1967. See Rock to Searle, May 22, 1967; Rock to Crosson, Jan. 2, 1970. All in JR-RA.

49. D. F. Gearing Associates, "An Analysis of the Rock Reproductive Clinic, Inc.," typescript, Dec. 1965, p. 8, JR-RA.

50. Ibid., 13. Rock did not want to abandon all clinical work. In 1966, for example, he wrote Aloys Naville, a Swiss fertility specialist who had been one of his former research fellows, about the Rock Clinic's results in testing clomiphene citrate. Rock to Naville, April 22, 1966, JR-RA.

51. Gearing Associates, "Analysis," 9–10.

52. Ibid., 17.

53. Ibid., 25.

54. Mulligan obituary, *Boston Globe*, Sept. 16, 1980, 45.

55. The Massachusetts legislature had to approve the merger, which it did in 1966. See Elmer Osgood Cappers, *History of the Free Hospital for Women, 1875–1975* (Boston: Boston Hospital for Women, 1975), 93–97, for the sanitized version. Loretta McLaughlin, having interviewed several of those involved, discusses the institutional politics involved. McLaughlin, *The Pill, John Rock, and the Church*, 195–201. Also, Gearing Associates, "Analysis."

56. For example, Rock to Searle, Dec. 4, 1962; Searle to Rock, Dec. 14, 1962; Searle to Rock, June 1, 1964; Rock to Searle, June 18, 1964, JR-RA.

57. McLaughlin, *The Pill, John Rock, and the Church*, 202, discusses Rock's financial plight.

58. Rachel Achenbach, interview by Margaret Marsh, July 6, 2007.

59. John G. Freymann, MD, General Director, Boston Hospital for Women, to Rock, Dec. 1, 1967. Negotiations dragged into the new year, with Rock's lawyer, James Storey, still attempting to negotiate in good faith, but by March, Rock had leased quarters elsewhere. See James M. Storey to Freymann, Jan. 22, 1968; Storey to Rock, March 15, 1968, JR-RA.

60. Tone, *Devices and Desires*, 239.

61. See, for example, "An Essay on Sex, Parenthood, and Contraception," draft of Pittsfield lecture, Oct. 18, 1966, JR-RA.

62. Tone, *Devices and Desires*, 273; Morton Mintz, *At Any Cost: Corporate Greed, Women, and the Dalkon Shield* (New York: Pantheon Books, 1985), 23, for Davis's lack of board certification. Nicole J. Grant, *The Selling of Contraception: The Dalkon Shield Case, Sexuality, and Women's Autonomy* (Columbus: Ohio State University Press, 1992), 40–43.

63. Elizabeth Siegel Watkins, *On the Pill*, 103–5, gives an excellent account of the feminist impulses behind Seaman's book.

64. We consulted the updated edition because we were interested in how much Seaman had or had not changed her views in the intervening years. This edition reprints the original as written and includes additional material and observations in separate chapters. Barbara Seaman, *The Doctors' Case Against the Pill: 25th Anniversary Updated Edition* (Alameda, Calif.: Hunter House, 1995). Quoted material on 107.

65. Please note that one of us, Marsh, has served on the board of trustees for a Planned Parenthood affiliate, and the other, Ronner, is a board-certified obstetrician and gynecologist.

66. Hugh J. Davis, MD, "A Public Scandal," introduction to Seaman, *The Doctors' Case Against the Pill*, 9–10. Emphasis in original.

67. Seaman, *The Doctors' Case Against the Pill*, 207–8.

68. Suzanne White Junod and Lara Marks, "Women's Trials: The Approval of the First Oral Contraceptive Pill in the United States and Great Britain," *Journal of the History of Medicine and Allied Sciences* 57, no. 2 (2002), 117–60.

69. Paul Starr, *The Social Transformation of American Medicine: The Rise of a Sovereign Profession and the Making of a Vast Industry* (New York: Basic Books, 1982), 391–92.

70. Watkins, *On the Pill*, 51.

71. "The Pill on Trial," *Time* 95 (Jan. 26, 1970), 60; United States Senate, "Competitive Problems in the Drug Industry," *Hearings Before the Subcommittee on Monopoly of the Select Committee*, 91st Cong., 2d sess. (1970), Hugh J. Davis statement, pp. 5925–26.

72. Ibid., 5938–39, 5941.

73. Ibid., Herbert Ratner statement, 6717–18, 6745, 6748.

74. "The Pill on Trial," 60.

75. Watkins, *On the Pill*, 110–13.

76. "Harvard Expert Insists Birth Pill Is Safe," *Boston Globe*, Jan. 16, 1970, 2, 19; Associated Press story clipped from the *Newark News*, Jan. 18, 1970 [n.p.], JR-RA.

77. Carl Djerassi, "Birth Control after 1984," *Science* 169 (Sept. 4, 1970), 941–51, quotation on 942.

78. "Poll Finds Shift in Views on Pill," *New York Times*, March 1, 1970, 49; "The Pill Trial (Contd.)," *Time* 95 (March 9, 1970), 32; "Poll on the Pill," *Newsweek* 75 (Feb. 9, 1970), 52–53; Watkins, *On the Pill*, 115; Tone, *Devices and Desires*, 249.

79. Tone, *Devices and Desires*, 273–83; Grant, *The Selling of Contraception*, 62–69.

80. "FDA Restricting Warning on Pill," *New York Times*, March 24, 1970, 8; Watkins, *On the Pill*, 126.

81. Djerassi, "Birth Control after 1984," 949–50.

82. Rock to Crosson, Jan. 2, 1970, JR-RA.

Chapter 10. A True Visionary

1. John Rock to Jack Searle, Nov. 25, 1974, JR-RA.

2. In early September 1971, Rock wrote with regret that "after two months uninterrupted stay here I start back to the office on Tuesday." John Rock diaries, Sept. 12, 1971. He found no joy in the idea of returning. John Rock diaries, March 1, 1972, JR-RA.

3. Clifford Grobstein, *From Chance to Purpose: An Appraisal of External Human Fertilization* (Reading, Mass.: Addison-Wesley, 1981), discusses the ethics board in considerable detail and reproduces its entire report.

4. See "Fertilization outside Womb," *Science Digest* 69 (Jan. 1971), 90.

5. See Naomi Pfeffer, *The Stork and the Syringe: A Political History of Reproductive Medicine* (Cambridge, UK: Polity Press, 1993), 165. Robert Edwards, *Life Before Birth* (New York: Basic Books, 1989), esp. 1–11.

6. Edwards, *Life Before Birth*, 7–8. The popular news sources that we used for this account of Louise Brown's birth are "The Test-Tube Baby," *Newsweek* 92 (July 24, 1978), 76; "The First Test-Tube Baby," *Time* 112 (July 31, 1978), 58; "Louise: Birth of a New Technology," *Science News* 114 (Aug. 5, 1978), 84; "Test-Tube Baby: It's a Girl," *Time* 112 (Aug. 7, 1978), 68; "All About that Baby," *Newsweek* 92 (Aug. 7, 1978), 66.

7. The Browns' life was cushioned by the financial deal that Steptoe arranged for them—exclusive rights to their story for a British tabloid, an arrangement that made the Browns at least a half million pounds wealthier. See Margaret Marsh and Wanda Ronner, *The Empty Cradle: Infertility in America from Colonial Times to the Present* (Baltimore: Johns Hopkins University Press, 1996), 236. There was an earlier claim of successful IVF, by Douglas Bevis, but Bevis refused to document it, saying shortly after making this claim that he planned to stop doing such research and would have no further comments on the matter. See "Test Tube Babies: Now a Reality?" *Science News* (July 20, 1974), 106; "The Baby Maker," *Time* 104 (July 30, 1974), 58; "Test Tube Babies: Reaction Sets In," *Science News* 106 (July 27, 1974), 53; "Test-Tube Babies?" *Newsweek* 84 (July 29, 1974), 70.

8. See "Hearings Asked on Va. Clinic for Test-tube Babies," *Washington Post*, Jan. 15, 1980, B2. See also Feb. 2, 1980, A3, and May 17, 1980, A2; Richard Cohen, "Test-tube Babies: Why Add to a Surplus?" *Washington Post*, Feb. 3, 1980, B1; Ellen Goodman, "The Baby Louise Clinic," *Washington Post*, Jan. 15, 1980, A15; editorial, *Washington Post*, Jan. 19, 1980, A14.

9. "Nation's First 'Test-tube' Baby Due Within Days . . ." *Washington Post*, Dec. 25, 1981, A6–A7; *New York Times*, Dec. 29, 1981, 1, C1.

10. R. G. Edwards, B. D. Bavister, and P. C. Steptoe, "Early Stages of Fertilization in vitro of Human Oocytes Matured in vitro," *Nature* 221 (Feb. 15, 1969), 632–35. See "In Vitro Fertilization of Human Ova and Blastocyst Transfer: An Invitational Symposium," *Journal of Reproductive Medicine* 11, no. 5 (Nov. 1973), 192–204, esp. 201–2.

11. Shulamith Firestone, *The Dialectic of Sex* (New York: William Morrow, 1970), 198–99, 11; Renate D. Klein, ed., *Infertility: Women Speak Out about Their Experiences of*

Reproductive Medicine (London: Pandora, 1989), cover quotation. See also Janice Raymond, *Women as Wombs: Reproductive Technology and the Battle over Women's Freedom* (San Francisco: HarperSanFrancisco, 1993), viii.

12. See, for example, "Reception and Dinner: Population Crisis Committee," brochure, printed [Sept. 1973]; Keith P. Russell (of ACOG) to Rock, May 31, 1974; Fernand G. Peron (of the WFEB) to Rock, Sept. 19, 1974; Rock to Peron, Nov. 25, 1974; Rock to Celso-Ramon Garcia, Dec. 12, 1974; Rock to Luigi Mastroianni, Dec. 12, 1974; Rock to A. Baird Hastings, Jan. 29, 1975, JR-RA.

13. For example, Garcia to Rock, May 6, 1976, and Rock's reply, May 26, 1976, JR-RA.

14. The articles were variously titled, "Father of the Pill: Man of Conscience," *Sunday Bulletin*, Oct. 7, 1983, 4:3; "Conscience Guided Developer of Birth Control Pill," *Cedar Rapids Gazette*, Oct. 7, 16A; and "Developer of the Pill Looks at Past, Future," *International Herald Tribune*, Oct. 12, 1973 [n. p.], JR-RA.

15. Richard P. McDonough to Rock, July 24, 1975, JR-RA. Rock's handwritten note on the bottom of the letter reads, "I tel[ephoned], left message with sec'y. If he thinks subject of letter is worth following up he'd better come and see me."

16. Rock to McDonough, Sept. 21, 1975; "The Quiet Years of Dr. Rock," *Boston Globe*, June 27, 1976, JR-RA; "Father of the Pill," *Newsweek* 88 (Aug. 30, 1976), 8–9.

17. "The Quiet Years of Dr. Rock" and "Father of the Pill."

18. James Reed, *From Private Vice to Public Virtue: The Birth Control Movement and American Society since 1830* (New York: Basic Books, 1978), 369, 373.

19. By the middle of the 1970s, survey research conducted by the University of Michigan's Institute for Social Research suggested that having children decreased marital happiness. Ann Landers said she was stunned that 70% of respondents to her said that if they could make their choices again, they would have remained childless. Unsigned article in *Look* 34 (Sept. 22, 1970), 17. See also "Make Love, Not Babies," *Newsweek* 75 (June 15, 1970), 111. A few "antichild" articles had appeared in the late 1960s, but in the 1970s they became pervasive, a trend that did not really moderate until the end of the decade and was evident in popular magazines as well as social science–oriented publications such as the *Journal of Marriage and the Family*. See "Childless Bliss," *Newsweek* 84 (Dec. 9, 1974), 87; "If You Had It to Do Over Again—Would You Have Children?" *Good Housekeeping* 182 (June 1976), 100–101ff; Tilla Vahanian and Sally Wendkos Olds, "Will Your Children Break . . . Or Make . . . Your Marriage?" *Parents* 49 (Aug. 1974), 79.

20. For NON membership, see e.g., Margaret Fisk, ed., *Encyclopedia of Associations*, 10th ed. (Detroit: Gale Research, 1976), 663; Nancy Yakes and Denise Akey, eds., *Encyclopedia of Associations*, 14th ed. (Detroit: Gale Research, 1980), 730; Denise Akey, ed., *Encyclopedia of Associations*, 16th ed. (Detroit, Gale Research, 1981), 767. In 1976 NON had two thousand members and forty-five local chapters. In an apparent attempt to increase membership, it enlarged its staff from four to eight in 1979 and produced more publications. This having failed, it changed its name to the National Alliance for Optional Parenthood in 1980. By 1982 the staff dropped to six, then to four in 1983. By

1984 the organization was defunct. For examples of coverage, see "Down with Kids," *Time* 100 (July 3, 1972), 35; "Kidding You Not," *Newsweek* 82 (Nov. 5, 1973), 82; "Childless Bliss," 87; "Those Missing Babies," *Time* 104 (Sept. 16, 1974), 54. The 1970s witnessed, as one scholar phrased it, a decline in "the taste for children." Susan Householder Van Horn, surveying such factors as the kinds of toys produced, the treatment of juvenile offenders in court, and the use of "contemptuous terminology such as 'rug rats' to describe young children," believes that children did become "less valued" in the 1970s. Van Horn, *Women, Work, and Fertility* (New York: New York University Press, 1988), 160. At the end of the 1970s, however, there was a move away from antichild attitudes. See e.g., "Wondering if Children Are Necessary," *Time* 113 (March 5, 1979), 42–43.

21. During the 1970s, a large body of scholarship appeared on voluntary childlessness, because some sociologists seemed to believe, as did the popular press, that a major cultural shift was under way. In fact, the 1970s were something of an antinatalist aberration. By the 1980s little scholarship was being done on the voluntarily childless.

22. Virginia Masters and William Johnson, "Advice for Women Who Want to Have a Baby," *Redbook* 144 (March 1975), 70.

23. Articles published in 1980 included one in the *Boston Globe* by Loretta McLaughlin (who was in the midst of writing a biography of Rock), headlined "I Would Do It All Again," *Boston Sunday Globe*, March 23, 1980, A1, A3; and Dennis L. Breo, "Proud of the Pill," *American Medical News* (Dec. 5, 1980), 1–3, 13. Obituary for William Mulligan, *Boston Globe*, Sept. 16, 1980, 45, JR-RA.

24. Jerome F. Strauss III and Luigi Mastroianni, Jr. "Celso-Ramon Garcia, M.D. (1922–2004), Reproductive Medicine Visionary," *Journal of Experimental and Clinical Assisted Reproduction* 2, no. 2 (2005). Text at www.jexpclinassistreprod.com/content/2/1/2.

25. Ibid.; also Luigi Mastroianni, interview by Wanda Ronner, July 5, 2007; biography of Luigi Mastroianni at www.med.upenn.edu/crrwh/faculty/Mastroianni/Mastroianni.html.

26. *First Annual John Rock Commemorative Symposium*, printed program, Oct. 21, 1980; Garcia to Rock, Sept. 22, 1980, and Oct. 24, 1980; Rock to Garcia, Oct. 31, 1980; Rock to "Alex and Cynny," Nov. 10, 1980; Rock to Winter, Nov. 6, 1980, and Winter to Rock, Nov. 18, 1980, JR-RA.

27. John Rock diaries, March 18, 1979, JR-RA.

28. Loretta McLaughlin, *The Pill, John Rock, and the Church: The Biography of a Revolution* (Boston: Little, Brown, 1982), 1–2.

29. For example, Mrs. L. L. to Rock, March 14, 1983; Mr. J. Q. to Rock, Feb. 9, 1983; Mrs. E. K. to Rock, Jan. 16, 1983; Mrs. H. G. to Rock, Jan. 30, 1983; Mrs. J. S. to Rock, July 28, 1983; Mrs. Milward (Tip) Martin to Rock, Feb. 27, 1983; and Somers Sturgis to Rock, Jan. 27, 1983, JR-RA.

30. Frederick E. Flynn to Rock, May 19, 1983, JR-RA.

31. Favorable reviews included "The Father of Pill Followed His Own Conscience," *Milwaukee Journal*, Jan. 16, 1983, Life/Style, 3; and Hilton A. Salhanick's review in the *New England Journal of Medicine* (July 21, 1983), 194.

32. Barbara Ehrenreich, "Bitter Pill," *New York Times Book Review*, March 6, 1983, 12; Gena Corea, *The Mother Machine: Reproductive Technology from Artificial Insemination to Artificial Wombs* (New York: Harper and Row, 1985), 101–3. Quotation on 102.

33. Luigi Mastroianni, interview by Wanda Ronner, July 5, 2007.

34. Elizabeth Siegel Watkins, *The Estrogen Elixir: A History of Hormone Replacement Therapy in America* (Baltimore: Johns Hopkins University Press, 2007), 132.

35. Paul Starr, *The Social Transformation of American Medicine: The Rise of a Sovereign Profession and the Making of a Vast Industry* (New York: Basic Books, 1982), 380–90. Quotations on 389, 380.

36. Watkins, *The Estrogen Elixir*, 132.

37. See, for example, Arthur Herbst, Howard Ulelfelder, and David Poskanzer, "Adenocarcinoma of the Vagina," *New England Journal of Medicine* 284, no. 16 (April 22, 1971), 878–81; *FDA Drug Bulletin, Diethylstilbestrol Contraindicated in Pregnancy*, Nov. 1971; "FDA Warns Ingestion of DES During Pregnancy May Cause Vaginal Cancer in Offspring Years Later," *BioMedical News* (Dec. 1971), 12; "DES Link to Vagina Cancer Questioned by California Ob.," *Ob/Gyn News* (Aug. 15, 1972), 1, 29; editorial, *Journal of the American Medical Association* 218, no. 10 (Dec. 6, 1971), 1564. By the late 1970s, data indicated that the cancer occurred in from 1/1000 to 1/10,000 of the exposed daughters.

38. Tone, *Devices and Desires*, 273–83; Grant, *The Selling of Contraception*, 62–69.

39. Watkins, *The Estrogen Elixir*, chap. 5, 93–108, discusses the medical findings, and chap. 6, 109–31, the response of feminist and other health activists to the findings.

40. Yes, it really is "the" difference, not "a" difference. Moffitt to Rock, July 1, 1983, JR-RA.

41. "It's as if Sara Davidson and her friends had invented sex and politics in 1961," John Leonard complained in the *New York Times*. Erica Jong found the author's experience to be "a touching story," even if the book did promote a "false sense of conveying history when it is really only dropping the names of historical events, as one might drop the names of famous people." John Leonard, "Books of the Times: Who Needs the 1960s?" May 17, 1977, 29. Erica Jong, "Coming of Age in the Sixties," *New York Times Book Review*, May 29, 1977, 20.

42. Sara Davidson, "Dr. Rock's Magic Pill," *Esquire* (Dec. 1983), 100–108. Elizabeth Siegel Watkins, *On the Pill: A Social History of Oral Contraceptives, 1950–1970* (Baltimore: Johns Hopkins University Press, 1998), conclusion, 132. By 1990, Watkins notes (p. 132), 80% of American women aged forty-five and younger had used the pill at some time in their lives. This cohort was just a bit younger than Davidson's. It was sterilization, not another form of reversible birth control, that edged out the pill in popularity in 1982 and 1983, however, as *Time* noted (Dec. 17, 1984), 79. *Time* also reported that "among unmarried women and women under 30, . . . the favored contraceptive is still the pill."

43. Davidson, "Dr. Rock's Magic Pill," quotations from 100–102.

44. McLaughlin, *The Pill, John Rock, and the Church*, 227, 232–33.

45. Davidson, "Dr. Rock's Magic Pill," 107.

46. Rachel Achenbach, interview by Margaret Marsh, July 6, 2007.

47. "John Rock, Developer of the Pill and Authority on Fertility, Dies," *New York Times*, Dec. 5, 1984, A29; "Dr. John C. Rock, at 94: 'Father of the Pill,'" *Boston Globe*, Dec. 5, 1984, 94.

48. Celso-Ramon Garcia and Luigi Mastroianni, "John Rock: A Memoriam," *Fertility News*, 10–11, JR-RA; Ellen Goodman, "Dr. Rock: His Pill Was the Start of a Social Revolution," *Boston Globe*, Dec. 6, 1984, 23.

49. Russell Shorto, "Contra-Contraception," *New York Times Magazine*, May 7, 2007, 48–55ff; Watkins, *On the Pill*, 137.

50. Peggy Orenstein, "Your Gamete, Myself," *New York Times Magazine*, July 15, 2007, 34–41ff. Quotation on 36. See also Marsh and Ronner, *The Empty Cradle*, epilogue.

51. Wanda Ronner witnessed the scene. We are preserving the anonymity of this particular doctor.

52. *The Early Show*, Aug. 2, 2005. The film clip is available at www.cbsnews.com/stories/2005/08/02/earlyshow/series/main713316.shtml. This infant became a political symbol for President George W. Bush in his opposition to stem cell research. We were unable to find any independent data on how many frozen embryos are donated yearly to infertile couples. For one source of embryo adoption, see www.nightlight.org/snowflakefaqsgp.htm.

53. In this article, the authors focus on the procurement of the uterus from local organ donor networks, and they consider techniques for the removal of the uterus from a donor. (In a cautionary note, however, the authors remind their colleagues that the only uterine transplant performed to date was controversial and unsuccessful.) Giuseppe Del Priore et al., "Human Uterus Retrieval from a Multi-Organ Donor," *Obstetrics and Gynecology* 109, no. 1 (Jan. 2007), 101–4.

54. Luigi Mastroianni, interview by Wanda Ronner, July 5, 2007.

Index